The

Speech and Hearing Anatomy

Course Companion

Workbook

Carole T. Ferrand PhD

This workbook can be ordered at:

Aplusanatomy.com

CTF PUBLICATIONS
2425 Trio Falls Drive
Loveland, Colorado 80538

ctfpublications@gmail.com   ISBN-978-0-578-80709-6

About the author

Dr. Carole Ferrand earned her BA in English Literature at the University of the Witwatersrand in Johannesburg, South Africa.

After immigrating to the United States, she obtained her MA and PhD in Communication Sciences and Disorders from Pennsylvania State University.

Dr. Ferrand taught in the Department of Speech-Language-Hearing Sciences at Hofstra University in New York for 28 years. Her research and teaching interests focused on the bioacoustic aspects of normal and disordered speech production.

She has authored two widely-used textbooks: "Speech Science: An Integrated Approach to Theory and Clinical Practice" now in its 4th edition, and "Voice Disorders: Scope of Theory and Practice", now in its 2nd edition.

In 2018 Dr. Ferrand moved to Colorado where she continues to explore bioacoustics in humans as well as in birds. In addition to writing textbooks, she is currently working on a book directed to the general public on the dinosaurian origins of bird song, and the close parallels between human speech and birdsong.

Dr. Ferrand enjoys travel, opera, hiking, biking and bird watching. Her interests have taken her to numerous countries throughout the world.

Contents

Preface

In an era when so great a portion of the educational material that students encounter is mediated through electronic devices, the idea of a physical workbook may at first seem to be an anachronism.

But the simple truth is that while pencils and paper may not have all the bells and whistles and digital pizazz of the internet and apps, nothing demands active engagement like drawing/coloring and writing with pencil and paper. No auto correct assists to guide one's hand along the contours of a drawing.

The visual exercises in this book require close attention. And by the very act of drawing with colored pencils, the activities create memories of the information on a different level. The brain/eye/hand coordination and engagement along with the tactile experience of drawing is different than the experience of looking at the all too familiar computer screen while pushing keys and moving a mouse around.

Having taught for many years in the Department of Speech-Language-Hearing Sciences at Hofstra University I came to realize that students were often able to memorize the names and descriptions of many anatomical features but sometimes had difficulty in forming an integrated visual concept of the anatomy they were studying.

Anatomical structures and relationships are inherently visual in nature, and using illustrations and models is essential to understanding these relationships. I duly inserted the clearest illustrations I could find into my PowerPoint slides, and brought in models of the lungs, the larynx, the vocal tract, the ear, and the brain.

No doubt these visual aids were helpful, but a critical element was still missing – meaningful interaction and engagement with the material.

I started thinking about how best to fill this need. I began by trying to create my own drawings of anatomical structures. I am no artist and the results were not works of art. But I soon discovered that by drawing, I found another pathway to teaching the material. What's more, I discovered that drawing and coloring in line drawings was enjoyable!

And so the idea for a visual activity course companion book for speech anatomy was born. It took years for the idea to become more fully fledged, as my time at Hofstra was consumed by teaching, research, administrative work, and writing textbooks ("Speech Science: An Integrated Approach to Theory and Clinical Practice", now in its 4th edition; and "Voice Disorders: Scope of Theory and Practice", now in its 2nd edition).

It is now a comprehensive workbook that includes narrative, reference illustrations, coloring illustrations, a wide array of self-assessment quizzes, an answer key, and a glossary.

It is my hope that students will find that using this Workbook will be a valuable learning experience.

Carole Ferrand, PhD
Professor Emerita
Department of Speech-Language-Hearing Sciences
Hofstra University, New York

Introduction

The Speech and Hearing Anatomy Course Companion Workbook follows the established model of the speech and hearing system most used in Speech and Hearing Anatomy courses. Reference and coloring illustrations, as well as "draw your own" pages are integrated within each unit. Following each unit is an extensive self-assessment section that includes multiple choice questions, true/false statements, fill-in-the blanks, matching, and crossword puzzles.

Standard Anatomical Position and Planes of Reference: presents basic information on the standard anatomical position, planes, and anatomical terminology. The information is important in helping the user to understand relationships between structures.

Section One- Cells and Tissues: introduces the cells and tissues that that make up organs involved in speech production.

Section Two- The Respiratory System: structures and muscles involved in inhalation and exhalation are described. Differences between breathing for life and breathing for speech are tabulated. Students are introduced to the classification of lung volumes and capacities.

Section Three - The Phonatory System: the outer framework of the larynx and the inner valves of the larynx are presented, followed by discussion of the laryngeal muscles. A description of the cover-body model and the myoelastic-aerodynamic theory of phonation concludes the unit.

Section Four - The Articulatory System: the vocal tract and its associated structures are described, including cranial and facial bones, muscles of expression and muscles of mastication. The muscles of pharynx, tongue, and velum are also explained.

Section Five - The Auditory System: the outer, middle, and inner ears are introduced, including the organ of Corti and the semicircular canals within the inner ear.

Section Six - The Nervous System: the unit opens with a description of nervous tissue, including neurons and glial cells. The structures of the brain and spinal cord are presented. Lobes of the brain are described and Brodmann's areas are introduced. Relevant cranial nerves are described. Blood supply to the brain is briefly discussed.

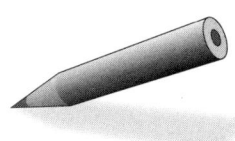

A note to students from the author and the illustrator about the "Draw your own" pages

We hope you will enjoy using this book!
Since learning anatomy is a highly visual endeavor, one of the best ways to help you remember the names and locations and forms of anatomical features is to **make the drawings yourself.**

"Works of Art" are not required. Cartoon style is just fine. Draw them over and over again and you will soon be able to recall much of what you have depicted.

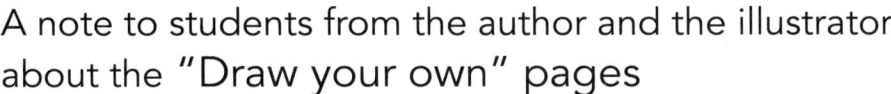

You can refer to the illustrations in this book and to other sources.

The BEST WAY to use drawing as a learning tool is to get yourself a **SKETCH BOOK** reserved just for anatomical drawings and fill it with your sketches.

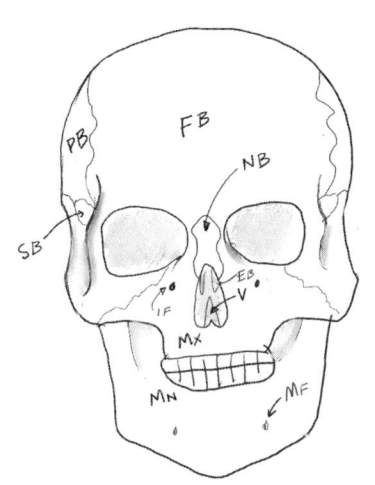

PS We would love to see your drawings and read your comments about this book!

C Ferrand & E Ferrand
CTFpublications@gmail.com

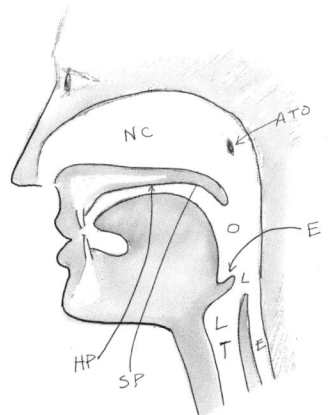

Anatomical Position
Directional Terms
Planes of Reference

Standardized anatomical positions, directional terms, and planes of reference provide a common basis for description, discussion and illustration of anatomical information across disciplines.

STANDARD ANATOMICAL POSITION AND DIRECTIONAL TERMS

When describing human anatomical structures, a standard anatomical position is used as a point of reference. In the standard anatomical position, the body is erect, feet together, the palms face forward, and the thumbs point away from the body. Directional terms describe the positions of structures relative to other structures or locations in the body.

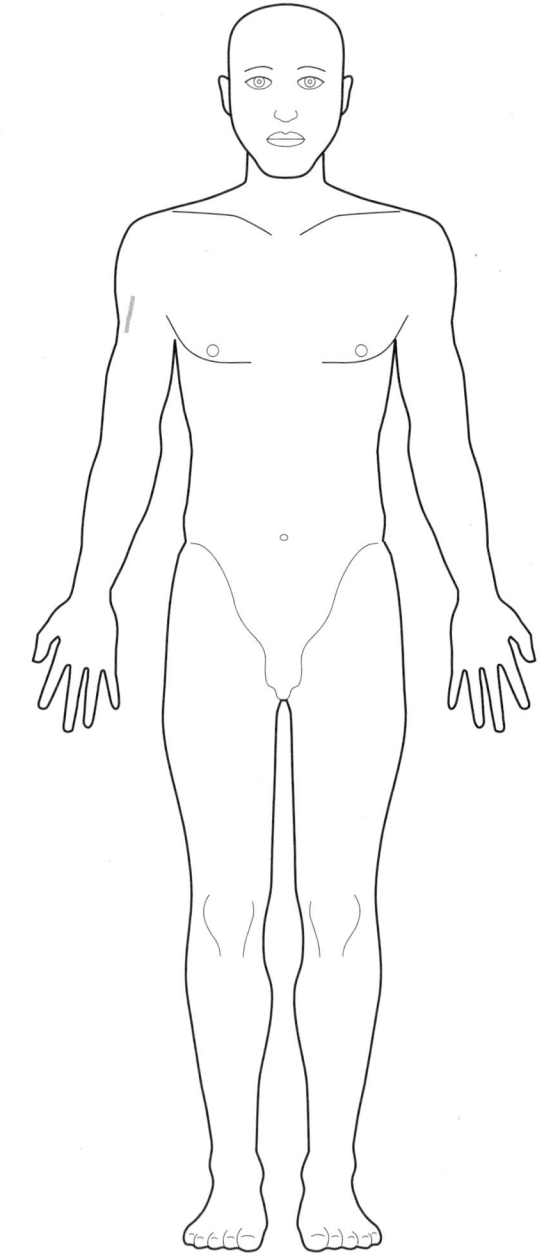

Superior/cranial/rostral - Toward the head; upper

Inferior/caudal - Away from the head; lower

Anterior/ventral Toward the front of the body

Posterior/dorsal -Toward the back of the body

Medial - Toward the midline of the body

Lateral - Away from midline; toward the side

Proximal - Toward or near the trunk or origin

Distal - Away from or farthest from

      the trunk or origin

Central - Toward the center

Peripheral - Toward the periphery

Deep - Away from the body surface

Superficial - Toward the body surface

External - On the outer surface

Internal - On the inner surface

Prone - Body lying face down

Supine - Body lying face up

Ipsilateral - On the same side

Contralateral - On the opposite side

PLANES OF REFERENCE

The body can be imaged in three different planes:

Sagittal

Coronal (also called frontal)

Transverse (also called horizontal)

These planes are used to
show structures
from different views

COLOR KEY
☐ 1 Sagittal plane
☐ 2 Coronal plane
☐ 3 Transverse plane

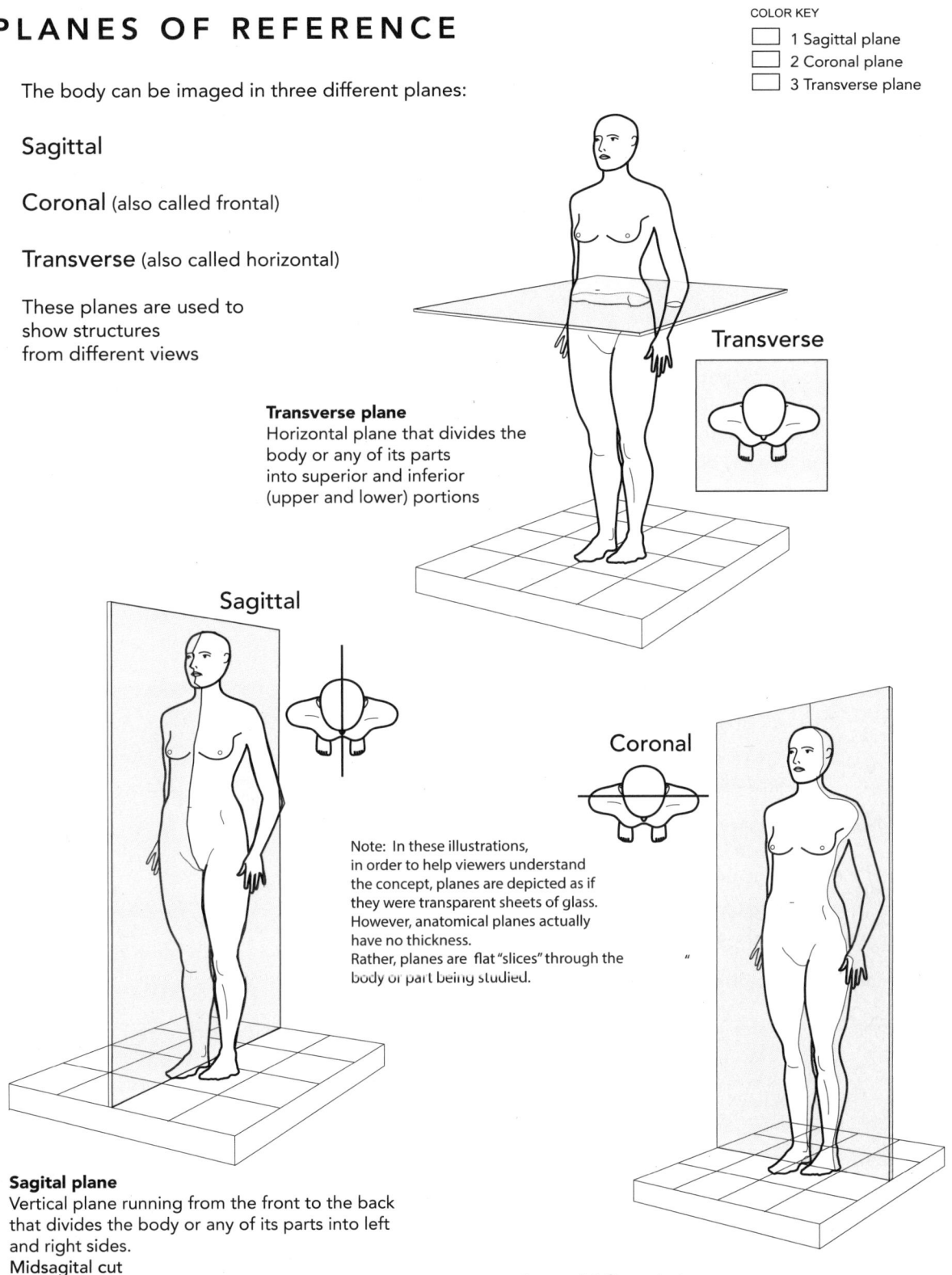

Transverse plane
Horizontal plane that divides the
body or any of its parts
into superior and inferior
(upper and lower) portions

Transverse

Sagittal

Coronal

Note: In these illustrations,
in order to help viewers understand
the concept, planes are depicted as if
they were transparent sheets of glass.
However, anatomical planes actually
have no thickness.
Rather, planes are flat "slices" through the
body or part being studied.

Sagital plane
Vertical plane running from the front to the back
that divides the body or any of its parts into left
and right sides.
Midsagital cut
Plane at the midline of the structure
Parasagittal cut
Plane away from the midline of the structure but
parallel to the sagittal plane

Coronal / Frontal plane
Vertical plane that divides the body or any of its parts
into front and back portions

TEST YOURSELF ANATOMICAL POSITION / PLANES OF REFERENCE

MULTIPLE CHOICE

1____   Which of the following planes divides the body into anterior and posterior parts?
  a.   Sagittal plane
  b.   Frontal plane
  c.   Median plane
  d.   Transverse plane

2 ____   In the standard anatomical position, the palmar surface of the hands
  a.   Faces anteriorly
  b.   Faces posteriorly
  c.   Faces superiorly
  d.   Can face any direction

3 ____   Which of the following planes divides the body into right and left parts?
  a.   Frontal plane
  b.   Transverse plane
  c.   Sagittal plane
  d.   Median plane

4 ____   Which best describes the relation between right hand and right foot?
  a.   They are medial
  b.   They are lateral
  c.   They are ipsilateral
  d.   They are contralateral

5 ____   If you are prone, you are
  a   Facing anteriorly
  b.   Lying face down
  c.   Lying face up
  d.   None of the above

6 ____   The relationship between your finger and your shoulder is
  a.   Distal
  b   Proximal
  c.   Central
  d.   Peripheral

TRUE/FALSE

1 _____ In the standard anatomical position, the body is erect, feet together, the palms face forward, and the thumbs point away from the body

2 _____ A coronal/frontal cut is at the midline of the structure

3 _____ A parasagittal cut is a vertical plane that divides the body or any of its parts into front and back portions

4 _____ A transverse cut divides the body into upper and lower portions

5 _____ The hand is inferior to the arm

6 _____ The head is caudal to the shoulders

7 _____ The right arm is contralateral to the left leg

MATCHING

Superior/cranial/rostral	1 Toward or nearest the trunk or the point of origin of a part
Posterior/dorsal	2 Toward the head end of the body; upper
Medial	3 Away from or farthest from the trunk or the origin of a part
Inferior/caudal	4 Toward the front of the body
Anterior/ventral	5 Away from the body surface
Lateral	6 Away from the head; lower
Proximal	7 Toward the midline of the body
Distal	8 Toward the back of the body
Central	9 On the outer surface
Peripheral	10 On the same side
Deep	11 Away from the midline of the body; toward the side
Superficial	12 On the opposite side
External	13 Body lying face down
Internal	14 Toward the center
Prone	15 Toward the body surface
Supine	16 On the inner surface
Ipsilateral	17 Toward the periphery
Contralateral	18 Body lying face up

FILL IN THE BLANK

1 The _____ plane divides the body into anterior

and posterior sections

2 The _____ plane divides the body into superior

and inferior sections

3 The _____ plane divides the body into right and left sides

4 Anterior is toward the _____ of the body

5 Farthest from the trunk or point of origin is called _____

6 Body lying face down is _____

7 Lateral is toward the _____

8 Nearest the point of origin is called _____

9 Toward the head of the body is _____

10 Toward the tail of the body is _____

11 A structure that is deep is _____

from the body surface

12 On the opposite side is _____

On the three lines below, write the name of the anatomical section that each plane creates

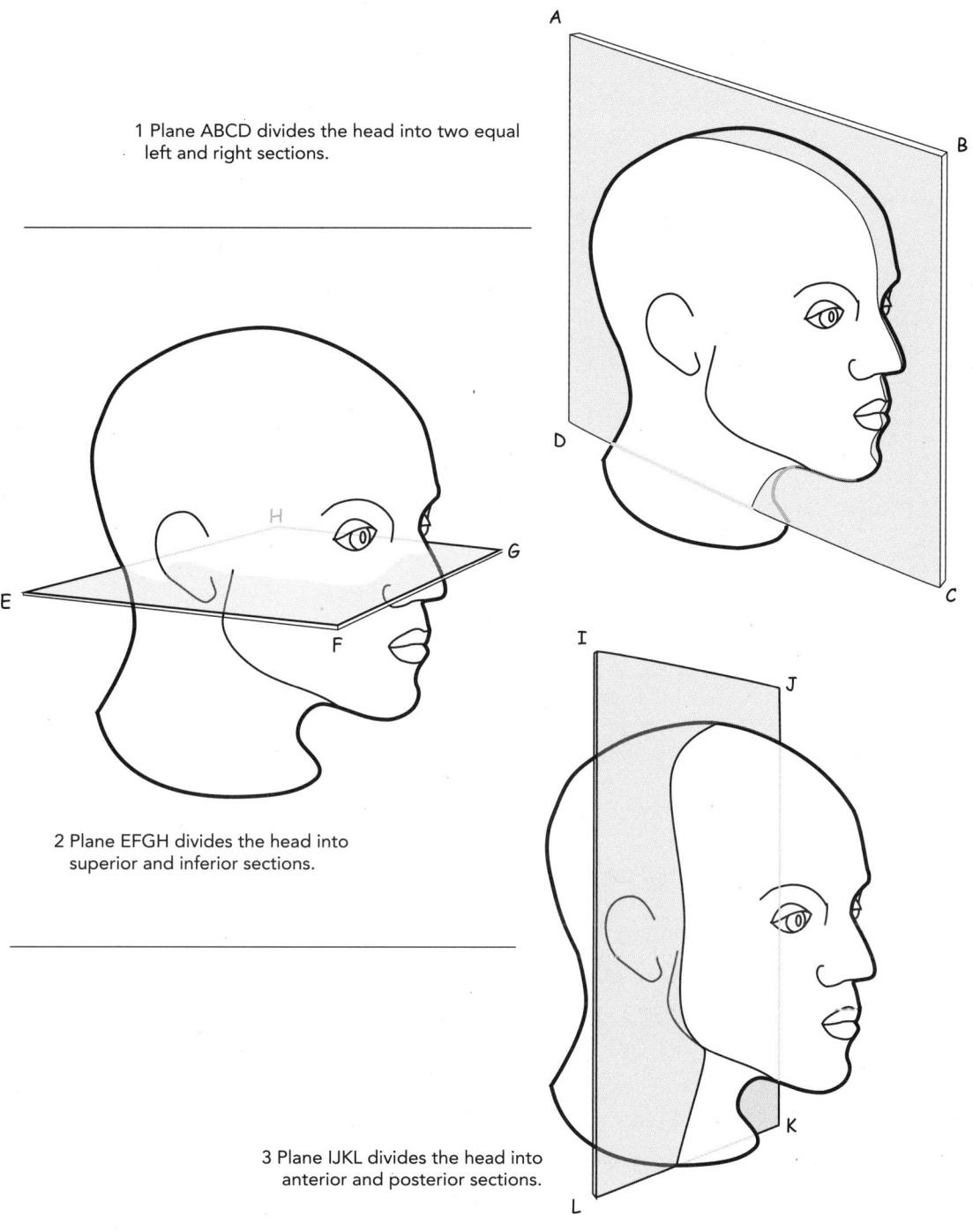

1 Plane ABCD divides the head into two equal left and right sections.

_____

2 Plane EFGH divides the head into superior and inferior sections.

_____

3 Plane IJKL divides the head into anterior and posterior sections.

_____

Planes and Terminology

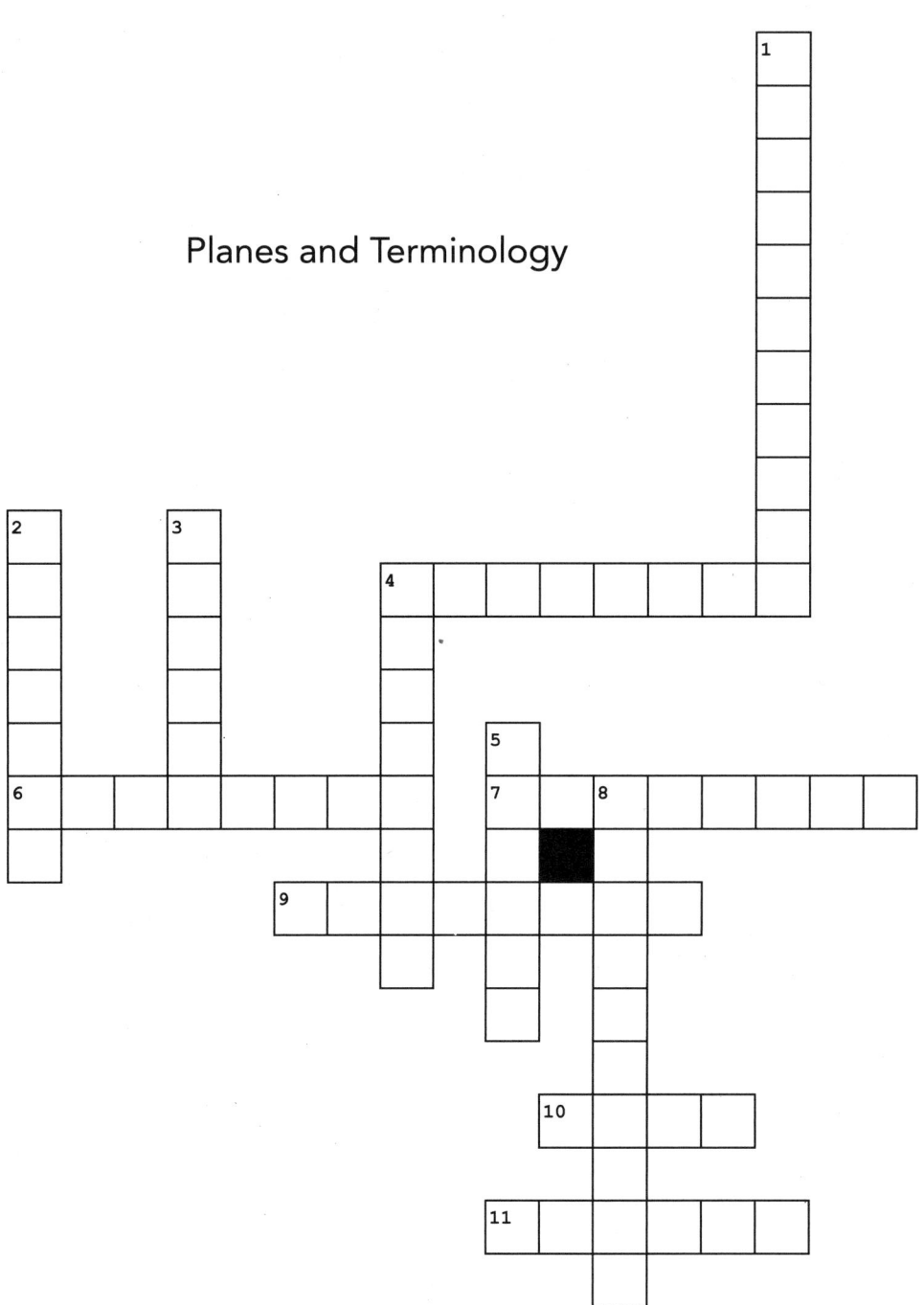

Across

4. This plane divides the body into right and left sides
6. Toward the front of the body
7. On the outer surface
9. Nearest the point of origin
10. Away from the body surface
11. Furthest from the origin

Down

1. On the same side
2. Divides body into front and back
3. Opposite of prone
4. Synonym for upper
5. Toward the midline of the body
8. This plane is also called the horizontal plane

Draw your own: Planes of reference

Cells and Tissues

Cells are the smallest structural and functional units of all organisms.

The human body is made up of more than 100 trillion cells. There are more than 200 types of cells specialized to perform different functions such as blood cell, nerve cell, muscle cell, fat cell, skin cell, and others.

Cells differ in size and shape depending on their function. Functions include external and internal linings of organs, storage, movement, communication, defense, and reproduction.

However, the basic structure of all cells is similar. Every cell is enclosed by a cellular membrane. Cells consist of cytoplasm (basic cellular material), a nucleus (the control center of the cell) as well as specialized organelles that carry out cellular functions.

During embryonic development, many cells are not yet specialized. These cells are called stem cells. Stem cells have the potential to develop into different types of cells and can also repair and replenish other cells. When a stem cell divides, each new cell has the potential either to remain a stem cell or become a cell with a more specialized function.

ORGANELLES

Cell membrane (plasma membrane): controls transfer into or out of the cell. The membrane is extremely flexible and can fuse with or absorb other membranes.

Cytoplasm: gel-like fluid substance that makes up the main mass of the cell.

Nucleus: the area of the cell containing deoxyribonucleic acid (DNA) and proteins. It is enclosed by a nuclear membrane which separates it from the cytoplasm. The membrane regulates the passage of molecules into and out of the nucleus.

Nucleolus: a mass of ribonucleic acid (RNA) with some DNA and proteins within the nucleus. It is involved in the formation of ribosomes.

Ribosomes: synthesize proteins by assembling amino acids into specific sequences.

Rough endoplasmic reticulum: series of membranes within the cytoplasm. It is studded with ribosomes and transports proteins synthesized at the ribosomes.

Smooth endoplasmic reticulum: series of membranes without attached ribosomes.

Golgi apparatus: flattened sacs that modifies, sorts, and packages proteins.

Mitochondria: convert carbohydrates, lipids, and protein molecules into a usable source of energy called adenosine triphosphate (ATP).

Peroxisomes: small vesicles within the cell that absorb nutrients and digest fatty acids.

Lysosomes: vesicles derived from the sacs of the Golgi apparatus. Lysosomes contain enzymes that break down unwanted material and recycle useful substances.

Centrioles: bundles of microtubules involved in cell division.

Microtubules and microfilaments: networks of protein fibers that provide structural support to the cell and allow internal cell parts to be transported within and outside of the cell.

Vacuoles/pinocytic vesicles: membrane-lined sacs that can fuse with one another or with the cell membrane. These structures act as transport vehicles for cellular material.

Chromatin: diffuse network of fine fibrils (small thin fibers) and proteins in the DNA of the nucleus.

COLOR KEY

☐ 1 Plasma membrane
☐ 2 Cytoplasm
☐ 3 Nucleus
☐ 4 Nucleolus
☐ 5 Rough endo. reticulum
☐ 6 Ribosomes
☐ 7 Smooth endo. reticulum
☐ 8 Golgi apparatus
☐ 9 Mitochondria
☐ 10 Centrioles
☐ 11 Peroxisomes
☐ 12 Lysosomes
☐ 13 Vacuoles

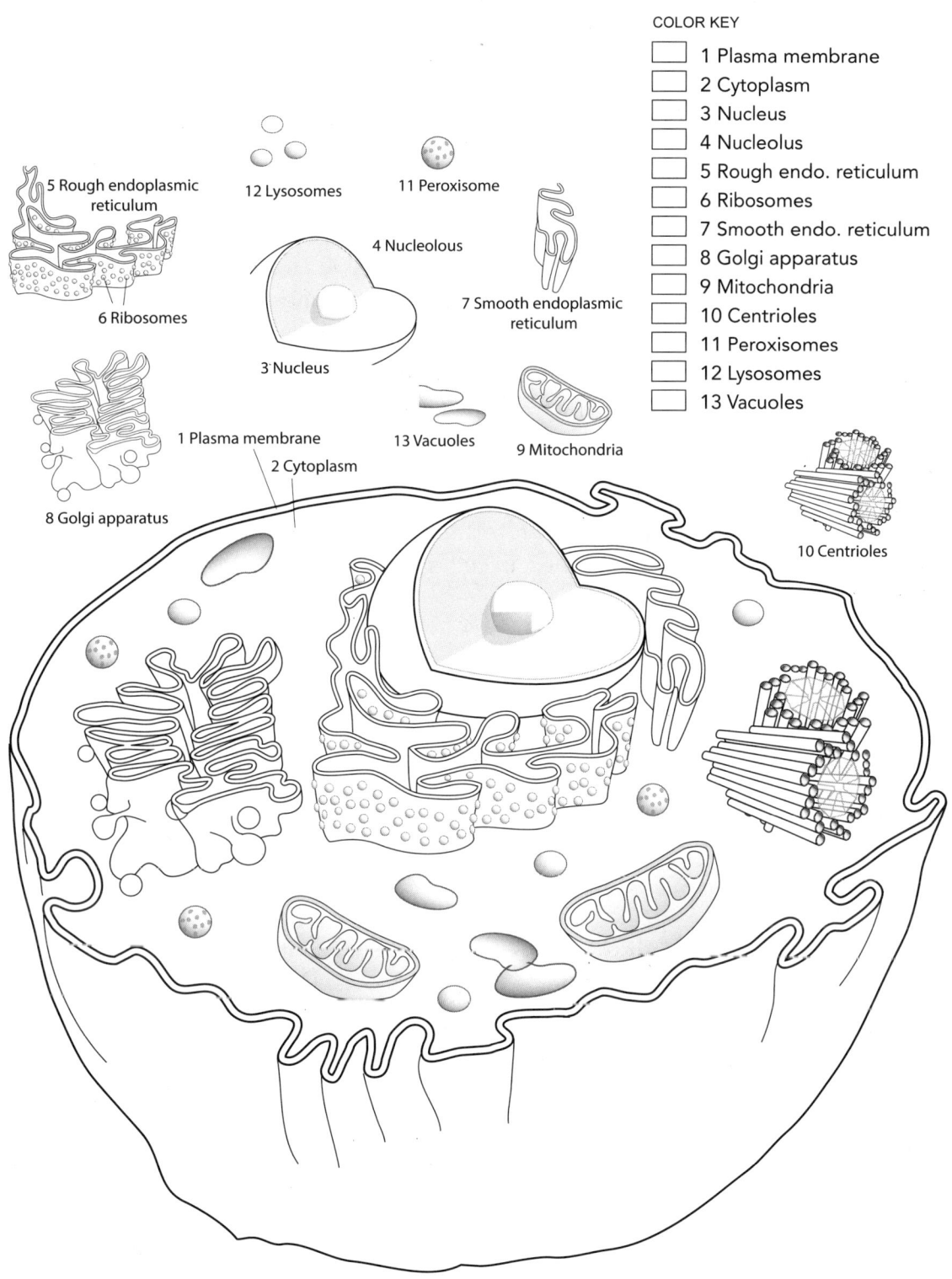

5 Rough endoplasmic reticulum

12 Lysosomes

11 Peroxisome

4 Nucleolous

7 Smooth endoplasmic reticulum

6 Ribosomes

3 Nucleus

1 Plasma membrane

2 Cytoplasm

13 Vacuoles

9 Mitochondria

8 Golgi apparatus

10 Centrioles

CHROMOSOMES AND MITOSIS

Chromosomes of all cells except egg and sperm occur in pairs called homologues which look alike and carry the same genes. Sex chromosomes are called X (female) and Y (male). A sex chromosome with two X's (XX) is female, and a sex chromosome with one X and one Y (XY) is male. All other chromosomes are called autosomes. Humans have 23 pairs of genes in every cell of the body, 22 of which are autosomes and 1 which is sex- linked.

A gene is the basic physical and functional unit of heredity. Genes are made up of deoxyribonucleic acid (DNA). Humans have between 20,000 and 25,000 genes, located on the chromosomes. DNA molecules consist of two chains wound about each other to form a double helix. The double helix is like a ladder with a vertical support on each side (backbone) and horizontal rungs. The horizontal rungs are formed by pairs of bases. A base pair is formed by two nucleotide bases attached to one another by hydrogen bonds.

Mitosis

Mitosis is the process of cell division that forms the trillions of cells in the human body and replaces the old, damaged, or dead ones. In cell division one cell divides into two identical daughter cells.

Interphase: time between cell divisions. This is the period during which the cell carries out its normal activities of obtaining nutrients, reading its DNA, and other necessary metabolic functions. In addition, the cell prepares for cell division by increasing in size and duplicating its DNA and centrioles. During interphase the DNA in the nucleus is composed of chromatin.

Mitotic phase: time when the cell divides into daughter cells. Composed of four stages: prophase, metaphase, anaphase, and telophase.

Prophase: dispersed fibrils of chromatin become condensed into short, thick, coiled chromosomes. Each chromosome contains two copies of its DNA. The two genetically identical sisters within each duplicated chromosome are called chromatids. The sister chromatids are joined at the centromere, which is a constricted region in the chromosome. The nucleolus breaks down and disappears and the centrioles migrate to opposite ends (poles) of the cell. Microtubules called asters project from each centriole. The nuclear membrane dissolves at the end of prophase, allowing the chromosomes to move freely into and through the cytoplasm.

Metaphase: spindle fibers grow from each centriole across the cell center toward the chromosomes. Some attach to the centromere of each chromosome. The spindle fibers allow the sister chromatids to line up in the center of the cell, with half (46) on one side and half (46) on the other side.

Anaphase: the spindle fibers shorten, pulling the sister chromatids apart at the centromere along the track of the spindle fiber. After the chromatids are pulled apart, each chromatid is called a single-stranded chromosome, with its own centromere. Each chromosome migrates to the opposite end of the cell resulting in 46 chromosomes at either pole. The cytoplasm and organelles undergo duplication.

Telophase: the cell pinches off in the center, forming two daughter cells. A new nuclear envelope forms around each set of chromosomes. The chromosomes begin to uncoil and return to the form of dispersed threads of chromatin. The mitotic spindle breaks up and disappears. Each new nucleus forms nucleoli. The two new daughter cells then enter the interphase of their life cycle, and the process begins again.

Proteins

The function of genes is to code for proteins. All proteins are composed of one or more chains of small molecules called amino acids. Proteins typically contain anywhere from 50 - 2,000 amino acids in many combinations and sequences. Each protein is characterized by a specific sequence of amino acids resulting in a characteristic shape, size, and function.

Proteins are the major structural components of skin, hair, fingernails, muscle, and organs; proteins also form enzymes and antibodies, and carry oxygen in blood to all cells of the body. Proteins are essential for growth, structural maintenance, repair, bodily defense, metabolism, and movement.

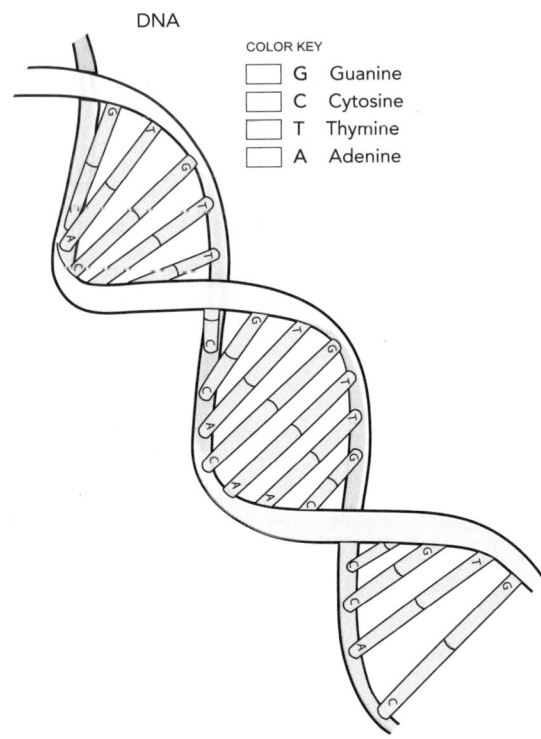

DNA

COLOR KEY

☐ G Guanine
☐ C Cytosine
☐ T Thymine
☐ A Adenine

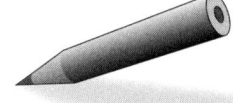

Proteins

COLOR KEY

- 1 Antigens
- 2 Antibodies
- 3 Amino acids
- 4 Collagen molecule
- 5 Polymerase III
- 6 DNA

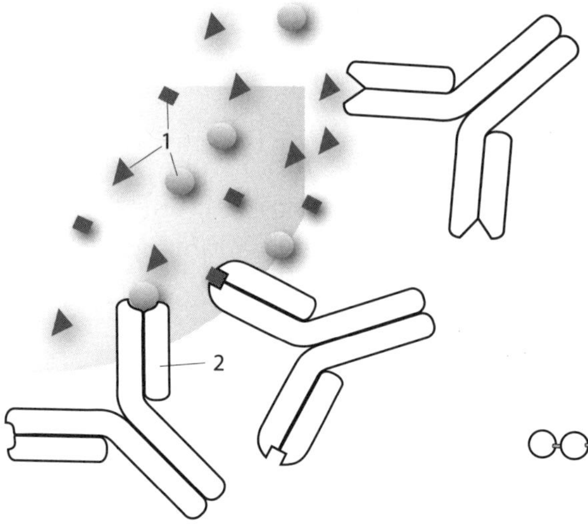

Antibodies are large Y shaped glycoproteins produced in response to invading foreign particles (antigens) such as microorganisms and viruses. They play a critical role in the immune system's defense against infection and disease.

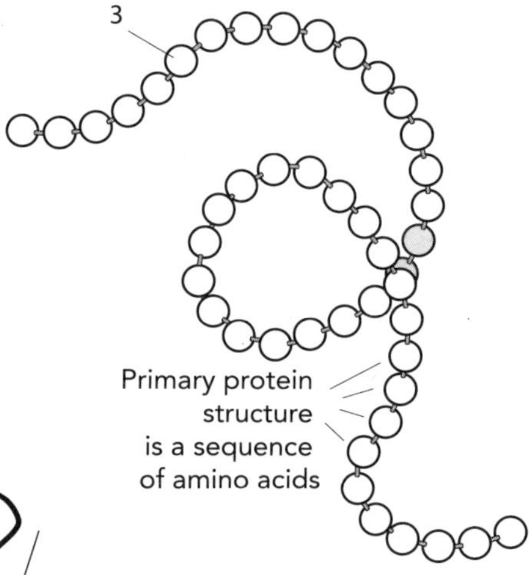

Primary protein structure is a sequence of amino acids

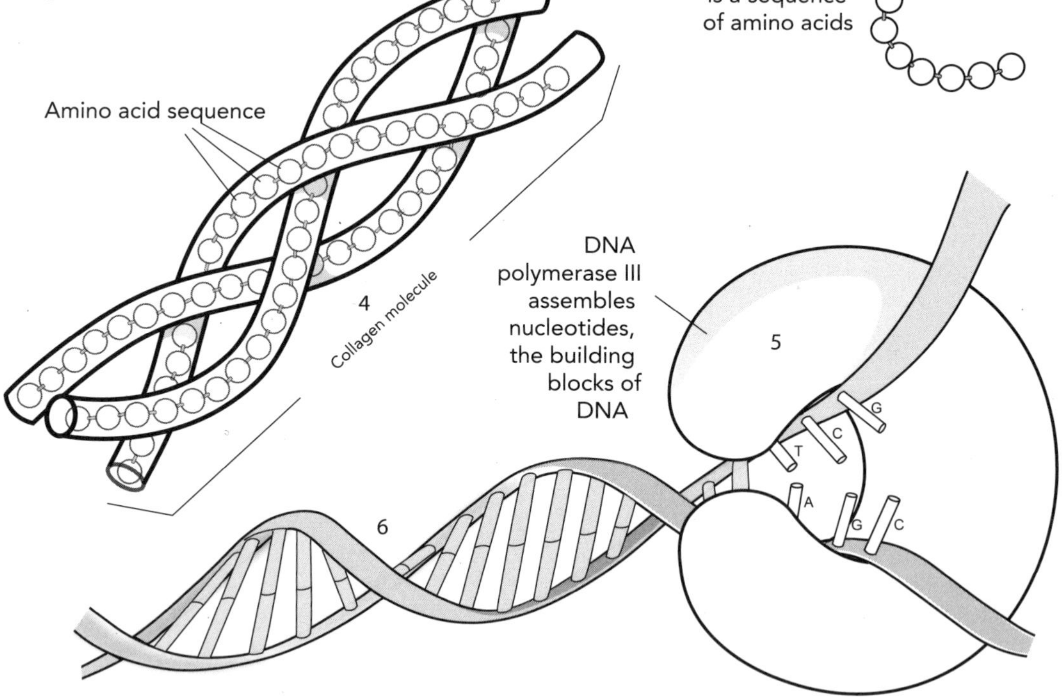

Amino acid sequence

4 Collagen molecule

DNA polymerase III assembles nucleotides, the building blocks of DNA

5

6

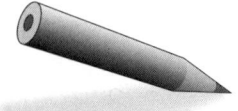

Mitosis

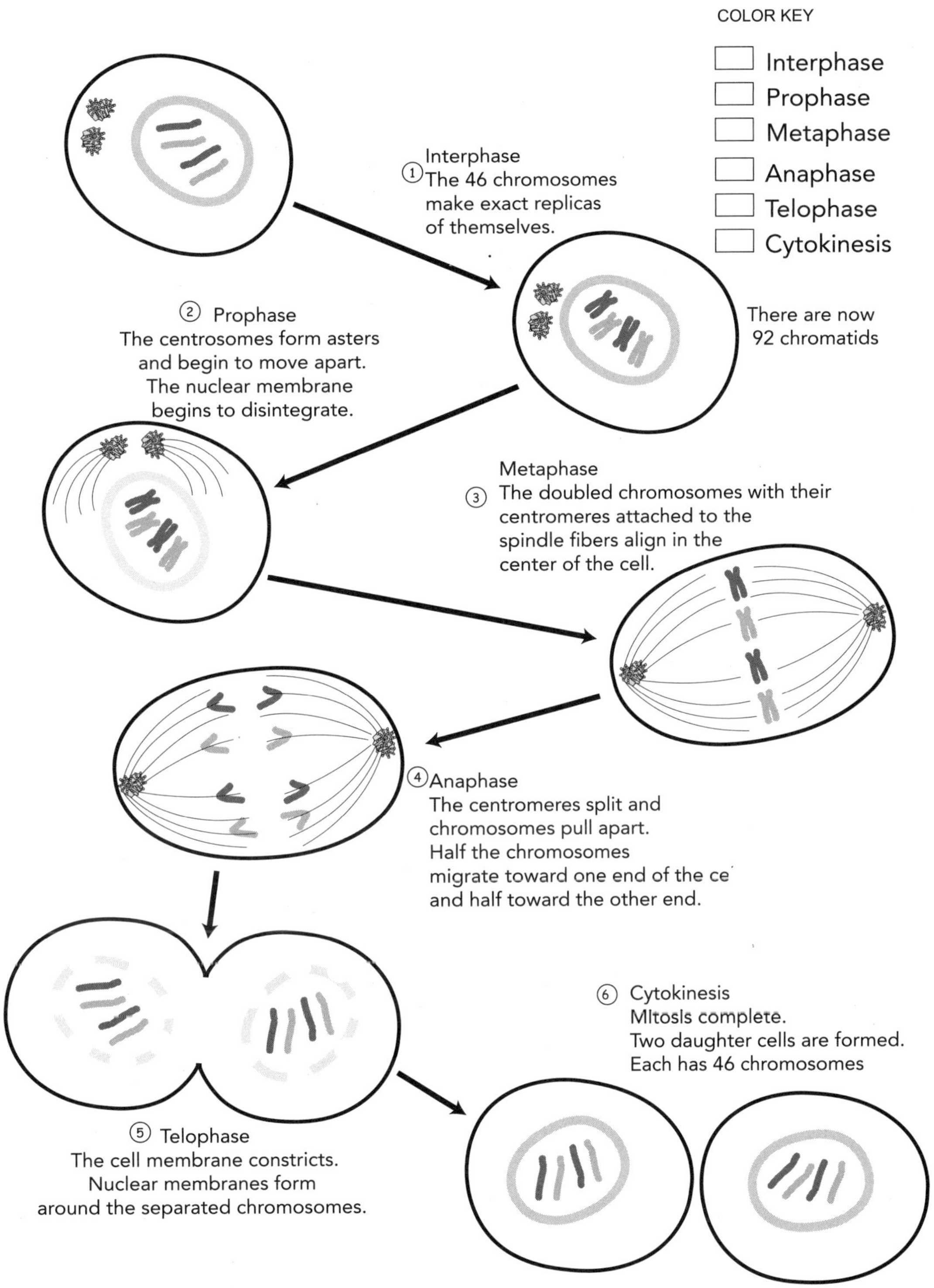

COLOR KEY

☐ Interphase
☐ Prophase
☐ Metaphase
☐ Anaphase
☐ Telophase
☐ Cytokinesis

① Interphase
The 46 chromosomes
make exact replicas
of themselves.

There are now
92 chromatids

② Prophase
The centrosomes form asters
and begin to move apart.
The nuclear membrane
begins to disintegrate.

Metaphase
③ The doubled chromosomes with their
centromeres attached to the
spindle fibers align in the
center of the cell.

④ Anaphase
The centromeres split and
chromosomes pull apart.
Half the chromosomes
migrate toward one end of the ce
and half toward the other end.

⑥ Cytokinesis
Mitosis complete.
Two daughter cells are formed.
Each has 46 chromosomes

⑤ Telophase
The cell membrane constricts.
Nuclear membranes form
around the separated chromosomes.

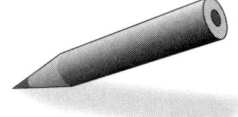

TISSUES

Tissues are groups of cells with a common structure and function. The four main tissue types in humans are epithelial tissue, connective tissue, muscle tissue, and nervous tissue. Nervous tissue will be covered in Section 6.

EPITHELIAL TISSUE

Epithelial tissue is characterized by cells which are packed very closely together. Epithelium forms a protective barrier that lines all the external and internal body surfaces of structures including the oral and nasal cavities, pharynx, and respiratory passages. It also forms a covering for external surfaces, such as skin. Epithelium is characterized by the shape of the cells and numbers of layers of cells. Shape can be squamous, cuboidal, or columnar. Squamous cells are thin and flat; cuboidal cells are about as tall as they are wide. Columnar cells are slender and taller than they are wide.

Simple epithelium consists of a single layer of cells, typically when the function is to absorb or filter substances. Stratified epithelium consists of more than one layer of cells, typically when the function is protection against abrasion. Pseudostratified epithelium looks stratified because the cells' nuclei are distributed at different levels but contains only one layer of cells. Epithelium can be ciliated or non-ciliated. Cilia are minute hair-like structures that project from the surface of the cell and move in a sweeping motion.

Different types of epithelium are specialized to perform different functions such as protection, absorption, filtration, and secretion. For example, ciliated columnar epithelium is found within the trachea and bronchi. This type of epithelium is involved in handling mucous secretions. Keratinized epithelium is found mainly in the skin and is highly waterproof. Squamous epithelium forms the lining of cavities such as the vocal tract, blood vessels, heart and lungs. Squamous epithelium also makes up the outer layers of the skin. All epithelial tissues rest on a basement membrane that connects the epithelium to the underlying connective tissue.

Epithelial tissue

COLOR KEY

☐ 1 Squamous cells
☐ 2 Cuboidal cells
☐ 3 Columnar cells
☐ 4 Ciliated columnar cells
☐ 5 Basement membrane

Squamous
epithelial cells

Cuboidal
epithelial cells

Columnar
epithelial cells

Basement membrane

Ciliated columnar
epithelial cells

Basement membrane

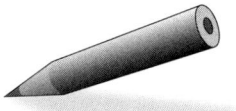

CONNECTIVE TISSUES

Connective tissue connects, supports, or separates different types of tissues and organs of the body. It is also involved in transportation, storage, and immune defense. Connective tissue forms the foundation for epithelial tissue. Blood vessels and nerves travel through connective tissue.

There are different types of fibers in connective tissue including collagen, elastin, and reticular fibers. Collagen fibers provide tensile strength; elastin fibers provide flexibility and tissue recoil; reticular fibers are thinner collagen fibers that provide strength.

Connective tissue is composed of a small number of different types of living cells embedded in a large amount of non-living substance called extracellular matrix (ECM).

Living cell types include

Fibroblasts: produce the fibers and other substances that make up the extracellular matrix.

Myofibroblasts: function like fibroblasts and are also capable of contraction.

Adipocytes (fat cells): store and release triglycerides (fat) and produce hormones and growth factors.

Macrophages: cells that eliminate damaged cells or pathogens by engulfing them.

Lymphocytes: main cells of the immune system.

Mast cells: involved in immune responses.

Plasma cells: synthesize antibodies.

Neutrophils: type of white blood cell that responds to injury and immune challenges.

Eosinophils: respond to allergens and parasitic infections.

Loose connective tissue

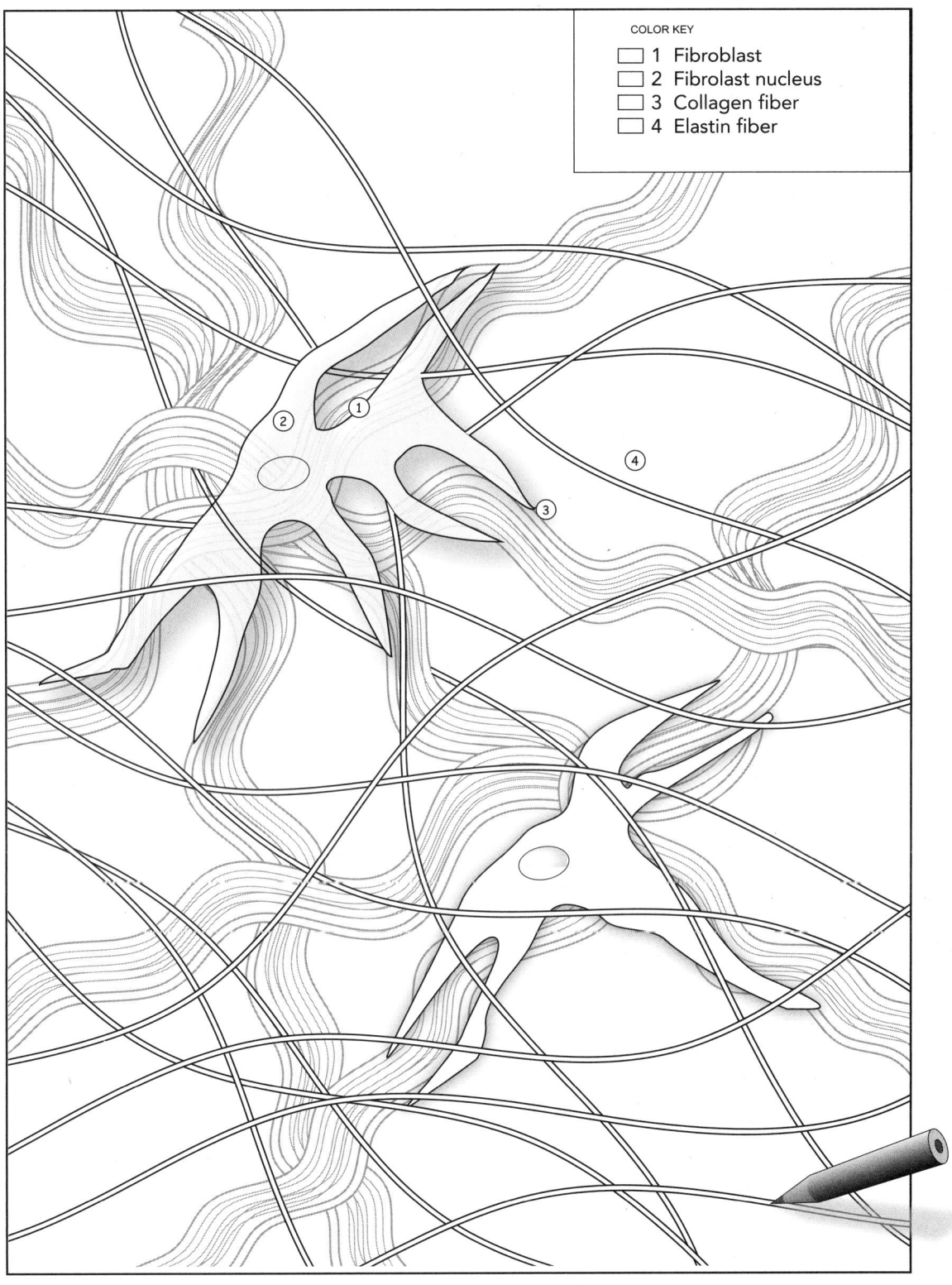

COLOR KEY
☐ 1 Fibroblast
☐ 2 Fibrolast nucleus
☐ 3 Collagen fiber
☐ 4 Elastin fiber

Connective tissue is categorized as
connective tissue proper OR specialized connective tissue

Connective tissue proper

Connective tissue proper is further divided into loose and dense types.

Loose connective tissue

Areolar: tissue consists of a loosely organized array of collagen and elastic fibers as well as many blood vessels. This type of tissue surrounds nerves, blood vessels, and individual muscle cells.

Adipose: tissue composed primarily of fat cells (adipocytes). This type of tissue serves as packing around structures which provides padding, cushions shocks, and acts as an insulator to slow heat loss through the skin.

Dense connective tissue

Regular dense connective tissue: is composed of tightly packed collagen fibers arranged parallel to each other. Tendons and ligaments are examples of this type of tissue. Tendons attach muscles to bones or cartilages. Ligaments attach bone to bone, bone to cartilage, or cartilage to cartilage. Ligaments hold structures together and stabilize joints.

Irregular dense connective tissue: comprises a scattered network of collagen fibers. This type of tissue forms supporting layers around cartilage and bone.

Elastic dense connective tissue: consists of branching elastic fibers as well as densely packed collagen fibers. It provides resilience and flexibility.

Specialized connective tissue

Specialized connective tissues include cartilage, bone, and blood.

Cartilage

Cartilage is characterized by a firm, gel-like extracellular matrix that provides strength and flexibility. It usually has a covering called the perichondrium. Cartilage supports soft tissues and provides a gliding surface at joints.

Hyaline cartilage: is the most common type of cartilage and is flexible and resilient. It has a bluish color and is somewhat translucent. It is found in many areas of the body, including the nose, trachea, most of the larynx, costal cartilage (the cartilage attached to the ribs), and the articular ends of long bones. At the articular ends of long bones, the cartilage allows the bones in a joint to move freely and easily.

Fibrocartilage: contains numerous coarse fibers in its extracellular matrix. Collagen fibers are also present making this type of cartilage extremely durable. It has no perichondrium but acts as a shock absorber and resists compression.

Elastic cartilage: contains numerous elastic fibers in its matrix creating a yellowish color which is more opaque than hyaline. Elastic cartilage is surrounded by a perichondrium and is even more resilient and flexible than hyaline. It is found in the epiglottis and in the external ear.

Bones

Bones are living tissues that constantly grow and repair themselves. They are nourished by blood vessels and have many functions. They protect and support the body; act as an anchor for muscles, tendons, and ligaments; maintain chemical balance in the blood through the storage of calcium; and produce blood cells through bone marrow.

The matrix in bone is rigid due to the presence of calcium and other minerals. There are two types of fibroblasts in bone: osteoblasts which form bone, and osteoclasts, which break it down via enzymes. This process is called remodeling. Throughout the lifespan bones are constantly remodeled as osteoblasts lay down bone tissue and osteoclasts selectively remove it.

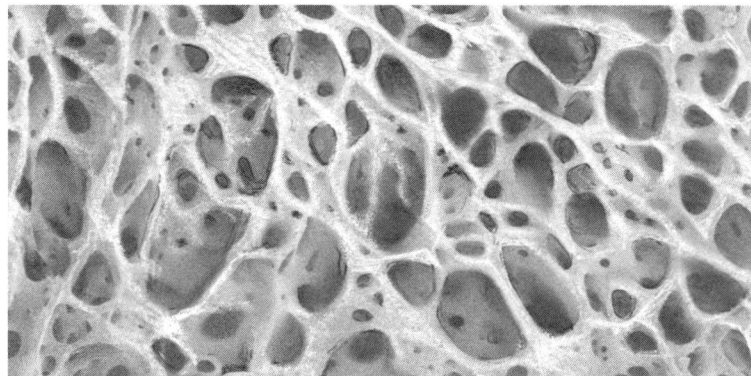

Bone matrix

Bones form and grow by the deposition of matrix that later becomes calcified, and by resorption of bone. Bones need a continual dietary source of vitamins in order to grow normally. For example, vitamin A activates osteoblasts, while vitamin C is required for normal synthesis of collagen. Vitamin D stimulates the absorption and transport of calcium and phosphate ions into the blood. Exercise is also important for normal bone remodeling. Bone can increase its strength in response to mechanical stress (i.e. exercise) over time. This occurs by increasing the amounts of mineral salts deposited and collagen fibers synthesized. Lack of mechanical stress weakens bone through both demineralization of the bone matrix and reduction of collagen formation.

Bones consist of outer and inner layers. The outer layer is made up of compact or dense bone tissue (also called cortical bone) which gives bones their smooth, white, and solid appearance.

The interior of the bone is composed of trabecular bone tissue (also called cancellous or spongy bone). This type of bone tissue is more porous than compact bone, allowing space for blood vessels and marrow. Red marrow produces blood cells; yellow marrow stores fat. Bones are covered by a membrane called the periosteum. The end of some bones that form joints with other bones is covered with a layer of cartilage.

Bones come in different sizes and four primary shapes: flat, long, short, and irregular.

Flat bones: include the scapula (shoulder blade), sternum and outer bones of the cranium.

Short bones: are nearly equal in length and width and include the carpals (wrist bones) and tarsals (ankle bones).

Irregular bones: have a complex shape, such as the vertebrae.

Long bones: are longer than they are wide, and include the femur (thigh), humerus (upper arm) and the bones of the fingers.

A typical long bone contains the following parts:
Diaphysis: the long shaft of the bone.

Epiphysis: the expanded end of the bone covered by a thin layer of hyaline cartilage called articular cartilage.

Metaphysis: the region in a bone between the diaphysis and the epiphysis.

Marrow cavity: a hollow, cylindrical space within the diaphysis. In adults, it contains yellow bone marrow. It also contains stem cells that produce blood cells.

Periosteum: a tough sheath of connective tissue that covers the outer surface of the bone, except for the areas covered by articular cartilage.

Bone structure

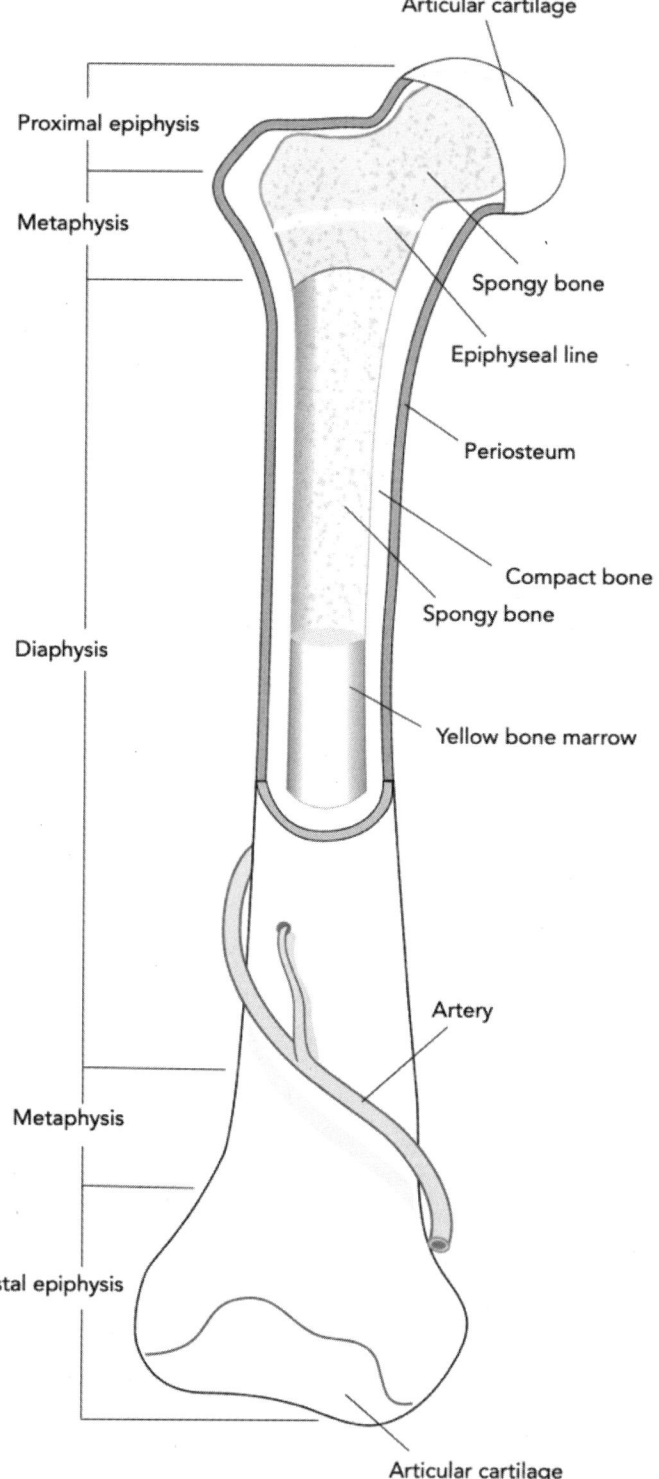

Articular cartilage

Proximal epiphysis

Metaphysis

Spongy bone

Epiphyseal line

Periosteum

Compact bone

Spongy bone

Diaphysis

Yellow bone marrow

Artery

Metaphysis

Distal epiphysis

Articular cartilage

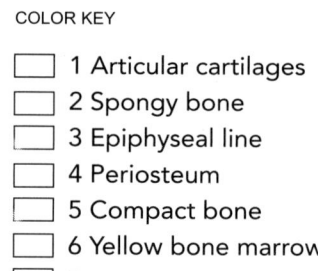

COLOR KEY

☐ 1 Articular cartilages
☐ 2 Spongy bone
☐ 3 Epiphyseal line
☐ 4 Periosteum
☐ 5 Compact bone
☐ 6 Yellow bone marrow
☐ 7 Artery

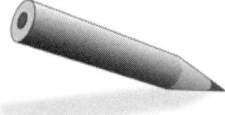

JOINTS

Joints form the connections between bones and cartilages and permit differing degrees of movements between them.

Functional classification of joints
Synarthrodial: immovable

Amphiarthrodial: partly movable

Diarthrodial: freely movable

Structural classification of joints
Fibrous: seam of tough connective tissue that fuses the adjoining bones together (e.g. cranium). This type of joint is also called a suture, and no movement is possible between the adjoining bones.

Cartilaginous: permit some movement, such as those between the vertebrae or between the ribs and sternum.

Synovial: permit a wide range of movements (e.g. wrist).
Synovial joints are composed of two bones encased within a synovial cavity. This allows considerable movement between them. The ends of the bones are covered with articular cartilage and held in place by ligaments. Within the joint is a capsule that encloses the ends of the bones that form the joint. The joint capsule is filled with synovial fluid, which lubricates the joint.

Synovial joints are classified into six groups according to the types of movement they allow.

Plane joints (gliding joints): connect flat bones. This type of joint allows the bones to glide past one another, but they cannot rotate. Example: hand bones below the wrist.

Ball and socket joints: ball-shaped head fits into the concave socket. These joints allow the greatest range of motion. Example: hips and shoulders.

Hinge joints: operate like a swinging gate, with a spool-shaped surface that fits into a concave surface. This type of joint only allows movement in one plane, which is flexion and extension. Examples: elbow and knee.

Pivot joints: formed by a ring of bone rotating about an axle of bone. Example: first and second cervical vertebrae.

Ellipsoidal joints: smaller versions of ball and socket joints. They are formed by the oval tip of one bone moving within an elliptical cavity formed by the other bone. This kind of joint allows flexion, extension, and some rotation. Example: temporomandibular joint.

Saddle joints: formed between a roughly U-shaped end of one bone into which the end of the other fits. Example: thumb.

Types of joint movement

Joints permit ten types of movement, depending on the structure of the joint, the ligaments that keep the joint in position, and the muscles associated with the joint. Joint movements are described in relation to the standard anatomical position.

Extension: movements are directed in the sagittal plane; angle between the bones is increased.

Flexion: movements are directed in the sagittal plane; angle between the bones is decreased.

Adduction: movements are directed medially; bone is moved toward the midline of the body or structure.

Abduction: movements are directed laterally; bone is moved away from the midline of the body or structure.

Circumduction: circular movement resulting from the movements of flexion, abduction, extension, and adduction performed in sequence.

Rotation: moving bone is turned about its axis; can be medial (internal) or lateral (external).

Inversion: turns the sole of the foot inward.

Eversion: turns the sole of the foot outward.

Supination: combines movements of inversion and adduction around a vertical axis (in the foot).

Pronation: combines movements of eversion and abduction around a vertical axis (in the foot).

BLOOD

Although blood is a fluid, it is classified as a connective tissue because it has living cells embedded in an extracellular matrix. Blood has many functions. It transports oxygen, carbon dioxide, and nutrients around the body; is involved in the body's immune response; prevents fluid loss through clotting; regulates pH and electrolyte balance; and regulates bodily heat by constricting and dilating blood vessels. Blood is composed of several elements including plasma, platelets, white blood cells and red blood cells.

Erythrocytes: also called red blood cells. These are the most common type of blood cell. Their main function is to deliver oxygen to every cell in the body through the circulatory system. The cytoplasm of red blood cells contains hemoglobin, a molecule that contains iron and gives the cell its red color.

Plasma: liquid portion of blood comprising about 55% of the blood volume. Plasma is composed primarily of water (92%), about 7% of plasma proteins (albumins, globulins, fibrinogen, enzymes, hormones, clotting proteins), and a small percentage of other solutes such as electrolytes, organic and inorganic molecules, and organic wastes. The red and white blood cells and platelets are suspended in plasma.

Platelets: cell fragments (i.e. without a nucleus) that can bind together in order to form clots and stop bleeding.

White blood cells: also called leukocytes. These are the cells of the immune system that are involved in defending the body against infectious diseases and foreign materials. Granular leukocytes have granules in their cells that contain digestive enzymes.
Agranular leukocytes do not contain these enzymes.
Types of granular leukocytes include
Neutrophils: function as phagocytes at sites of inflammation.
Eosinophils: phagocytes that respond to allergic reactions.
Basophils: function in immune, allergic, and inflammatory reactions.
Types of agranular leukocytes include
Lymphocytes: produce circulating antibodies, involved in immune responses.
Monocytes: involved in immune function.

Types of cells

COLOR KEY

- ☐ 1 Neutrophil
- ☐ 2 Lymphocyte
- ☐ 3 Monocyte
- ☐ 4 Macrophage
- ☐ 5 Basophil
- ☐ 6 Eosinophil
- ☐ 7 Erythrocytes
- ☐ 8 Bacteria

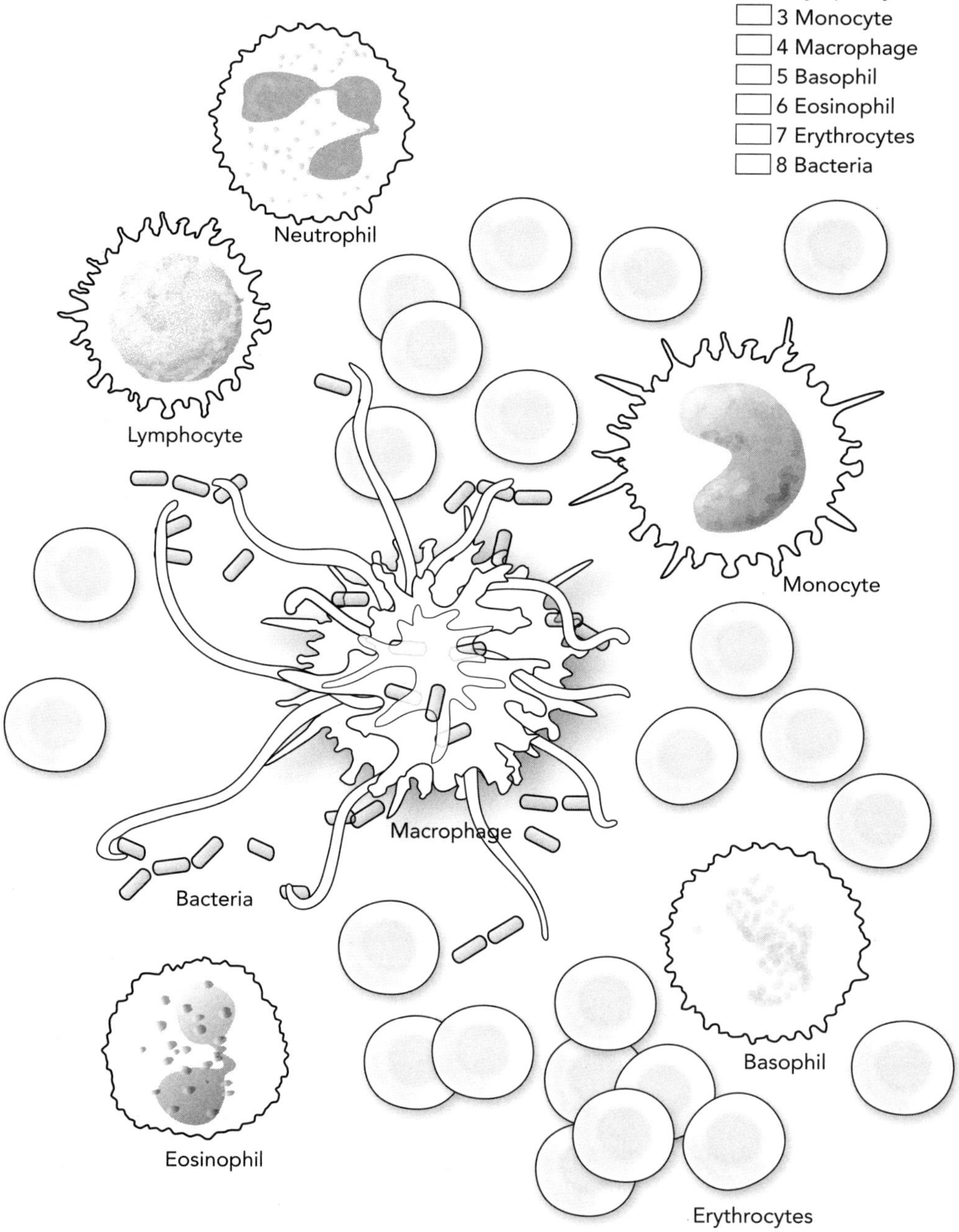

Neutrophil

Lymphocyte

Monocyte

Bacteria

Macrophage

Eosinophil

Basophil

Erythrocytes

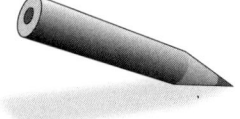

MUSCLE TISSUE

Muscle tissue is composed of specialized cells called fibers that respond to stimulation by contracting and becoming shorter. Contraction can produce movements, maintain posture, produce changes in shape, or propel substances through tissues or organs. There are three types of muscle in the body: skeletal muscle (voluntary muscle), cardiac muscle, and smooth muscle (involuntary muscle).

Skeletal muscle

Skeletal muscle fibers, also called myofibers, are long and thin. They contain contractile proteins called myofilaments. The myofilaments are arranged in alternating light and dark striations. Fibers are enclosed by a cell membrane called sarcolemma. Depending on its size and function a skeletal muscle may contain hundreds to thousands of individual fibers. Skeletal (striated) muscles are voluntary and thus under conscious control. They attach to the bones of the skeleton and produce movement at the joints. Upon contraction, one of the bones moves while the other bone usually remains fixed. The less mobile attachment of a muscle is called its origin. The more mobile attachment of the muscle is its insertion. When contracted, the insertion is pulled toward the origin. Skeletal muscles may also attach to the skin in some areas such as the muscles of facial expression. Skeletal muscle cells are arranged into bundles (called fascicles) surrounded by thin layers of connective tissue. The fascicles are arranged into larger bundles, which form the muscular organ (e.g., the biceps). The connective tissue surrounding the fascicles extends as dense regular connective tissue to anchor the muscle to the bone in the form of a tendon.

Structures of skeletal muscle

Muscle fiber: long, thin cells within muscle tissue.

Myofilament: contractile protein within myofibers, composed of myosin and actin molecules.

Fascicle: contains a bundle of muscle fibers.

Muscle: composed of many fascicles.

Endomysium: thin sheet of connective tissue separating individual muscle fibers.

Perimysium: sheet of connective tissue between the fascicles.

Epimysium: connective tissue surrounding fascicles.

Structure of a skeletal muscle

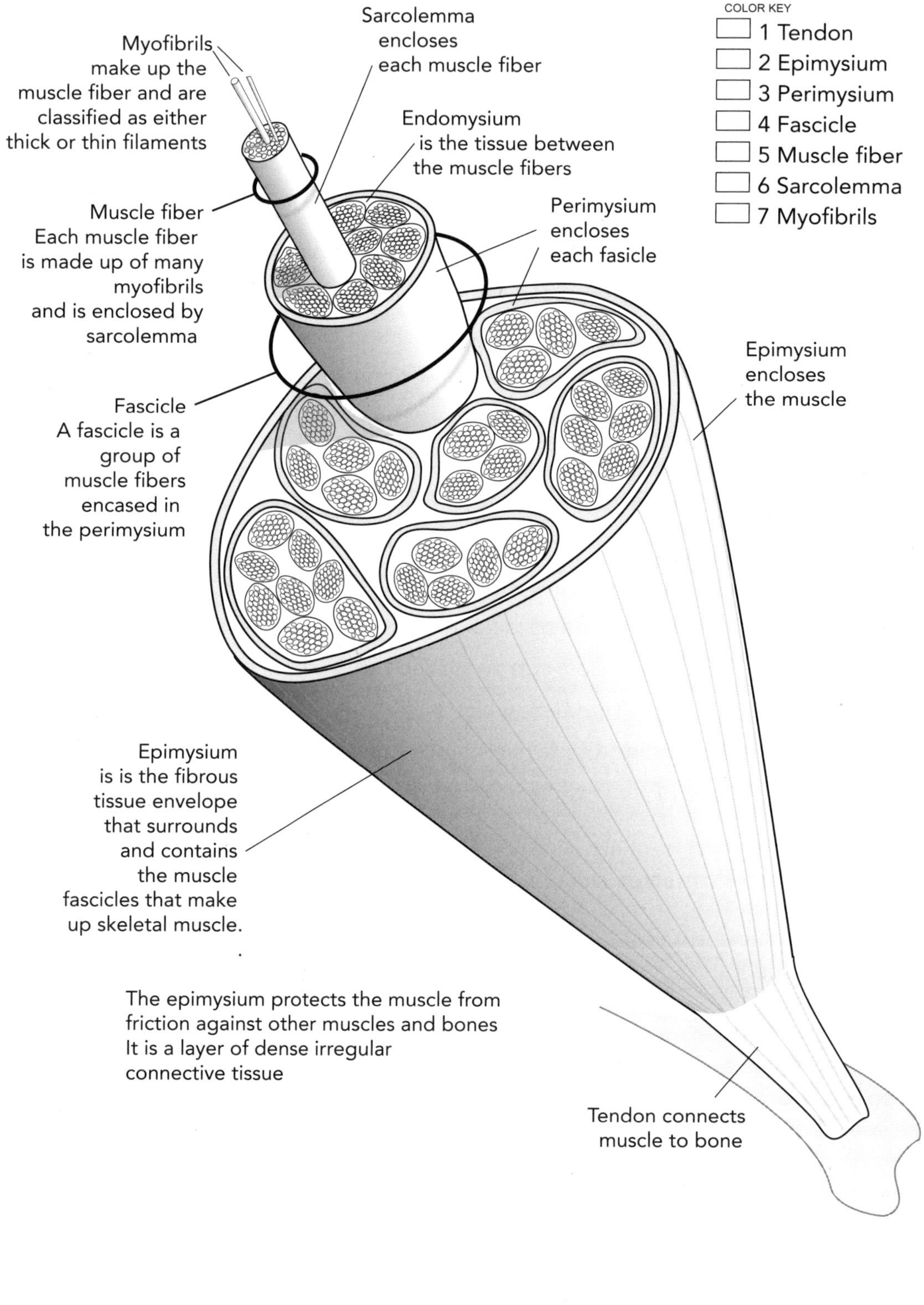

Myofibrils make up the muscle fiber and are classified as either thick or thin filaments

Sarcolemma encloses each muscle fiber

Endomysium is the tissue between the muscle fibers

Muscle fiber
Each muscle fiber is made up of many myofibrils and is enclosed by sarcolemma

Perimysium encloses each fascicle

Fascicle
A fascicle is a group of muscle fibers encased in the perimysium

Epimysium encloses the muscle

Epimysium is is the fibrous tissue envelope that surrounds and contains the muscle fascicles that make up skeletal muscle.

The epimysium protects the muscle from friction against other muscles and bones It is a layer of dense irregular connective tissue

Tendon connects muscle to bone

COLOR KEY
- [ ] 1 Tendon
- [ ] 2 Epimysium
- [ ] 3 Perimysium
- [ ] 4 Fascicle
- [ ] 5 Muscle fiber
- [ ] 6 Sarcolemma
- [ ] 7 Myofibrils

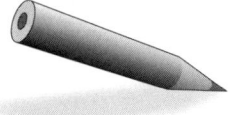

Skeletal muscles can be classified based on their gross appearance.

Fusiform: thick in the center and tapered at the ends.

Quadrate: four-sided.

Flat: fibers are arranged parallel to each other.

Circular: fibers form a sphincter that closes off tubes.

Pennate: looks feathered, like the wing of a bird. May be unipennate, bipennate, or multipennate.

Cardiac muscle

Cardiac muscle forms the thick middle layer of the heart wall. Although cardiac muscle is striated and possesses myofilaments it is involuntary because the cells do not require voluntary nervous system activity to initiate a contraction.

Smooth muscle

Smooth muscle lacks striation and is involuntary. Smooth muscle cells are called myocytes. Smooth muscle is controlled by the autonomic nervous system. This type of muscle is found in the walls of organs such as the esophagus.

Draw your own: skeletal muscle

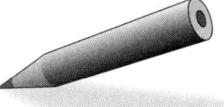

TEST YOURSELF: CELLS AND TISSUES

MULTIPLE CHOICE CELLS

1 _____   The _____ of the cell directs its overall activities and contains its genetic material
    a. Nucleolus
    b. Endoplasmic reticulum
    c. Nucleus
    d. Centrosome

2 _____   The transport system that moves molecules throughout the cell is/are
    a. Mitochondria
    b. Microtubules and microfilaments
    c. Ribosomes
    d. Peroxisomes

3 _____   In what part of the nucleus does ribosome production occur?
    a. Within the nuclear membrane
    b. In the chromatin
    c. In the area of the nucleolus
    d. Ribosome production does not occur in the nucleus

4 _____   The _____ of a cell has a function directly related to the synthesis of proteins
    a. Mitochondrion
    b. Lysosome
    c. Ribosome
    d. Centriole

5 _____   The __ is a system of membrane lined sacs that transport molecules within and out of cells
    a. Vacuole
    b. Chromatin
    c. Nucleolus
    d. Endoplasmic reticulum

6 _____   The rough ER is so named because it has an abundance of
    a. Mitochondria
    b. Lysosomes
    c. Golgi bodies
    d. Ribosomes

7 _____   The Golgi apparatus is involved in
    a. Transporting proteins that are to be released from the cell
    b. Packaging proteins into vesicles
    c. Altering or modifying proteins
    d. All of the above

8 ____   The control center of a cell is the
        a. Nucleus
        b. Cytoplasm
        c. Chromosome
        d. Cell membrane

9 ____   The structure that contains the genetic material (DNA) is
        a. The cell membrane
        b. Ribosomes
        c. Nucleus
        d. Mitochondria

10 ____   Which organelle digests old matter that is no longer useful to the cell?
        a. Ribosomes
        b. Mitochondria
        c. Lysosomes
        d. Chromatin

TRUE/FALSE CELLS

1 ____   All cells consist of cytoplasm and a nucleus surrounded by a membrane.

2 ____   Cell inclusions refer to all the organelles within the cell.

3 ____   Stem cells have the potential to develop into different types of cells and can also repair

and replenish other cells in a living organism.

4 ____   The human body is made up of more than 100 trillion cells.

5 ____   Each new stem cell has the potential either to remain a stem cell or become a

cell with a more specialized function.

6 ____   The cell membrane regulates which substances enter and exit the cell.

7 ____   The nucleus contains ribonucleic acid (RNA).

8 ____   Rough and smooth endoplasmic reticulum are both studded with ribosomes.

9 ____   Mitochondria are the flattened sacs that modify, sort, and package proteins for use

in the cell or for export.

10 ____   Lysosomes contain enzymes that break down unwanted material and

recycle useful substances.

11 ____   The bundles of microtubules involved in cell division are called centrioles.

12 ____   Chromatin refers to a diffuse network of fine fibrils and proteins in the DNA in the nucleus.

FILL IN THE BLANK CELLS

1.   _____ are not yet specialized to perform specific functions.

2.   Nonliving components within a cell are called _____.

3.   The _____ separates the interior of the cell from the outside environment.

4.   Proteins are synthesized by _____.

5.   The main mass of the cell is made up of_____.

6.   The _____ is a series of flattened sacs that modifies, sorts, and packages proteins.

7.   Nutrients are absorbed, and fatty acids are digested by _____.

8.   The _____ is a series of membranes studded with ribosomes.

9.   Carbohydrates, lipids, and protein molecules are converted into ATP by _____.

10.   The _____ contains DNA and proteins.

11.   The _____ is a mass of RNA with some DNA and proteins within the nucleus.

12.   The series of membranes without attached ribosomes is the _____.

13.   _____ contain enzymes that break down unwanted material and recycle useful substances.

14.   _____ are bundles of microtubules involved in cell division.

15.   The diffuse network of fine fibrils in the nuclear DNA is called _____.

16.   The two networks of protein fibers that provide structural support to the cell and allow internal cell parts to be transported within and outside of the cell

      are_____ and _____.

MATCHING CELLS

Ribosomes	1 Sacs that modify, sort, and package proteins
Mitochondria	2 Controls what can pass in/out the cell
Golgi apparatus	3 Synthesize proteins by assembling amino acids
Rough endoplasmic reticulum	4 Convert carbohydrates, lipids, protein molecules into ATP
Nucleus	5 Series of membranes studded with ribosomes
Plasma membrane	6 RNA and proteins involved in formation of ribosomes
Smooth endoplasmic reticulum	7 Vesicles that absorb nutrients and digest fatty acids
Microtubules/microfilaments	8 Area of the cell containing DNA and proteins
Chromatin	9 Series of membranes without attached ribosomes
Cytoplasm	10 Networks of protein fibers that support the cell
Nucleolus	11 Sacs that can fuse with other sacs or cell membrane
Vacuoles/pinocytic vesicles	12 Network of fine fibrils in the DNA in the nucleus
Lysosomes	13 Bundles of microtubules involved in cell division
Cell inclusions	14 Gel-like substance that makes up the main cell mass
Centrioles	15 Vesicles with enzymes that break down unwanted material
Peroxisomes	16 Nonliving components not bounded by membranes

Draw your own: cell

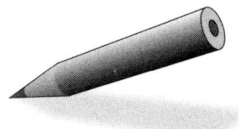

MULTIPLE CHOICE   MITOSIS

1_____ Each duplicated chromosome prior to division is held together at the

      a. Synapsis

      b Chromosome articulation

      c. Chromatid

      d. Centromere

2_____ Prior to division, each chromosome is composed of two genetically identical pairs called

      a. Centromeres

      b. Dyads

      c. Sister chromatids

      d. Genetic partners

3_____ The phase in which a cell spends most of its life is

      a. Interphase

      b. Metaphase

      c. Prophase

      d. Anaphase

4_____ Which fibers shorten during anaphase and pull the chromosomes apart?

      a. Centriolar fibers

      b. Metaphasal fibers

      c. Polar fibers

      d. Asters

5_____ When does DNA replication occur in the cell cycle?

      a. Interphase

      b. Prophase

      c. Anaphase

      d. Telophase

6_____ Which structure in the cell brings about chromosomal movement?

      a. Mitochondria

      b. Golgi apparatus

      c. Centromeres

      d. Spindle fibers

7_____ When a cell begins to divide, when do organelles such as centrioles, duplicate?

      a. Interphase

      b. Prophase

      c. Metaphase

      d. Telophase

8_____ Which of the following is the correct sequence of mitotic phases?

      a. Metaphase, anaphase, telophase, prophase

      b. Anaphase, prophase, metaphase, telophase

      c. Prophase, anaphase, metaphase, telophase

      d. Prophase, metaphase, anaphase, telophase

9____ During ____, spindle fibers attach to the centromeres of each chromosome
      a. Prophase
      b. Metaphase
      c. Anaphase
      d. Telophase

10____ At the start of ____, the sister chromatids separate, and the daughter chromosomes move up to the poles of the spindle
      a. Metaphase
      b. Anaphase
      c. Prophase
      d. Telophase

11____ A centromere refers to
      a. A chromosome
      b. A constricted region of a chromosome
      c. The point to which daughter chromosomes migrate
      d. A spindle fiber

12____ What is a chromatid?
      a. A chromosome outside the nucleus
      b. A special region that holds two centromeres together
      c. A duplicated chromosome
      d. None of the above

FILL IN THE BLANK   MITOSIS

1. Somatic cells undergo _____.

2. Sex cells undergo _____.

3._____ is the time between divisions.

4. The cell divides into daughter cells during the _____ phase.

5. The cell carries out metabolic functions during _____.

6. Chromatin is found in the nuclear DNA during _____.

7. Sister chromatids are pulled apart during _____.

8. During _____ spindle fibers grow from each

centriole across the cell center toward the chromosomes.

9. Chromatin become condensed into chromosomes during _____.

10. The cell pinches off in the center and forms two daughter cells during

_____.

11. During _____ each chromosome contains two copies of its DNA.

12. The cell prepares for cell division by increasing in size and duplicating its DNA

and centrioles during _____.

MATCHING MITOSIS

	Metaphase	1 Time between cell divisions
	Interphase	2 Chromatin becomes condensed into chromosomes
	Telophase	3 Spindle fibers grow from each centriole
	Anaphase	4 Cell pinches off in the center forming two daughter chromosomes
	Prophase	5 Sister chromatids are pulled apart as the spindle shortens

TRUE/FALSE MITOSIS

1.____   All the cells in the body undergo mitosis during which one cell divides

into two identical daughter cells

2.____   There are two major phases of cell division called interphase and

the mitotic phase

3.____   Most cells are in the mitotic phase during most of their lives

4.____   The cell prepares for cell division by increasing in size and duplicating

its DNA and centrioles during interphase

5.____   Dispersed fibrils of chromatin become condensed into short, thick,

coiled chromosomes during prophase

6.____   Duplicated chromosomes consist of two sister chromatids,

joined together at a constricted region called the centromere

7.____   Sister chromatids line up in the center of the cell during anaphase

8.____   The nuclear membrane dissolves at the end of metaphase

9.____   Two daughter cells form during telophase

10.____   The two new daughter cells enter the interphase of their life cycle at the end of telophase

MULTIPLE CHOICE TISSUES

1 ____ A group of cells that performs a specific function is organized as a/an
     a. Organ
     b. Tissue
     c. System
     d. Organelle

2 ____ Which type of tissue lines body areas?
     a. Epithelial
     b. Connective
     c. Muscle
     d. Nervous

3 ____ Epithelial tissue is characterized by all the following except
     a. It can be simple or stratified
     b. It functions in secretion, absorption, and excretion
     c. Epithelial cells are loosely packed and have much intercellular material
     d. It is anchored to a basement membrane

4 ____ Epithelium that appears layered because cell nuclei are distributed at different levels, but which is not actually layered is called
     a. Transitional epithelium
     b. Squamous epithelium
     c. Pseudosimple epithelium
     d. Pseudostratified epithelium

5 ____ The primary purpose of stratification in epithelial tissue is for increased
     a. Protection
     b. Secretion
     c. Absorption
     d. Thickening of the basement membrane

6 ____ Squamous cells are
     a. Tall and circular
     b. Thin and flat
     c. As wide as they are long
     d. Tall and thin

7 _____   Ciliated columnar epithelium is found in
    a. Skin
    b. Vocal tract
    c. Trachea and bronchi
    d. All the above

8 _____   Connective tissues
    a. Occur throughout the body
    b. Serve many different functions
    c. Contain a few living cells and much extracellular material
    d. All the above

9 _____   Substance that living cells of connective tissue cells are embedded in is called
    a. Ground substance
    b. Extracellular matrix
    c. Fiber network
    d. Stroma

10 _____   Which fibers cause tissue to return to its original shape after being displaced?
    a. Collagen
    b. Elastin
    c. Reticular
    d. Muscular

11 _____   Fibers that provide tensile strength are
    a. Collagen
    b. Elastin
    c. Reticular
    d. Muscular

12 _____   Loose connective tissue includes
    a. Regular
    b. Elastic
    c. Irregular
    d. Areolar

13 _____   Blood is classified as a _____ tissue because it has cells embedded in a matrix
    a. Epithelial
    b. Muscle
    c. Nervous
    d. Connective

14 _____ Cells that produce the fibers and ground substance components of the extracellular matrix are
   a. Mast cells
   b. Neutrophils
   c. Fibroblasts
   d. Eosinophils

15 _____ The cells that store and release triglycerides are
   a. Macrophages
   b. Lymphocytes
   c. Mast cells
   d. Adipocytes

16 _____ Tendons and ligaments are composed of which type of connective tissue?
   a. Adipose
   b. Regular
   c. Irregular
   d. Elastic

17 _____ Which type of connective tissue surrounds nerves and blood vessels?
   a. Adipose
   b. Areolar
   c. Elastic
   d. Collagen

TRUE/FALSE TISSUES

1 _____ Epithelium is characterized by the shape of the cells and numbers of layers of cells.

2 _____ Epithelium can be ciliated or non-ciliated.

3 _____ Epithelium can be squamous, cuboidal, or columnar.

4 _____ Keratinized epithelium is highly waterproof.

5 _____ Simple epithelium typically protects against abrasion.

6 _____ Connective tissue contains blood vessels and nerves.

7 _____ Types of fibers in connective tissue include collagen, elastin, and reticular.

8 _____ Connective tissue is characterized by many living cells

surrounded by small amounts of extracellular matrix.

9 _____ Fibroblasts produce the fibers and other substances of

the extracellular matrix and are also capable of contraction.

10 _____ Damaged cells within the extracellular matrix are engulfed by lymphocytes.

11 _____ Macrophages store and release triglycerides and produce hormones and growth factors.

12 _____ Mast cells and neutrophils are both involved in immune response.

13 ____ Areolar tissue consists of a loosely organized array of collagen and elastic

fibers and many blood vessels.

14 ____ Regular dense connective tissue is composed primarily of adipocytes and acts

as a shock absorber.

15 ____ Elastic tissue also contains collagen fibers.

FILL IN THE BLANK TISSUES

1   Epithelial cells that are thinner and taller than they are wide

are called _____.

2   _____ epithelial cells are thin and flat.

3   _____ is found within the trachea and bronchi.

4   _____ epithelium is found primarily in the skin.

5   The lining of the vocal tract is formed by _____ epithelium.

6   Epithelial tissues rest on a _____ membrane.

7   The nonliving substance in connective tissue is called _____.

8   _____ remove damaged cells or pathogens in connective tissue.

9   Hormones and growth factors are produced by _____.

10   _____ produce the fibers and ground substance

components of the extracellular matrix array of collagen and elastic fibers.

11   _____ function like fibroblasts and are also capable of contraction.

12   _____ tissue is composed of a loosely organized array of

collagen and elastic fibers.

13   Tendons and ligaments are made up of _____ fibers.

14   Fibers that provide resilience and flexibility are _____.

15   _____ fibers form supporting layers around cartilage and bone.

MATCHING TISSUES

	Fibroblasts	1 Provides padding and acts as an insulator
	Myofibroblasts	2 Store and release triglycerides and produce hormones and growth factors
	Adipocytes	3 Branching elastic fibers together with packed collagen fibers
	Macrophages	4 Respond to allergens and parasitic infections
	Lymphocytes	5 Produce extracellular matrix
	Mast cells	6 Tightly packed collagen fibers arranged in parallel
	Plasma cells	7 Synthesize antibodies to fight diseases
	Neutrophils	8 Responds to injury and immune challenges
	Eosinophils	9 Produce extracellular matrix and can also contract
	Areolar	10 Secrete heparin and histamine
	Adipose	11 Scattered network of collagen fibers
	Regular	12 Phagocytize damaged cells or pathogens
	Irregular	13 Primary cells of the immune system
	Elastic	14 Loosely organized array of elastin and collagen fibers

MULTIPLE CHOICE   CARTILAGE, BONE, AND BLOOD

1 _____   The outer layer of cartilage is called
   a. Periosteum
   b. Perichondrium
   c. Perifibrous
   d. None of the above

2 _____   The most common type of cartilage is
   a. Hyaline
   b. Elastic
   c. Resilient
   d. Fibrous

3 _____   Fibrocartilage
   a. Allows the bones in a joint to move freely and easily
   b. Provides support through flexibility and resilience
   c. Has a bluish color
   d. Acts as a shock absorber and resists compression

4 ____   The fibrous connective tissue that forms the outer covering of the bone is the

    a. Epiphysis

    b. Diaphysis

    c. Articular cartilage

    d. Periosteum

5 ____   Surrounding the diaphysis of a long bone is

    a. Compact bone

    b. Spongy bone

    c. Cartilage

    d. Yellow marrow

6 ____ The cells that tear down and remodel bone are the

    a. Osteoblasts

    b. Osteocytes

    c. Osteoclasts

    d. Macrophages

7 ____ The part of the bone covered by articular cartilage is the

    a. Diaphysis

    b. Endosteum

    c. Epiphysis

    d. Periosteum

8 ____ The primary cell in cartilage is called a

    a. Fibroblast

    b. Chondrocyte

    c. Osteocyte

    d. Osteoblast

9 ____ Tissue that is translucent is most likely

    a. Bone

    b. Elastic cartilage

    c. Hyaline cartilage

    d. Fibrocartilage

10 ____ The flexibility of the outer ear is due mainly to

    a. Hyaline cartilage

    b. Elastic cartilage

    c. Fibrocartilage

    d. Epithelium

11 ____ Which of the following statements is NOT true?

    a. Bone is where most blood cells are made

    b. Bone serves as a storehouse for various minerals

    c. Bone is a dry and non-living supporting structure

    d. Bone protects and supports the body and its organs

12 ____ What makes bones so strong?
   a. Silicone
   b. Cartilage
   c. Blood and marrow
   d. Calcium and phosphorus

13 ____ What is the difference between cartilage and bone?
   a. Bone is flexible, and cartilage is inflexible
   b. Cartilage is flexible, and bone is inflexible
   c. Bone is a more primitive tissue than cartilage
   d. Bone is inside the body and cartilage is outside

14 ____ Which type of bone is the scapula?
   a. Flat
   b. Long
   c. Short
   d. Irregular

15 ____ Which of the following does not make up the interior of the bone?
   a. Compact bone tissue
   b. Spongy bone tissue
   c. Red marrow
   d. Yellow marrow

16 ____ The liquid portion of blood is referred to as
   a. Whole blood
   b. Hematocrit
   c. Plasma
   d. Serum

17 ____ Which of the following is involved in the transportation of oxygen?
   a. Hemoglobin
   b. Oxyhemoglobin
   c. Reduced hemoglobin
   d. None of the above

Draw your own: Long bone

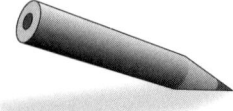

Tissues and Joints

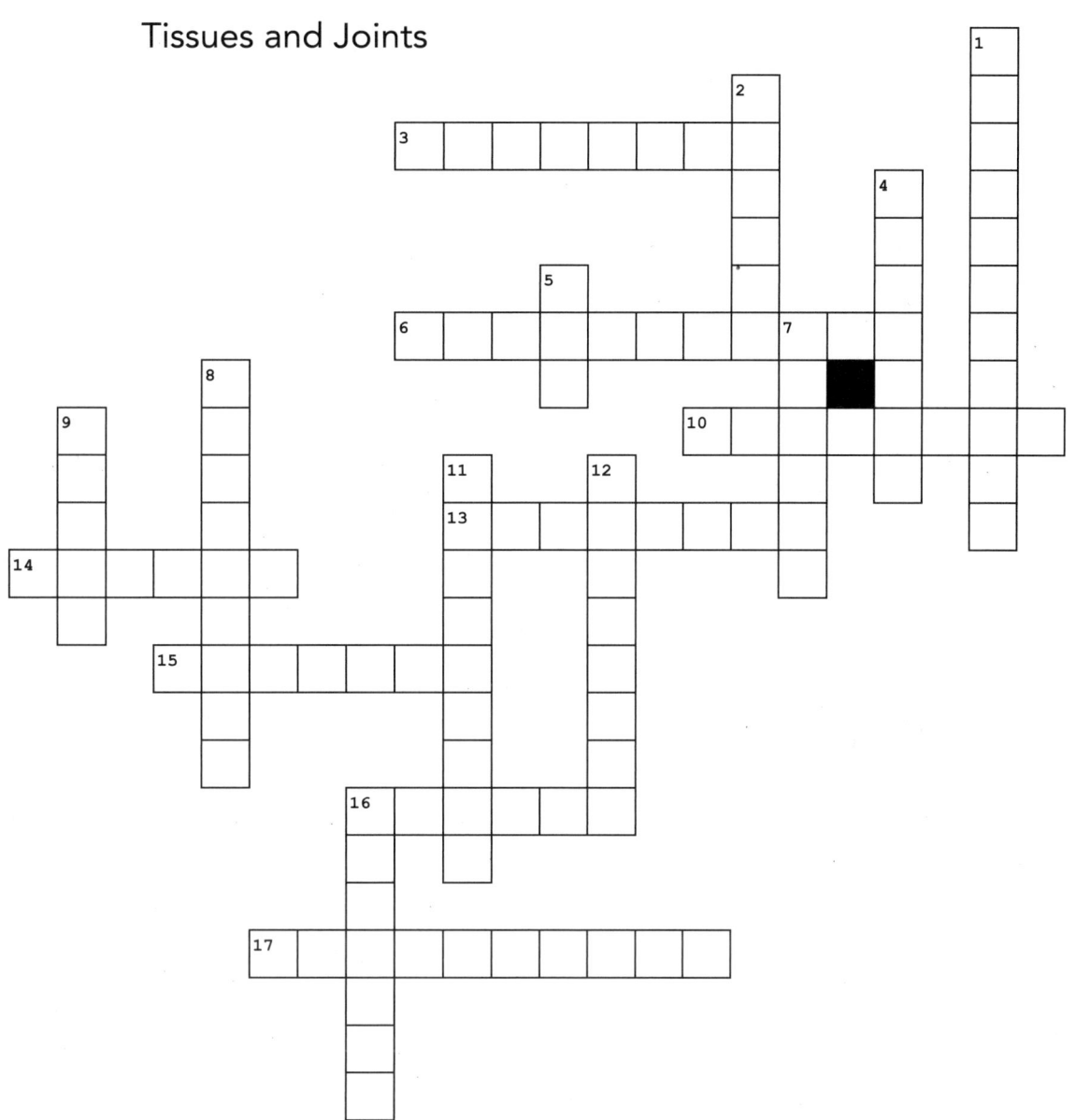

Across

3. Freely movable joint
6. These break down bone
10. Name for a skeletal muscle fiber
13. Connects bone to bone
14. Attaches muscle to bone or cartilage
15. Translucent and flexible
16. Synonym for a fibrous joint
17. Covers bones

Down

1. A contractile protein
2. Liquid portion of blood
4. Cartilage in the epiglottis
5. Most common type of blood cell
7. Type of muscle found in the esophagus
8. Synonym for white blood cell
9. Protect and support the body
11. Can bind together to stop bleeding
12. Bundle of muscle fibers
16. Example of a flat bone

TRUE/FALSE   CARTILAGE, BONE, AND BLOOD

1 _____ The extracellular matrix in cartilage is firm and gel-like allowing for flexibility

2 _____ The most common type of cartilage is hyaline

3 _____ Elastic cartilage is found in many areas of the body, including the nose, trachea, and most of the larynx

4 _____ Fibrocartilage acts as a shock absorber and resists compression

5 _____ Elastic cartilage and fibrocartilage both are characterized by densely intertwined strands of collagen fibers

6 _____ The matrix in bone is rigid due to the presence of calcium and other minerals

7 _____ Bone is remodeled via osteoclasts which form bone, and osteoblasts, which break it down

8 _____ Vitamins and exercise are very important in bone health

9 _____ The outer layer of bone is made up of compact bone tissue; the interior is composed of spongy bone

10 _____ Red marrow produces blood cells; yellow marrow stores fat

11 _____ The end of bones that form joints with other bones is called the diaphysis

12 _____ Articular cartilage covers the metaphysis of the bone

13 _____ The long shaft of the bone is called the diaphysis

14 _____ Plasma comprises more than half of blood volume

15 _____ Proteins make up the major portion of plasma

16 _____ White blood cells can bind together in order to form clots and stop bleeding

17 _____ Granular leukocytes contain digestive enzymes

18 _____ Monocytes are a type of granular leukocyte

19 _____ Erythrocytes are the most common type of blood cell

20 _____ Red blood cells deliver oxygen to every cell in the body

21 _____ Neutrophils and eosinophils act as phagocytes

FILL IN THE BLANK   CARTILAGE, BONE, AND BLOOD

1   Cartilage usually has a covering called the _____.

2   _____ cartilage is found in the nose, trachea, and most of the larynx.

3   _____ cartilage is durable due to its densely packed collagen fibers.

4   _____ cartilage has a yellowish color.

5   _____ is the most common type of cartilage.

6   The matrix in bone contains _____ and _____.

7   Fibroblasts in bone include _____ and _____.

8   Vitamin _____ stimulates the absorption of calcium and phosphate ions into the blood.

9   The outer layer of bone is made up of _____.

10   _____ forms the interior of the bone.

11   The sternum is an example of a _____ bone.

12   The _____ is the long shaft of the bone.

13   The _____ refers to the expanded ends of the bone.

14   The region in a bone between the _____ and the _____

        is the _____.

15   _____ bind together in order to form clots and stop bleeding.

16   White blood cells are also called _____.

17   _____ produce circulating antibodies and can kill virus-infected cells.

18   _____ are phagocytes that respond to allergic reactions.

19   The most common type of blood cell is _____.

20   The liquid portion of blood is _____.

21   _____ is a molecule that contains iron and gives the cell its red color.

22   _____ leukocytes contain digestive enzymes.

MATCHING CARTILAGE, BONE, AND BLOOD

Diaphysis	1 Tough sheath of connective tissue that covers the outer surface of the bone
Epiphysis	2 Region in a bone between the diaphysis and the epiphysis
Metaphysis	3 Responds to injury and immune challenges
Marrow cavity	4 Long shaft of the bone
Periosteum	5 Red blood cells
Neutrophils	6 Expanded ends of the bone covered by a thin layer of hyaline cartilage
Plasma	7 Hollow, cylindrical space within the diaphysis
Platelets	8 Do not contain digestive enzymes
Lymphocytes	9 Liquid portion of blood
Eosinophils	10 Contain digestive enzymes
Granular leukocytes	11 Cell fragments without a nucleus
Erythrocytes	12 Phagocytes that respond to allergic reactions
Agranular leukocytes	13 Main cells of the immune system

MULTIPLE CHOICE JOINTS

1____   What is a joint?
   a. The cushion between two bones
   b. Where two bones meet and move
   c. The outer coating of the bone
   d. The hard part of a skeleton

2 ____   Which is not a type of human joint?
   a. Hinge
   b. Ball and socket
   c. Pivot
   d. Swinging

3 ____   Where might you find a gliding joint?
   a. Neck
   b. Spine
   c. Hand
   d. Hip

4 _____   What connects bones to each other at the joints?
    a. Ligaments
    b. Tendons
    c. Filaments
    d. None of the above

5 _____   All the following are structural classifications of joints, except
    a. Cartilaginous
    b. Osseous
    c. Fibrous
    d. Synovial

6 _____   The type of joint that has a fluid-filled joint cavity is
    a. Fibrous
    b. Cartilaginous
    c. Synovial
    d. Amphiarthrodial

7 _____   In a _____ joint, an oval surface fits into a concave depression
    a. Hinge
    b. Saddle
    c. Ellipsoidal
    d. Pivot

8 _____   The temporomandibular joint is
    a. Ellipsoidal
    b. Plane
    c. Saddle
    d. Hinge

9 _____   The movement of the sole of the foot outward or laterally is
    a. Inversion
    b. Eversion
    c. Retraction
    d. Elevation

10 _____   The joints in the cranium are
    a. Fibrous
    b. Diarthrodial
    c. Cartilaginous
    d. Synovial

11 ____ Movement of a limb towards the midline of the body is called
   a. Inversion
   b. Abduction
   c. Adduction
   d. Extension

12 ____ A synovial joint is an example of a(n)
   a. Diarthrosis
   b. Amphiarthrosis
   c. Synarthrosis
   d. None of the above

13 ____ An immovable joint is a(n)
   a. Diarthrosis
   b. Amphiarthrosis
   c. Synarthrosis
   d. None of the above

MATCHING JOINTS

Hinge	1 Movements directed in the sagittal plane; angle between the bones is increased
Plane	2 Smaller versions of ball and socket joints
Saddle	3 Combines movements of eversion and abduction around a vertical axis (in the foot)
Ellipsoidal	4 Turns the sole of the foot inward
Pivot	5 Formed by a ring of bone rotating about an axle of bone
Ball and socket	6 Bone is moved away from the midline of the body or structure
Adduction	7 Operates like a swinging gate
Rotation	8 Allow the greatest range of motion
Circumduction	9 Formed between a roughly U-shaped end of one bone into which the end of the other fits
Abduction	10 Circular movement of flexion, abduction, extension, and adduction performed in sequence
Pronation	11 Allows bones to glide past one another, but they cannot rotate
Extension	12 Bone is moved toward the midline of the body or structure
Inversion	13 Movements are directed in the sagittal plane; angle between the bones is decreased
Flexion	14 Moving bone is turned about its axis; can be medial (internal) or lateral (external)
Supination	15 Turns the sole of the foot outward
Eversion	16 Combines movements of inversion and adduction around a vertical axis (in the foot).

TRUE/FALSE JOINTS

1 ____   Joints are classified functionally as synovial, cartilaginous, or fibrous

2 ____   A suture is an example of a synovial joint

3 ____   Synovial joints are diarthrodial

4 ____   Synovial joints are composed of two bones encased within a synovial cavity

5 ____   The ends of the bones in a synovial joint are held in place by ligaments

6 ____   Plane joints allow the greatest range of motion

7 ____   Examples of pivot joints are the first and second cervical vertebrae

8 ____   Ellipsoidal joints are smaller versions of ball and socket joints

9 ____   The types of movement permitted by a joint depends its structure

as well as its associated ligaments and muscles

10 ____   In abduction movements are directed medially so that the bone

is moved toward the midline of the body or structure

11 ____   Rotation is circular movement resulting from the movements of

flexion, abduction, extension, and adduction performed in sequence

12 ____   Flexion occurs when the angle between the bones is decreased

FILL IN THE BLANK JOINTS

1.   _____ joints have a seam of tough connective tissue that fuses the

adjoining bones together.

2.   Joints that permit a wide range of movements are _____.

3.   _____ joints are composed of two bones encased within a cavity.

4.   A joint formed by a ring of bone rotating about an axle of bone is a _____ joint.

5.   _____ joints connect flat bones.

6.   The hips and shoulders are examples of _____ joints.

7.   _____ joints operate like a swinging gate.

8.   The temporomandibular joint is an example of a _____ joint.

9.   _____ results from the movements of flexion, abduction, extension,

and adduction performed in sequence.

10.   In _____ the angle between the bones is decreased.

11.   In adduction the bone is moved _____ the midline of the body/structure.

12.   _____ turns the sole of the foot inward.

13.   The angle between the bones is increased in _____.

14.   _____ allows movements to be directed laterally.

MULTIPLE CHOICE MUSCLE

1.   Layer of connective tissue that separates the muscle tissue into individual fibers is the
   a. Fascicle
   b. Epimysium
   c. Perimysium
   d. Endomysium

2.   Which term is the smallest subdivision in this group?
   a. Fiber
   b. Fibril
   c. Myofilament
   d. Actin

3.   The cell membrane that encloses the myofibers is the
   a. Fascicle
   b. Sarcolemma
   c. Epimysium
   d. None of the above

4.   The more mobile attachment of a muscle is called its
   a. Attachment
   b. Joint
   c. Insertion
   d. Articulation

5.   What happens when a skeletal muscle contracts?
   a. The origin is pulled away from the insertion
   b. The origin is pulled toward the insertion
   c. The origin may be pulled toward or away from the insertion depending
      on the muscle
   d. All the above statements are true

6.   Which of the following statements (if any) is NOT true of cardiac muscle?
   a. Cardiac muscle is striated and is therefore under conscious control
   b. Cardiac muscle forms the middle layer of the heart wall
   c. Cardiac muscle possesses myofilaments
   d. All the above statements are true

7.   The esophagus contains
   a. Skeletal muscle
   b. No muscle
   c. Smooth muscle
   d. Striated muscle

8.   Skeletal muscle looks striated because
    a. The myofilaments are arranged in alternating light and dark areas
    b. Myofilaments are enclosed by a cell membrane that varies in darkness
    c. Individual fibers vary in darkness
    d. All the above

9.   Fusiform muscles
    a. Are thick in the center and tapered at the ends
    b. Are four-sided
    c. Fibers form a sphincter
    d. Look feathered

10.   The type of muscle that closes off tubes is
    a. Quadrate
    b. Flat
    c. Circular
    d. Pennate

11.   Myocytes are cells of which type of muscle?
    a. Striated
    b. Cardiac
    c. Voluntary
    d. Smooth

12.   The connective tissue that surrounds multiple fascicles to form a complete muscle "belly" is
    a. Epimysium
    b. Endomysium
    c. Perimysium
    d. None of the above

TRUE/FALSE MUSCLE

1 ____   Muscle tissue is composed of fibers that respond to stimulation by becoming longer.

2 ____   Myofilaments are arranged in alternating light and dark striations.

3 ____   The less mobile attachment of a muscle is called its origin and the more mobile attachment is its insertion.

4 ____   Skeletal muscles can only attach to bones or cartilages.

5 ____   Myofilaments are arranged into fascicles surrounded by thin layers of connective tissue.

6 _____ The thin layer of connective tissue surrounding the fascicles

develops into a tendon that attaches to a bone.

7 _____ The epimysium is a sheet of connective tissue between the fascicles.

8 _____ The endomysium is a thin sheet of connective tissue

separating individual muscle fibers.

9 _____ Circular muscles form a sphincter that closes off tubes.

10 _____ Flat muscles are typically four sided.

11 _____ Fusiform muscles are thicker in the center and thinner at the ends.

12 _____ Cardiac muscle is voluntary because it is striated and possesses myofilaments.

13 _____ Smooth muscle is found in the walls of organs such as the esophagus and stomach.

FILL IN THE BLANK MUSCLE

1.   Skeletal muscle fibers are called _____.

2.   The contractile element in a skeletal muscle fiber is the _____.

3.   The less mobile attachment of a muscle is the _____ and the more

mobile   attachment of the muscle is its _____.

4.   The _____ encloses each individual muscle fiber.

5.   Groups of muscle cells are arranged into _____.

6.   Muscles are attached to bones by _____.

7.   The sheet of connective tissue between the fascicles is called _____.

8.   _____ surrounds multiple fascicles to form a complete muscle "belly".

9.   Myofilaments are composed of _____ and

_____ molecules.

10.   Fibers are arranged parallel to each other in _____ muscles.

11.   _____ muscles have a feathery look.

12.   Muscles that are thick in the center and tapered at the ends are

called _____.

13.   _____ muscles form a sphincter that closes off tubes.

MATCHING   MUSCLE

Flat	1 Connective tissue surrounding multiple fascicles forming a muscle "belly"
Muscle	2 Long, thin cells within muscle tissue
Muscle fiber	3 Thick in the center and tapered at the ends
Circular	4 Sheet of connective tissue between the fascicles
Perimysium	5 Four-sided
Fusiform	6 Fibers are arranged in parallel
Fascicle	7 Thin sheet of connective tissue separating individual muscle fibers
Endomysium	8 Fibers form a sphincter that closes off tubes
Pennate	9 Composed of many fascicles
Myofilament	10 Looks feathered, like the wing of a bird
Quadrate	11 Contractile protein within myofibers
Epimysium	12 Contains a bundle of muscle fibers

Cells

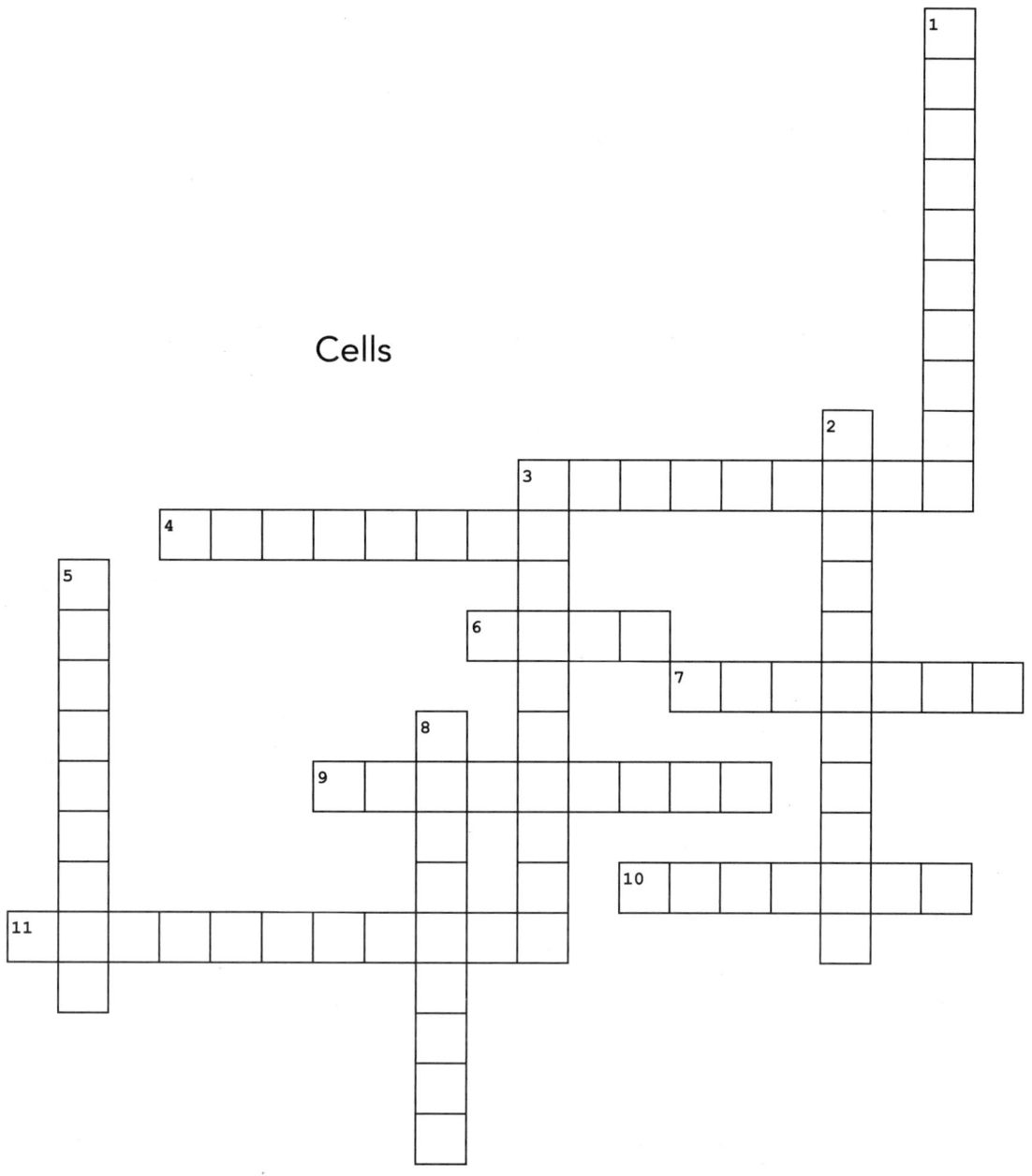

Across

3. Fluid gel-like substance within a cell
4. Breaks down unwanted material
6. Cells which are not yet specialized
7. Tissue composed primarily of fat cells
9. Stores fat
10. It contains DNA
11. Produce extracellular matrix

Down

1. Cells can be cuboidal, squamous, or columnar
2. Eliminate damaged or dead cells
3. These are involved in cell division
5. Diffuse network of fine fibrils in DNA
8. Synthesizes proteins

The Respiratory System

The respiratory system provides oxygen to every cell of the body and eliminates carbon dioxide. A respiratory cycle includes inhalation and exhalation. Exhalation provides the airstream that forms the basis of all voice and speech production. The respiratory system encompasses the oral and nasal cavities, pharynx, larynx, trachea, bronchi, bronchioles, alveolar sacs, and the lungs. The oral and nasal cavities and pharynx form the upper respiratory tract; the trachea and bronchial structures comprise the lower respiratory tract. The larynx is located at the junction of the upper and lower tracts.

THORACIC CAVITY

The lungs are located within the thoracic cavity. The thoracic cavity is bounded by the sternum (breast bone) and rib cage on the front and sides, the spinal column and vertebrae at the back, and the diaphragm muscle at the bottom. The rib cage is composed of 12 ribs on either side, which are attached by means of costal cartilage to the sternum.

Body cavities

COLOR KEY

☐ 1 Pleural cavities
☐ 2 Pericardial cavity
☐ 3 Abdominal cavity
☐ 4 Pelvic cavity

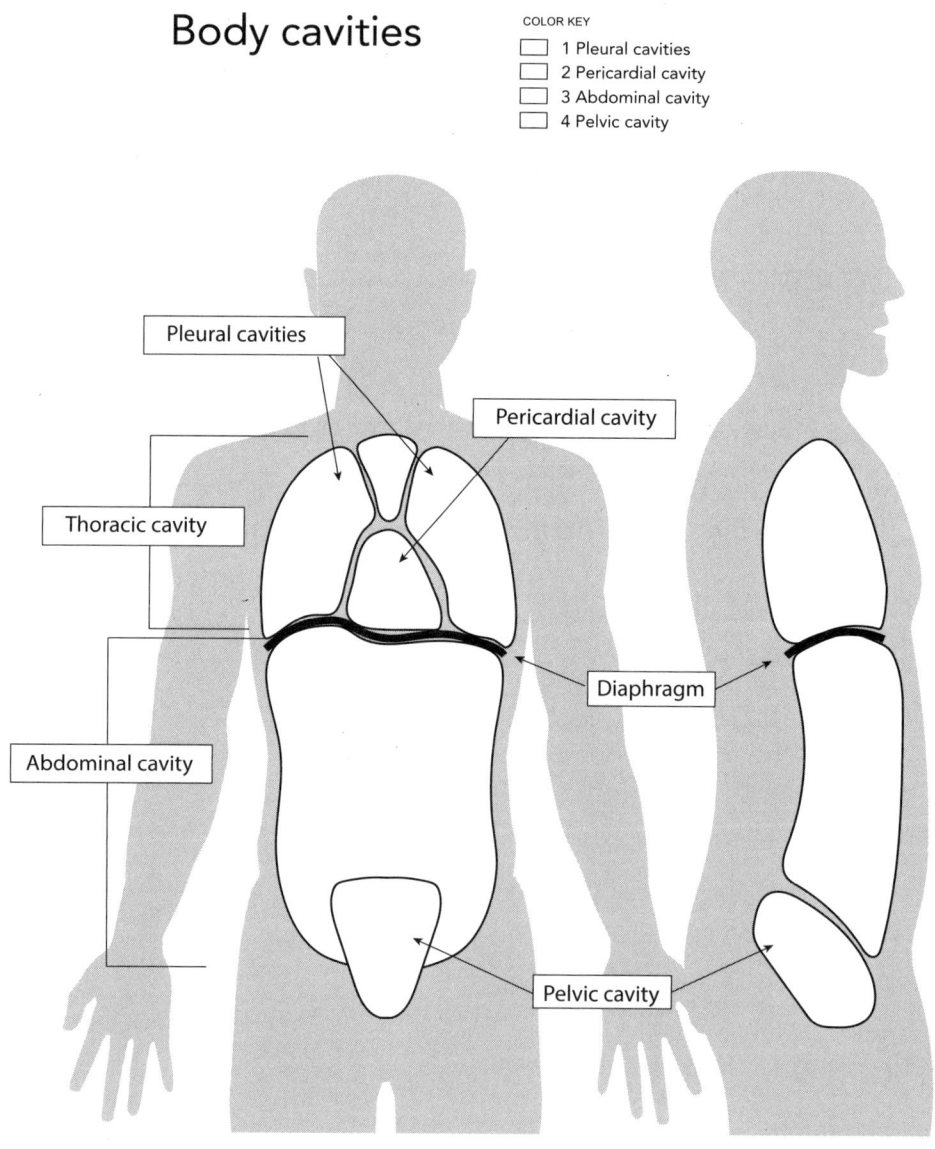

Pleural cavities

Pericardial cavity

Thoracic cavity

Diaphragm

Abdominal cavity

Pelvic cavity

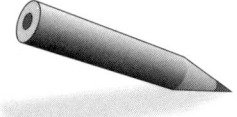

The pectoral girdle also forms part of the rib cage. This structure includes the two collar bones (clavicles) in front and two shoulder blades (scapulae) at the back. Many muscles attach to the rib cage and to the pectoral girdle. The diaphragm muscle forms the floor of the thoracic cavity, separating it from the abdominal cavity. The chest wall forms an integral part of the respiratory system, and is made up of the ribcage, the diaphragm, the abdominal wall, and the abdominal contents.

TRACHEOBRONCHIAL TREE

The tracheobronchial tree is an air conducting system formed by the trachea, bronchi, bronchioles, and alveolar sacs.

Trachea: hollow tube formed by 16-20 C-shaped rings of hyaline cartilage. The cartilages are closed anteriorly and open posteriorly. The cartilage is covered by layers of smooth muscle and mucous membrane which serve to close the tube posteriorly and are also present between the cartilages. The inside of the tube (lumen) is lined with pseudostratified ciliated columnar epithelium. The epithelium contains goblet cells that secrete mucous. The mucous traps particles of dust and bacteria, and the cilia move in a wave-like fashion to sweep this matter upwards and out of the airways. Air traveling to the lungs is thereby cleaned and filtered.

Bronchi: trachea divides into two primary (mainstem) bronchi which each enter a lung. Within each lung the primary bronchi further divide into secondary and tertiary bronchi. The secondary bronchi supply the lobes of the lungs (two lobes in the left lung, three in the right); the tertiary bronchi supply the segments of the lungs (eight segments in the left lung, ten in the right). Each primary bronchus is slightly less than one half the diameter of the trachea, and the secondary and tertiary bronchi become increasingly smaller and narrower. The tertiary bronchi continue to branch and divide into smaller and smaller tubes.

Bronchioles: tertiary bronchi eventually branch into microscopic bronchioles. Bronchioles are composed solely of smooth muscle and mucous membrane. The bronchioles continue the branching pattern and finally terminate in respiratory bronchioles. The respiratory bronchioles open into alveolar ducts which end in alveolar sacs.

Alveolar sacs: microscopic, thin-walled air-filled structures surrounded by a network of microscopic blood capillaries. The alveolar sacs form the location of gas exchange between oxygen and carbon dioxide.

Lungs: composed of the branching bronchi, bronchioles, and alveoli, in addition to blood vessels and nerves. The lungs are cone shaped structures housed within the thoracic cavity. Because it needs to accommodate the heart, the left lung is smaller than the right, with two lobes and eight segments. The larger right lung consists of three lobes and ten segments. The lungs are porous and elastic structures enabling them to be easily expanded and contracted.

Pleural linkage

The lungs contain very little muscle tissue and are unable to spontaneously generate movement. They are, however, highly compliant. This means that they can be easily moved by an external source. Each lung is encased in an airtight membrane called the visceral pleura. The inside surface of the thoracic cavity is lined by a membrane called the parietal pleura. Between these pleurae is a potential space known as the pleural space. The pleural space contains pleural fluid. This fluid has a permanent negative pressure. Because of the negative pressure the visceral and parietal pleurae are tightly coupled to each other. This pleural linkage allows the thorax and lungs to act as an integrated unit. Thus, whenever the thoracic cavity is moved by active or passive forces, the lungs are moved as well.

Lungs

COLOR KEY

- [ ] 1 Thyroid cartilage
- [ ] 2 Cricoid cartilage
- [ ] 3 Trachea
- [ ] 4 Right superior lobe
- [ ] 5 Left superior lobe
- [ ] 6 Middle lobe
- [ ] 7 Right inferior lobe
- [ ] 8 Left inferior lobe
- [ ] 9 Parietal pleura
- [ ] 10 Visceral pleura
- [ ] 11 Pleural space

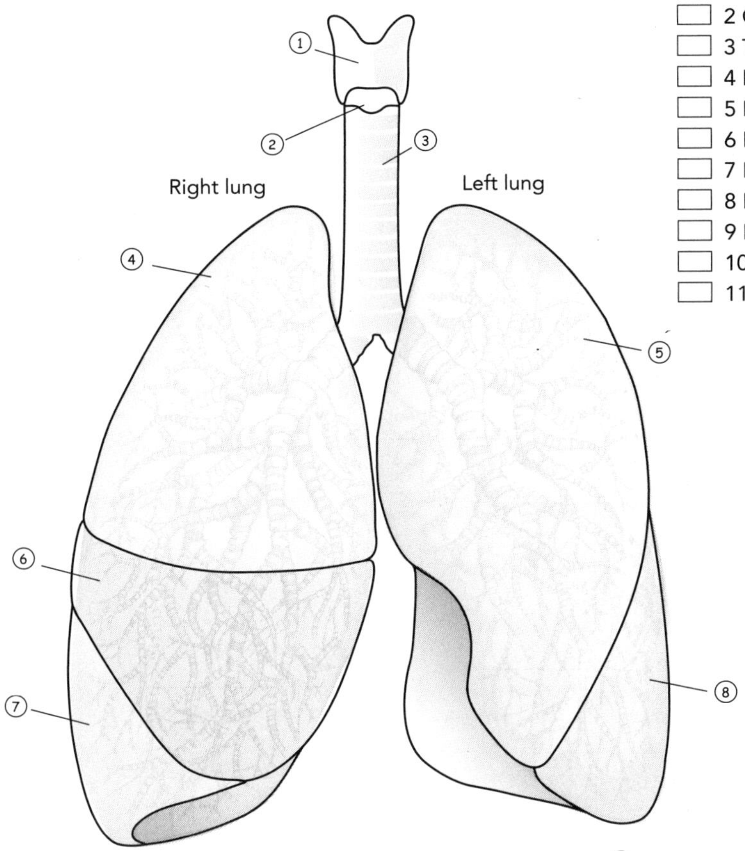

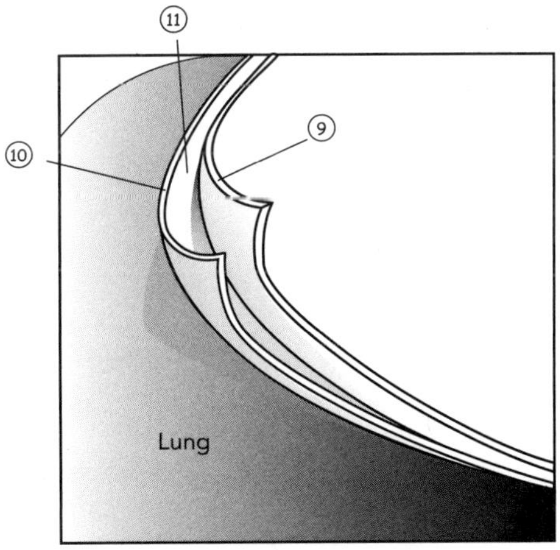

Right lung

Left lung

Lung

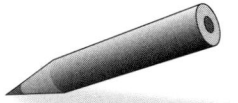

The bronchial tree

The trachea divides into finer and finer branches and terminates in the alveolar sacs where the oxygen and carbon dioxide exchange takes place

Trachea
↓
Primary bronchi
↓
Secondary bronchi
↓
Tertiary bronchi
↓
Bronchioles
↓
Terminal bronchioles
↓
Respiratory bronchioles
↓
Alveoli

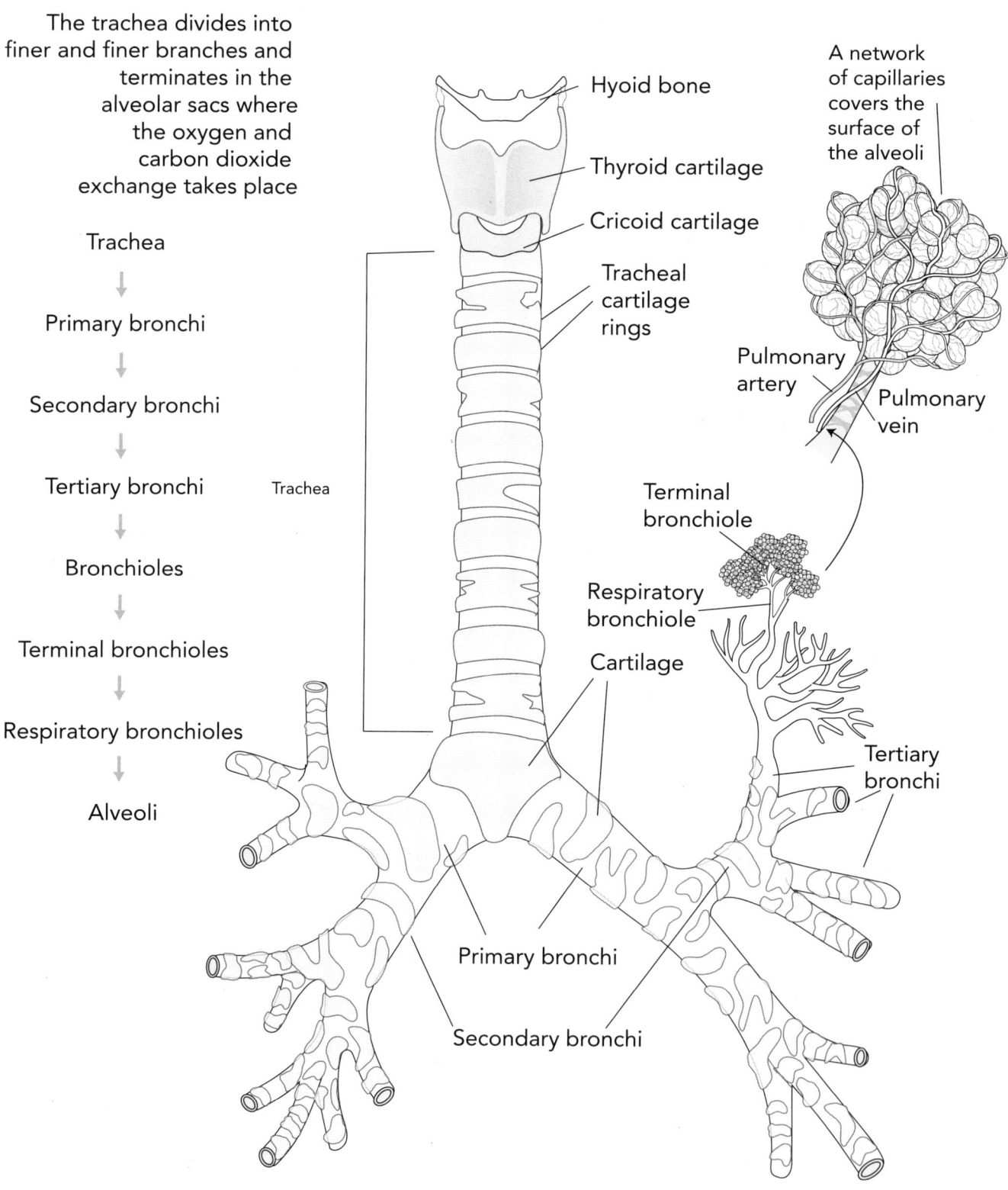

A network of capillaries covers the surface of the alveoli

Hyoid bone

Thyroid cartilage

Cricoid cartilage

Tracheal cartilage rings

Pulmonary artery

Pulmonary vein

Trachea

Terminal bronchiole

Respiratory bronchiole

Cartilage

Tertiary bronchi

Primary bronchi

Secondary bronchi

The bronchial tree

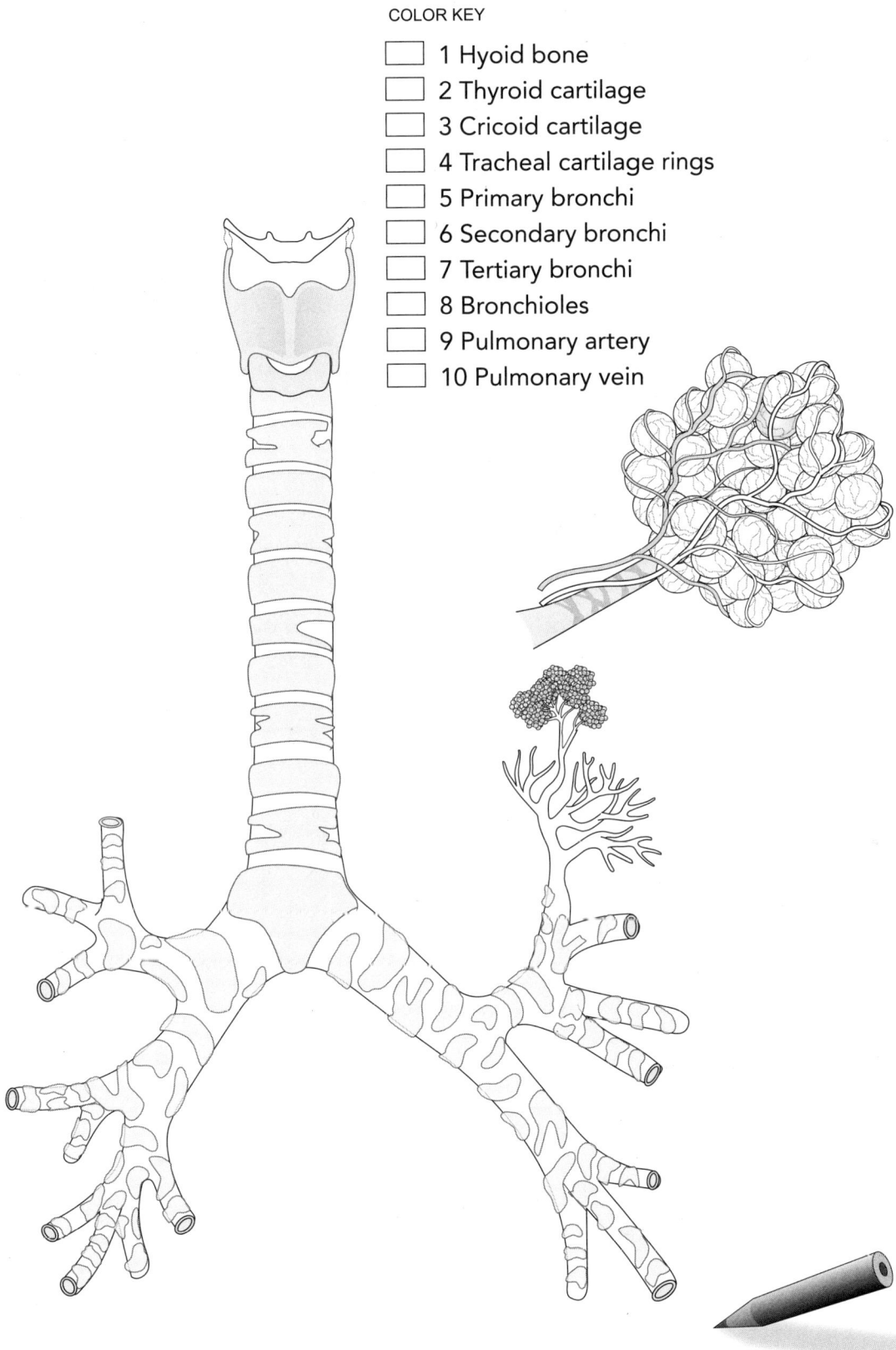

COLOR KEY

- 1 Hyoid bone
- 2 Thyroid cartilage
- 3 Cricoid cartilage
- 4 Tracheal cartilage rings
- 5 Primary bronchi
- 6 Secondary bronchi
- 7 Tertiary bronchi
- 8 Bronchioles
- 9 Pulmonary artery
- 10 Pulmonary vein

Muscles of Respiration

Diaphragm: large muscle that attaches to the bottom six ribs on either side of the ribcage. At rest the muscle is shaped like an inverted bowl. Upon contraction the muscle flattens out. This increases the vertical dimension of the thoracic cavity.

External intercostals: 11 pairs that run between the ribs. Each pair originates on the lower surface of the rib, and the fibers course downward and forward at an oblique angle, inserting into the upper border of the rib below. When these muscles contract, each one raises the rib below, elevating portions of, or the entire, rib cage. The volume of the thoracic cavity is therefore increased in the front-to-back and lateral directions. Contraction also stiffens the tissues in the spaces between the ribs, which prevents them from being sucked inward or pushed outward by changing pressures.

Internal intercostals: 11 pairs which are similar in structure to the external intercostals. The internal intercostals lie deep to the external intercostals and run at an opposite angle (downward and backward) to that of the external intercostals. When contracted, the internal intercostals pull down on the rib immediately above, which lowers portions of, or the entire, rib cage. The volume of the thoracic cavity is decreased by this action.

Accessory muscles of respiration

Sternocleidomastoid: elevates rib cage

Scalene (anterior, medial, posterior): elevates ribs 1 and 2

Serratus anterior: elevates ribs 1 to 9

Pectoralis major: elevates rib cage

Pectoralis minor: depresses ribs 3 to 5

Costal levators: elevate rib cage

Subcostals: lower rib cage

Serratus posterior inferior: depresses ribs 9 to 12

Transverse thoracic: depresses rib cage

Subclavius: elevates rib cage

The diaphragm muscle

The diaphragm separates the thoracic cavity, containing the heart and lungs, from the abdominal cavity

As the diaphragm contracts, the volume of the thoracic cavity increases and creates negative pressure which draws air into the lungs.

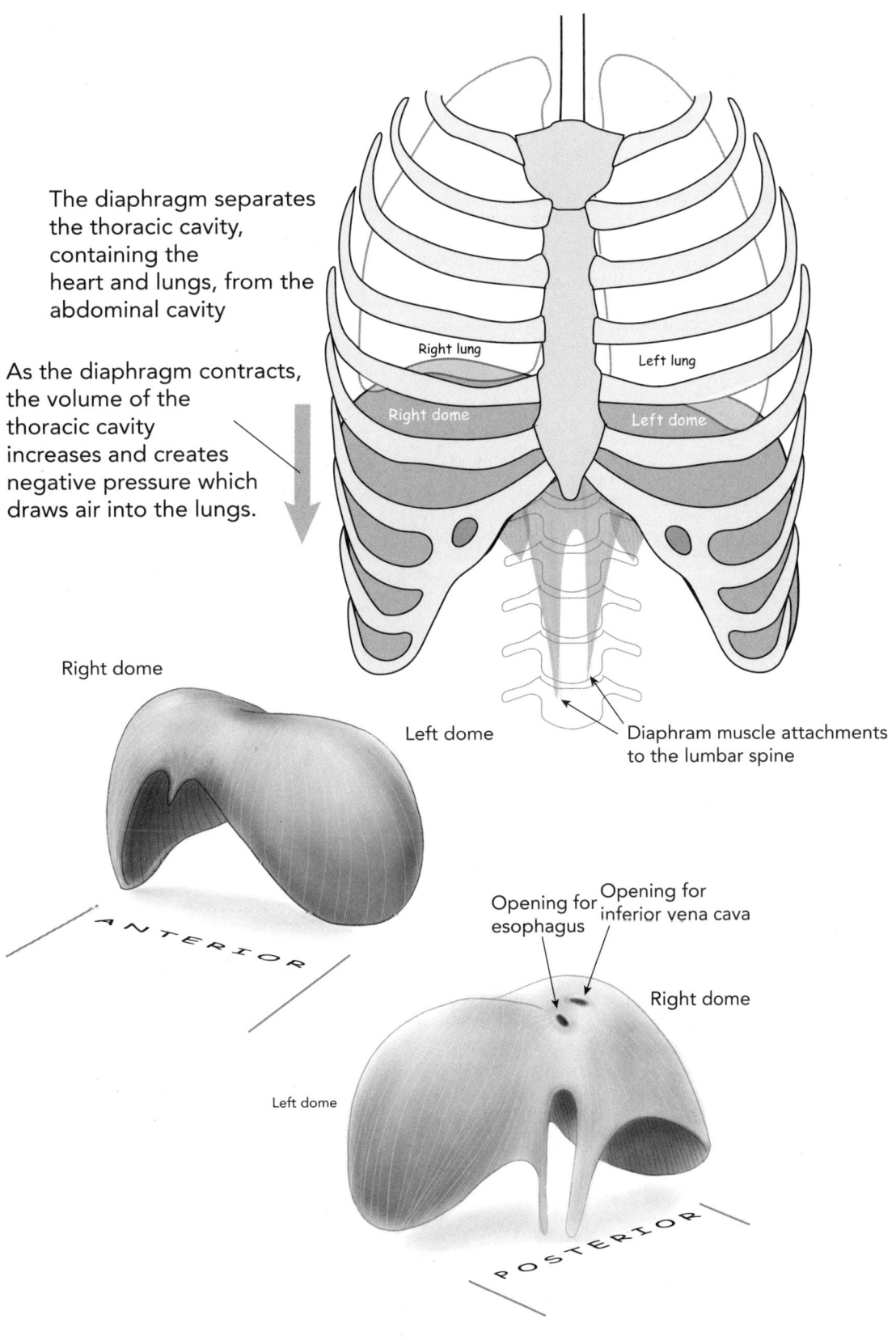

Right lung

Left lung

Right dome

Left dome

Right dome

Left dome

Diaphram muscle attachments to the lumbar spine

ANTERIOR

Opening for esophagus

Opening for inferior vena cava

Right dome

Left dome

POSTERIOR

The scalene muscles

COLOR KEY

- 1 Sternocleidomastoid
- 2 Anterior scalene
- 3 Middle scalene
- 4 Posterior scalene

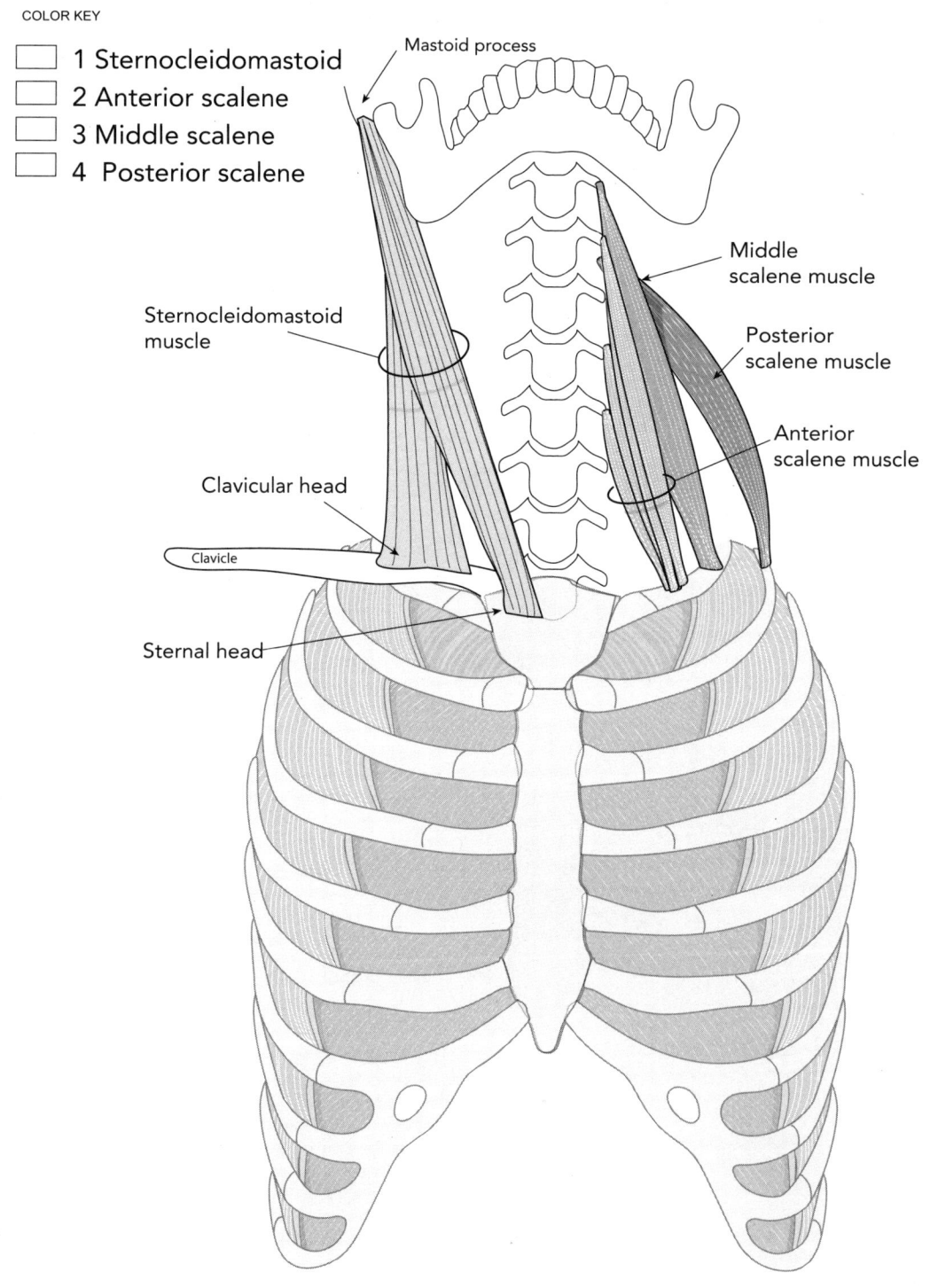

Mastoid process

Middle scalene muscle

Posterior scalene muscle

Anterior scalene muscle

Sternocleidomastoid muscle

Clavicular head

Clavicle

Sternal head

The intercostal muscles

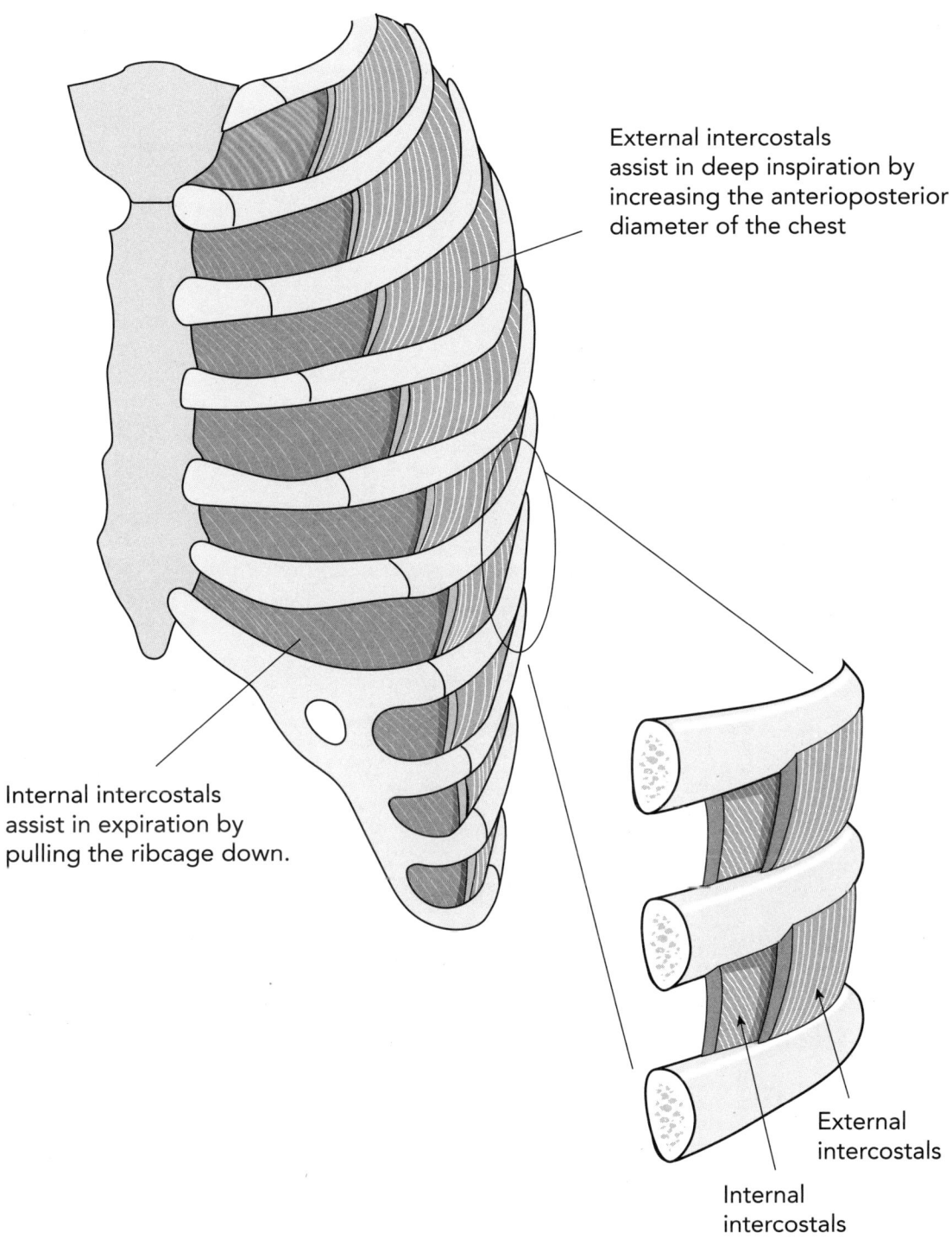

External intercostals assist in deep inspiration by increasing the anterioposterior diameter of the chest

Internal intercostals assist in expiration by pulling the ribcage down.

External intercostals

Internal intercostals

Muscles of expiration (abdominal muscles)

The muscles of the abdomen play an important part in respiration. The four muscles of the abdomen work as a unit to compress the contents of the abdominal cavity. This has the effect of exerting upward pressure on the diaphragm. In turn, the volume of the thoracic cavity is decreased.

Rectus abdominis
External oblique
Internal oblique
Transversus abdominis

Cycles of respiration

One cycle of respiration includes an inhalation and an exhalation phase. Inhalation depends on active muscle forces. In order to inhale, the thoracic cavity and lungs must expand using the external intercostal and diaphragm muscles. This causes the lung pressure (alveolar pressure) to decrease, and air therefore flows into the lungs. To exhale the thoracic cavity and lungs must contract, raising the pressure within the lungs, and forcing air out of the respiratory system. In quiet breathing exhalation is passive and does not require active muscle force.

COLOR KEY

1 Platysma
2 Pectoralis major
3 Serratus anterior
4 Transversus abdominis
5 Internal oblique
6 External oblique
7 Rectus abdominis

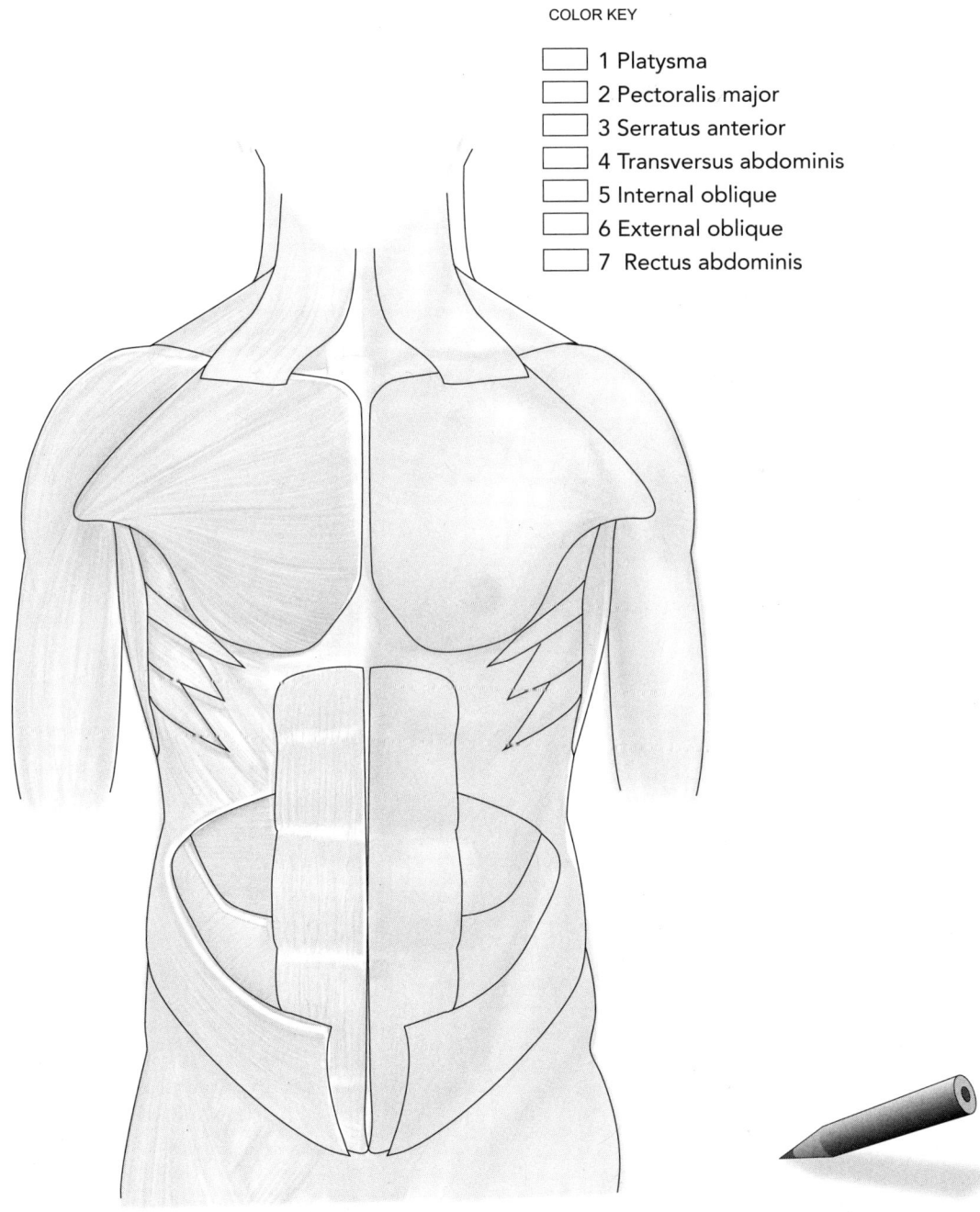

THE PULMONARY CIRCUIT

The pulmonary circuit consists of the pulmonary arteries and pulmonary veins that transport blood between the heart and lungs. The right side of the heart pumps deoxygenated blood to the lungs. Once gas exchange has occurred, the freshly oxygenated blood is transferred to the left side of the heart. The left side of the heart then pumps the oxygenated blood to every cell in the body

COLOR KEY
☐ 1 Oxygen poor blood
☐ 2 Oxygen rich blood

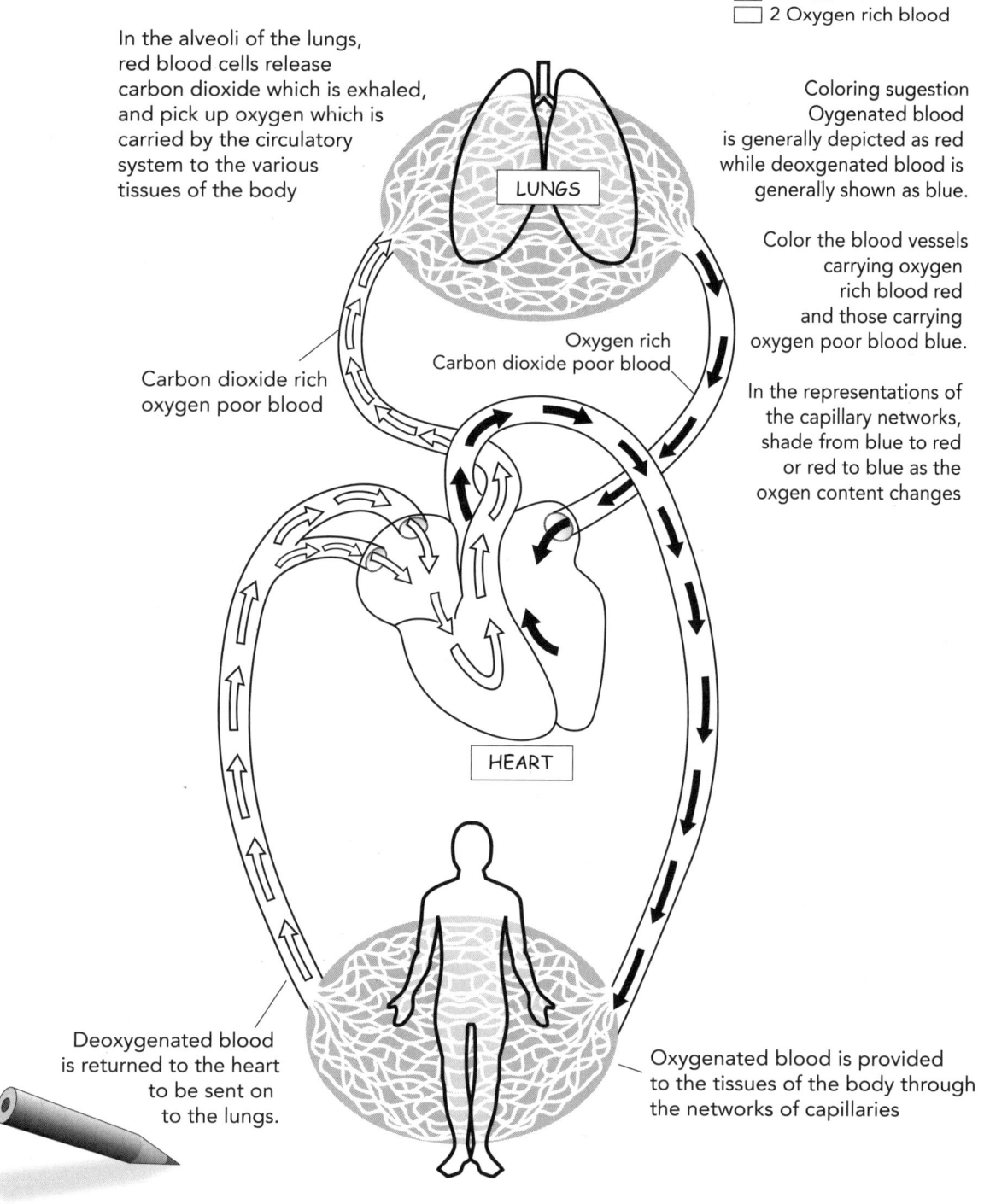

In the alveoli of the lungs, red blood cells release carbon dioxide which is exhaled, and pick up oxygen which is carried by the circulatory system to the various tissues of the body

Coloring sugestion
Oygenated blood is generally depicted as red while deoxgenated blood is generally shown as blue.

Color the blood vessels carrying oxygen rich blood red and those carrying oxygen poor blood blue.

In the representations of the capillary networks, shade from blue to red or red to blue as the oxgen content changes

Carbon dioxide rich oxygen poor blood

Oxygen rich
Carbon dioxide poor blood

LUNGS

HEART

Deoxygenated blood is returned to the heart to be sent on to the lungs.

Oxygenated blood is provided to the tissues of the body through the networks of capillaries

LUNG VOLUMES AND CAPACITIES

Resting expiratory level (REL) refers to a state of equilibrium in the respiratory system in which alveolar pressure and atmospheric pressure are equalized, so air does not enter or exit the system. This occurs at the end of every inspiration and expiration. The endpoint of a quiet expiration is also called the end-expiratory level (EEL). Lung volumes and capacities provide a way of categorizing volumes of air inhaled and exhaled through the respiratory system in relation to REL. Volumes and capacities are measured with a spirometer in units of milliliters (ml) or liters (l). Volumes are single non-overlapping quantities: capacities are composed of two or more volumes.

Lung volumes

Tidal volume (TV): volume of air inhaled and exhaled during a cycle of respiration. Tidal volume varies, depending on age, build, and degree of physical activity.
On average, TV is 500 mL.

Inspiratory reserve volume (IRV): amount of air that can be inhaled above TV.

Expiratory reserve volume (ERV): amount of air that can be exhaled below TV.

Residual volume (RV): volume of air remaining in the lungs after a maximum exhalation.

Lung capacities

Vital capacity (VC): maximum amount of air that a person can exhale after having inhaled as deeply as possible. It is the combination of tidal volume, inspiratory reserve volume, and expiratory reserve volume (TV + IRV + ERV). On average, VC is 5000 mL.

Functional residual capacity (FRC): amount of air remaining in the lungs and airways at the end-expiratory level. It combines expiratory reserve volume and residual volume (ERV + RV).

Inspiratory capacity (IC): amount of air that can be inhaled from end-expiratory level. It combines tidal volume plus inspiratory reserve volume (TV + IRV).

Total lung capacity (TLC): total amount of air that the lungs can hold. It combines tidal volume, inspiratory reserve volume, expiratory reserve volume, and residual volume (TV + IRV + ERV + RV). On average this amount is 6000 mL.

Vital capacity expended

Volumes and capacities are often described in terms of the percentage of vital capacity expended. VC is the maximum amount of air one can voluntarily breathe in and out, and therefore corresponds to 100%. REL occurs at around 35-40% VC. At that point one can inhale 60-65% more air to fill the lungs to their maximum capacity (100%) and can continue to exhale below REL to 0% VC. Tidal volume for quiet breathing is around 10% VC. Normal conversational speech uses approximately 20% VC.

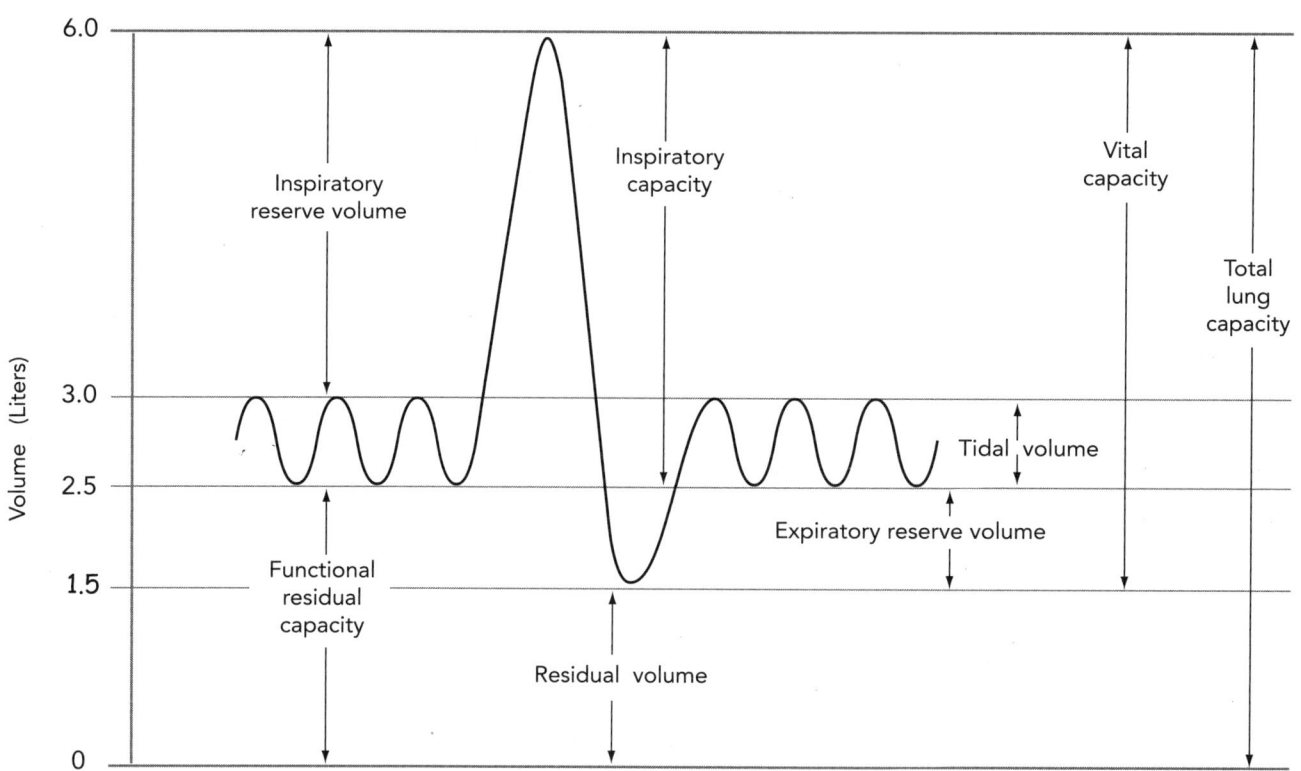

DIFFERENCES BETWEEN LIFE AND SPEECH BREATHING

Change	Life	Speech
Location of air intake	Nose	Mouth
Ratio of time for inhalation versus exhalation	Inhale: 40% Exhale: 60%	Inhale: 10% Exhale: 90%
Volume of air	500 mL; 10% VC	Variable depending on length and volume of utterance; around 20% VC
Muscle activity for exhalation	Passive: muscles of thorax and diaphragm relax	Active: thoracic and abdominal muscles contract to regulate recoil of ribcage and diaphragm
Chest wall position	Abdomen displaced outward relative to rib cage	Abdomen displaced inward relative to rib cage

Location: for life breathing air is inhaled through the nose where it is warmed, moistened, and filtered before entering the tracheobronchial tree. Air is inhaled through the mouth for speech breathing, which is more efficient.

Ratio of inhalation to exhalation: for life breathing the inhalation and exhalation durations per cycle are almost equal. For speech, a quick inhalation is followed by an extended exhalation. This allows the speaker to produce conversationally appropriate numbers of words and phrases per exhalation.

Volume of air inhaled and exhaled: life breathing uses approximately 10% of the total VC. Inhalation begins at REL (40% VC) and goes up only to around 50% VC. Depending on the length and loudness of the upcoming utterance, speech breathing typically uses around 20% VC, extending from REL to 60% VC. Singers who need to sustain long phrases may extend to 80% or even 100% VC.

Muscle activity for exhalation: to exhale, the volume of the thoracic cavity and lungs must decrease to force air out of the respiratory system. For life breathing the thorax and lungs recoil back to their original positions after the inhalation, without needing additional muscular activity. For speech breathing, however, the duration of the recoil must be extended. To achieve this, the muscles of inhalation (diaphragm and external intercostals) continue to contract. This prevents the lungs from collapsing too quickly to their original position after the inhalation.

Chest wall position: for life breathing the abdomen is positioned outward relative to the rib cage. For speech breathing the abdomen is positioned inward relative to the ribcage. This is a more efficient posture for speech production.

TEST YOURSELF: THE RESPIRATORY SYSTEM

MULTIPLE CHOICE   STRUCTURE

1 _____ The nasal cavities, oral cavity, and pharynx are part of the
   a. Lower respiratory system
   b. Bronchial tree
   c. Upper respiratory system
   d. None of the above

2 _____ The pectoral girdle includes
   a. The diaphragm and ribcage
   b. The sternum and spinal column
   c. The clavicles and scapulae
   d. All the above

3 _____ Which of the following is NOT a part of the lower respiratory system?
   a. Lungs
   b. Trachea
   c. Alveolar sacs
   d. Pharynx

4 _____ The units involved in the exchange of oxygen and carbon dioxide are
   a. Lobules
   b. Alveoli
   c. Bronchioles
   d. None of the above

5 _____ The bronchi branch into smaller passages called
   a. Bronchioles
   b. Alveoli
   c. Connective tissue sacs
   d. Lungs

6 _____ The right lung has ___ lobes and the left lung has ___ lobes
   a. 4, 6
   b. 3, 2
   c. 3, 4
   d. 4, 2

7 _____ The ___ forms the floor of the thoracic cavity
   a. Sternum
   b. Ribcage
   c. Diaphragm
   d. Abdominal wall

8 _____ Which of the following statements (if any) is NOT true of the trachea?
   a. It is lined with ciliated pseudostratified columnar epithelium
   b. It is formed of cartilage, smooth muscle, and membrane
   c. The cilia serve to filter incoming air
   d. All the above are true

9 ____   Which statement best characterizes the bronchi?
a. They are composed solely of smooth muscle and membrane
b. They open into alveolar sacs
c. They divide into secondary and tertiary branches
d. They have the same diameter as the trachea

10 ____   The lungs are enclosed by the
a. Visceral pleura
b. Parietal pleura
c. Bronchial membranes
d. All the above

11 ____   What is the function of the visceral and parietal pleurae?
a. To serve as a passageway for air entering the lungs
b. To produce mucous
c. To protect and lubricate the lungs
d. None of the above

12 ____   The pleural space lies between the lung and the
a. Visceral pleura
b. Parietal pleura
c. Heart
d. Alveolar sacs

13 ____   The pressure within the pleural space
a. Is always positive
b. Is always negative
c. Changes from negative to positive depending on the phase of breathing
d. Equals atmospheric pressure

14 ____   What is the force that causes air to flow into the lungs during inspiration and out of the lungs during expiration?
a. Muscle contraction
b. Surface tension
c. Diaphragmatic movement
d. Changes in the lung pressures

15 ____   During exhalation
a. Alveolar pressure is positive
b. Alveolar pressure is negative
c. The thoracic cavity expands
d. The diaphragm contracts and flattens

16 ____   The muscles of the abdomen
a. Contract to decrease the volume of the thoracic cavity
b. Relax to decrease the volume of the thoracic cavity
c. Contract to increase the volume of the thoracic cavity
d. None of the above

TRUE/FALSE   STRUCTURE

1 _____   The upper respiratory tract is formed by the trachea, bronchi, and lungs.

2 _____   The boundaries of the thoracic cavity are the sternum, rib cage, spinal column,

vertebrae, and diaphragm muscle.

3 _____   Positive pressure in the pleural space keeps the lungs and thorax connected

and allows them to function as one unit.

4 _____   During inspiration the pressure in the lungs increases.

5 _____   The bronchioles are composed solely of smooth muscle and mucous membrane.

6 _____   The chest wall is made up of the ribcage, the diaphragm, the

abdominal wall, and the abdominal contents.

7 _____   The lumen of the trachea is lined with pseudostratified ciliated

columnar epithelium.

8 _____   The secondary and tertiary bronchi become increasingly wider as they branch.

9 _____   The left lung contains three lobes and ten segments and the right lung contains two lobes and

eight segments.

10 _____   The respiratory bronchioles open into alveolar ducts which terminate n alveolar sacs.

11 _____   Each lung is encased in a visceral pleura and the inside surface of the

thoracic cavity is lined by a parietal pleura.

12 _____   When the diaphragm contracts it raises and decreases the volume of the thoracic cavity.

13 _____   The external intercostal muscles raise the ribcage and the internal intercostal muscles lower the ribcage.

14 _____   The external intercostals lie deep to the internal intercostals.

FILL IN THE BLANK   STRUCTURE

1   The lumen of the trachea is lined with _____

2   The trachea divides into two _____

3   There are_____ lobes and_____ segments in the left lung;_____ lobes and _____ segments in the right lung

4   The _____ are composed solely of smooth muscle and mucous membrane

5   The respiratory bronchioles open into _____

6   Gas exchange between oxygen and carbon dioxide takes places in the _____

7   The _____ encases each lung; the _____ lines

the inside of the thoracic cavity

8   The pressure between the lungs and thorax is always _____

9   The internal intercostal muscles _____ the rib cage

10   The_____ muscles increase the front-to-back volume of the thoracic cavity

11   The vertical dimension of the thoracic cavity is increased when the

_____ contracts

12   Contraction of the abdominal muscles _____ the volume of the thoracic cavity

13   Inhalation occurs when alveolar pressure _____

14   Exhalation occurs when alveolar pressure_____

MATCHING   STRUCTURE

	Sternocleidomastoid	1 Compress the abdominal contents
	Serratus posterior inferior	2 Run between the ribs on either side
	Pectoralis major	3 Elevates ribs 1 and 2
	External intercostals	4 Depresses ribs 9 to 12
	Scalene (anterior, medial, posterior)	5 Elevates rib cage
	Subcostals	6 Depresses ribs 3 to 5
	Serratus anterior	7 Flattens to enlarge the thoracic cavity
	Internal intercostals	8 Elevates ribs 1 to 9
	Costal levators	9 Elevate rib cage
	Abdominal muscles	10 Lowers rib cage
	Subclavius	11 Elevates rib cage
	Transverse thoracic	12 Depress rib cage
	Pectoralis minor	13 Run deep to the external intercostals
	Diaphragm	14 Elevate rib cage

MULTIPLE CHOICE LUNG VOLUMES AND CAPACITIES, LIFE VS SPEECH BREATHING

1 ____ Which statement is true of resting expiratory level?
   a. State of equilibrium in the respiratory system
   b Moment when alveolar pressure equals atmospheric pressure
   c. Occurs at the end of every exhalation
   d. All the above statements are true

2 ____ The volume of air that can be inhaled above tidal volume is known as
   a. Inspiratory reserve volume
   b. Residual volume
   c. Expiratory reserve volume
   d. None of the above

3 ____ Inspiratory capacity is
   a. The amount of air that can be inhaled from end-expiratory level.
   b. The amount of air that can be inhaled above vital capacity.
   c. The combination of tidal volume plus expiratory reserve volume (TV + ERV)
   d. None of the above

4 ____ Which statement (if any) is true of resting expiratory level?
   a. Occurs at around 80% of VC
   b. Occurs for life breathing but not for speech breathing
   c. Occurs in adults but not in children
   d. None of the above statements is true

5 ____ The volume of air that can be exhaled below tidal volume is known as
   a. Inspiratory reserve volume
   b. Residual volume
   c. Expiratory reserve volume
   d. None of the above

6 ____ Normal adult quiet breathing and conversational speech use approximately what percent of vital capacity, respectively?
   a. 10, 15 %
   b. 10, 20 %
   c. 15, 20 %
   d. 15, 30 %

7 ____ Which statement (if any) best describes functional residual capacity?
   a. Volume of air expelled during exhalation
   b. Expiratory reserve volume plus residual volume
   c. State during which air neither enters nor exits the respiratory system
   d. None of the above

8 _____   Resting tidal breathing
     a. Employs all the muscles of the thoracic cavity and neck
     b. Uses approximately 10% of VC
     c. Typically begins and ends below REL
     d. All the above

9 _____   The amount of air that enters the lungs during normal breathing is called
     a. Vital capacity
     b. Tidal volume
     c. Total lung capacity
     d. Inspiratory reserve volume

10 _____   The amount of air that cannot be exhaled is the
     a. Residual volume
     b. Tidal volume
     c. Expiratory reserve volume
     d. Total lung volume

11 _____   Which of these is the sum of the other three?
     a. Tidal volume
     b. Expiratory reserve volume
     c. Vital capacity
     d. Inspiratory reserve volume

12 _____   Exhalation for life breathing is
     a. Active
     b. Passive
     c. Neutral
     d. None of the above

13 _____   In speech breathing the abdomen is
     a. Displaced inward relative to the rib cage
     b. Displaced outward relative to the rib cage
     c. In a neutral position
     d. None of the above

TRUE/FALSE   LUNG VOLUMES AND CAPACITIES, LIFE VS SPEECH BREATHING

1 ____   Volumes are single non-overlapping quantities: capacities are composed of two or more volumes.

2 ____   The endpoint of a quiet expiration is also called the functional residual capacity.

3 ____   Resting expiratory level (REL) is a state in which alveolar pressure equals atmospheric pressure.

4 ____   Tidal volume varies depending on age, build, and degree of physical activity.

5 ____   IRV, ERV, and TV together make up the VC.

6 ____   IC combines TV plus RV.

7 ____   TLC includes all the volumes and capacities excluding RV.

8 ____   At REL one can inhale 60-65% more air to fill the lungs to maximum capacity.

9 ____   Even after a maximum exhalation there is always some air left in the lungs.

10 ____   The total amount of VC ranges from 0-100%.

11 ____   Inhalation ratio for speech breathing changes from 40% to 10%.

12 ____   Air is inhaled through the nose for speech and through the mouth for life breathing.

FILL IN THE BLANK   LUNG VOLUMES AND CAPACITIES, LIFE VS SPEECH BREATHING

1   The state of equilibrium in which alveolar pressure and atmospheric pressure are

     equalized is called _____.

2   _____ refers to the endpoint of a quiet expiration.

3   Lung _____ are composed of two or more volumes.

4   The volume of air inhaled and exhaled during a cycle of

     respiration is called _____.

5   The volume of air remaining in the lungs even after a maximum exhalation

     is called _____.

6   The amount of air that can be exhaled below tidal volume

     is called _____.

7 _____ is the combination of tidal volume, inspiratory reserve volume, and expiratory reserve volume.

8 REL occurs at around _____% VC.

9 The average amount of VC is _____ mL.

10 The average amount of tidal volume is _____ mL.

11 _____ is the combination of expiratory reserve volume and residual volume.

12 Tidal volume for quiet breathing is around _____% VC.

13 Normal conversational speech uses approximately _____% VC.

14 _____ is the combination of tidal volume plus inspiratory reserve volume.

15 Muscle activity for exhalation is _____ for life and _____ for speech.

MATCHING   LUNG VOLUMES AND CAPACITIES, LIFE VS SPEECH BREATHING

	Total lung capacity	1 Amount of air that can be inhaled above TV
	Resting expiratory level	2 Air remaining in lungs and airways at the end-expiratory level
	Functional residual capacity	3 Amount of air that can be exhaled below TV
	Expiratory reserve volume	4 Amount of air that can be inhaled from end-expiratory level
	Residual volume	5 State of equilibrium in the respiratory system
	Vital capacity	6 Air remaining in the lungs after a maximum exhalation
	Inspiratory reserve volume	7 Air inhaled and exhaled during a cycle of respiration
	Inspiratory capacity	8 Total amount of air that the lungs can hold
	Tidal volume	9 Maximum amount of air that can be exhaled following a maximum inhalation

Draw your own: Muscles of respiration

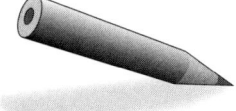

Respiration

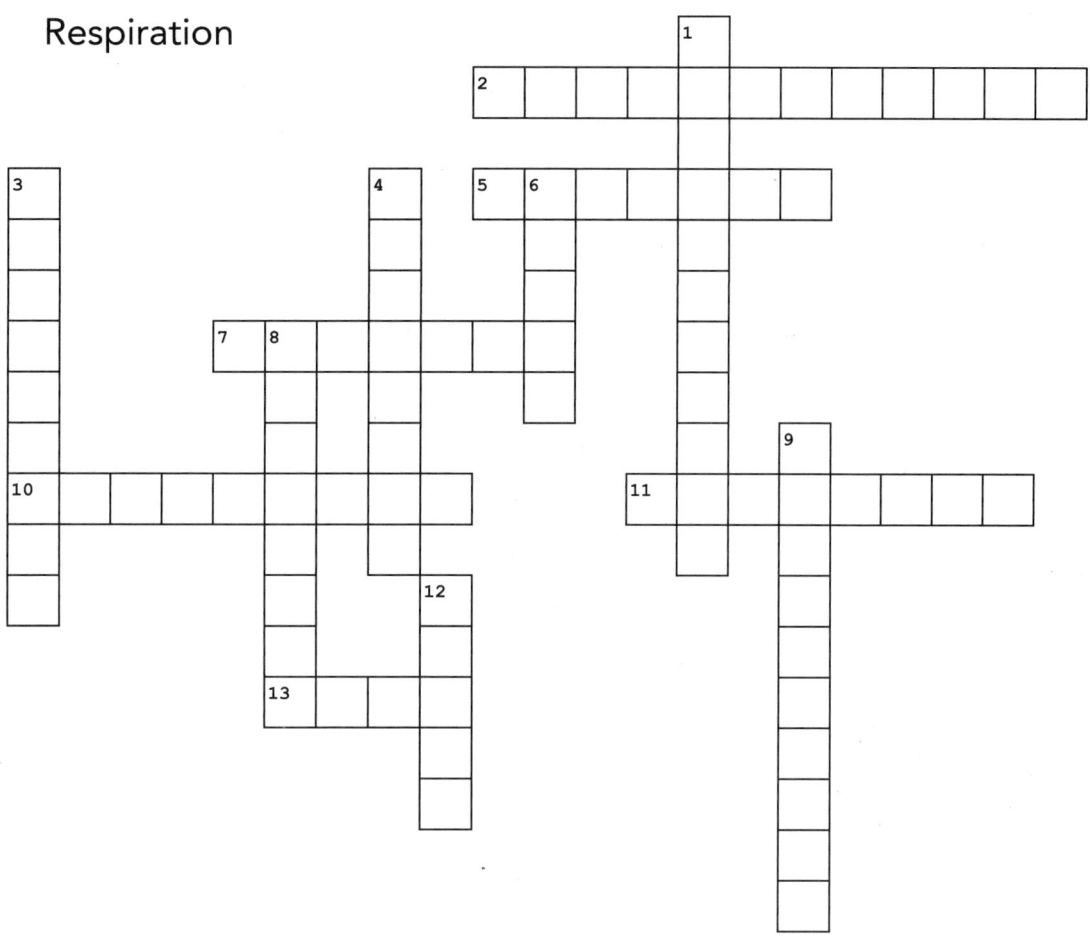

Across

2. In between each rib

5. Another word for breastbone

7. Hollow tube formed by 16-20 rings of cartilage

10. These muscles help to exert upward pressure on the diaphragm

11. Air enters the lungs when pressure is ___

13. Smaller of the two lungs

Down

1. Smallest division of the tertiary bronchi

3. Shaped like an inverted bowl

4. Pleura surrounding each lung

6. Volume of air inhaled and exhaled during a cycle of respiration

8. Volume of air remaining in the lungs after a maximum exhalation

9. Composed or two or more lung volumes

12. Maximum capacity that can be exhaled after a maximum inhalation

The Phonatory System

The larynx is a complex structure formed by interlinked cartilages, membranes and ligaments, muscles, and soft tissues. While the larynx is the major structure involved in voice production, it also plays a crucial role in many biological functions. The larynx is continuous with both the trachea and the pharynx, and is involved in respiration, in swallowing, and in airway protection, as well as in phonation.

FRAMEWORK OF THE LARYNX

The supporting framework of the larynx is composed of one bone, nine cartilages, and two joints.

Hyoid bone: consists of a body anteriorly, major horns which form the sides of the bone, and minor horns, which are small protrusions extending superiorly. The larynx is suspended from the hyoid bone by a sheet of membrane, the hyothyroid membrane.

Thyroid cartilage: is formed by two sheets of hyaline cartilage which are fused in the front and open in the back. The cartilage protrudes at an angle at the fusion, forming the "Adam's apple". Directly above the prominence is the v-shaped thyroid notch. Superior horns project upward and connect the thyroid cartilage to the hyoid bone by means of the thyrohyoid ligament. This ligament is formed by the thickening of the lateral portions of the thyrohyoid membrane that connects the thyroid cartilage to the hyoid bone. The inferior horns project downward and form a joint with the cricoid cartilage. A slight ridge is visible along the side of the thyroid lamina. This is called the oblique line, and two of the extrinsic laryngeal muscles have their points of attachment here. The true vocal folds are attached to the inner surface of the thyroid immediately below the thyroid notch. The point at which they attach is called the anterior commissure.

Cricoid cartilage: is a complete ring of hyaline cartilage. It is narrow in the front (the arch) and broader and wider in the back (quadrate lamina). The cricoid is located immediately superior to the trachea. It connects to the trachea by means of the cricotracheal membrane. The cricoid cartilage also attaches to the thyroid cartilage by way of the cricothyroid membrane. The interior of the cricoid cartilage forms the narrowest point of the larynx.

Epiglottis: is a leaf shaped, elastic cartilage. It is attached to the thyroid cartilage by the thyroepiglottic ligaments. It is also attached to the hyoid bone by the hyoepiglottic ligaments. The base of the epiglottis is narrow and is called the petiole. The space between the base of the tongue and the epiglottis forms the vallecula.

Framework of the Larynx

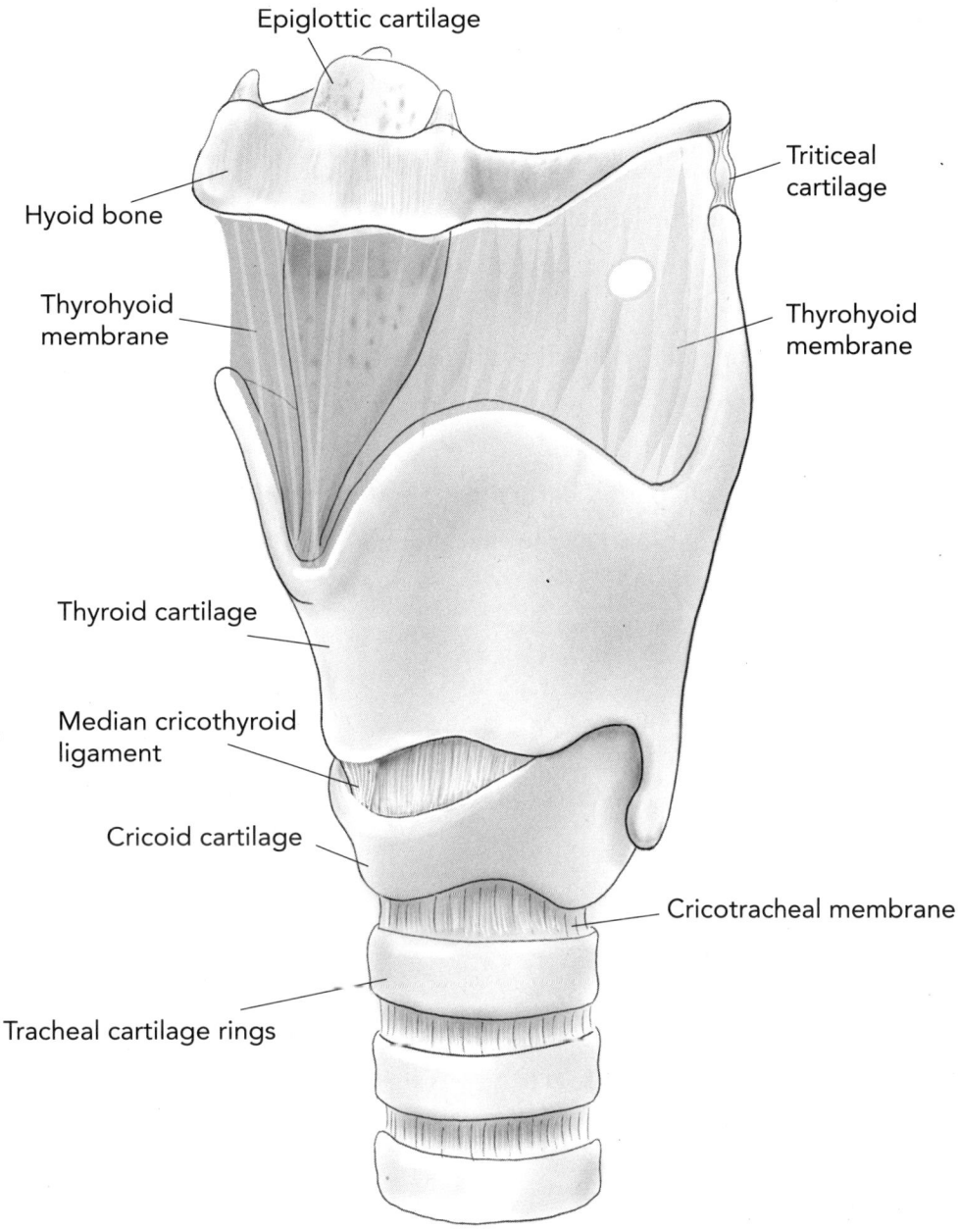

Epiglottic cartilage

Triticeal cartilage

Hyoid bone

Thyrohyoid membrane

Thyrohyoid membrane

Thyroid cartilage

Median cricothyroid ligament

Cricoid cartilage

Cricotracheal membrane

Tracheal cartilage rings

Arytenoid cartilages: are paired small, cone shaped cartilages. They are located on the superior surface of the quadrate lamina. The base of each arytenoid has a vocal process and a muscular process. The vocal process projects anteriorly and attaches to the vocal folds. The muscular process projects posterolaterally. This process forms the point of attachment for muscles which adduct and abduct the vocal folds to open and close the glottis. The base of the arytenoid and the superior portion of the quadrate lamina forms a joint between the cartilages.

Corniculate cartilages: are small elastic cartilages located on the apex of each arytenoid cartilage.

Cuneiform cartilages: are small, paired cartilages embedded within the aryepiglottic folds.

Triticeal cartilages: are small, paired cartilages found within the thyrohyoid membrane. They are present in some individuals and absent in others.

Hyoid bone and thyroid cartilage

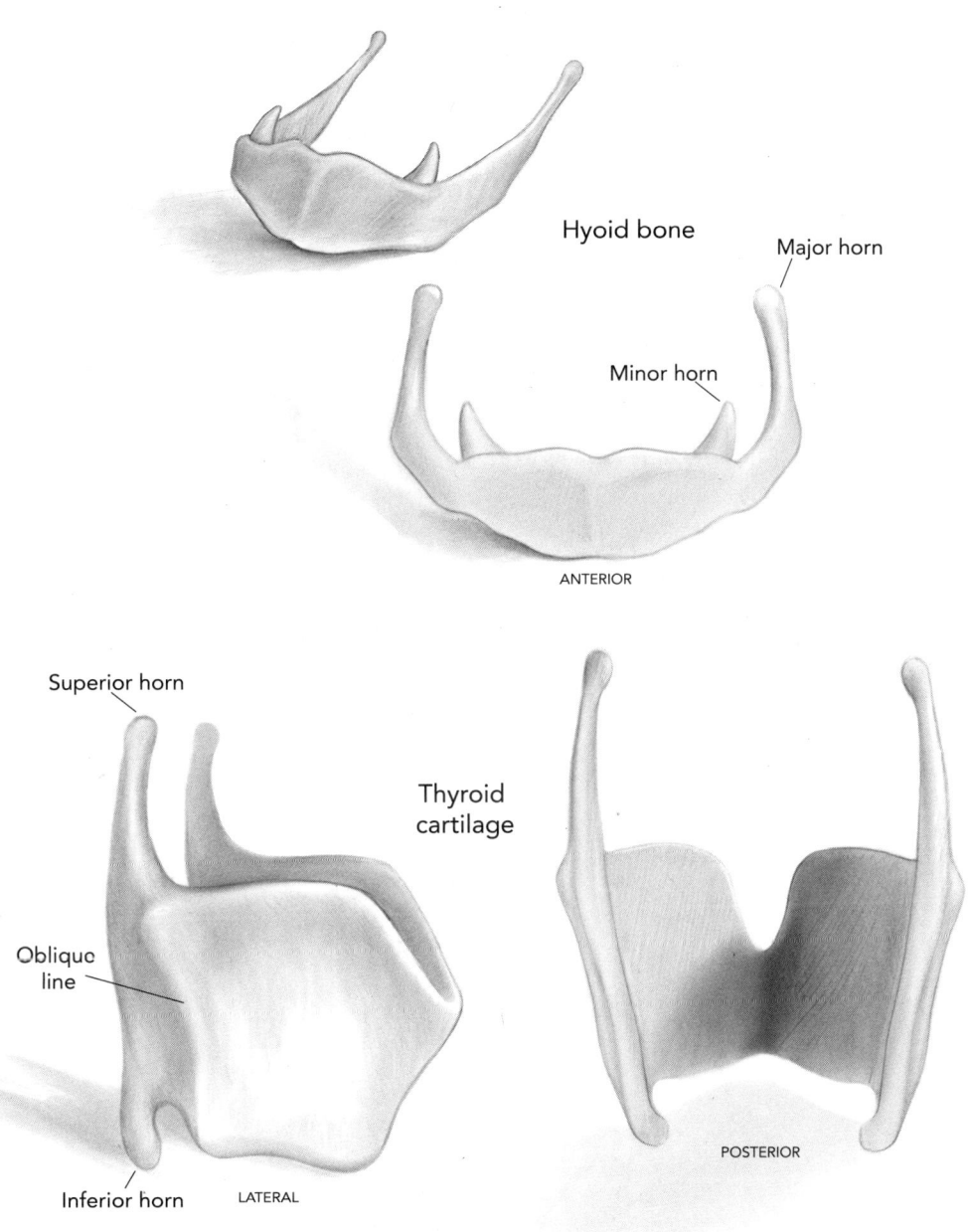

Hyoid bone

Major horn

Minor horn

ANTERIOR

Superior horn

Thyroid
cartilage

Oblique
line

Inferior horn   LATERAL

POSTERIOR

Corniculate, arytenoid, and cricoid cartilages

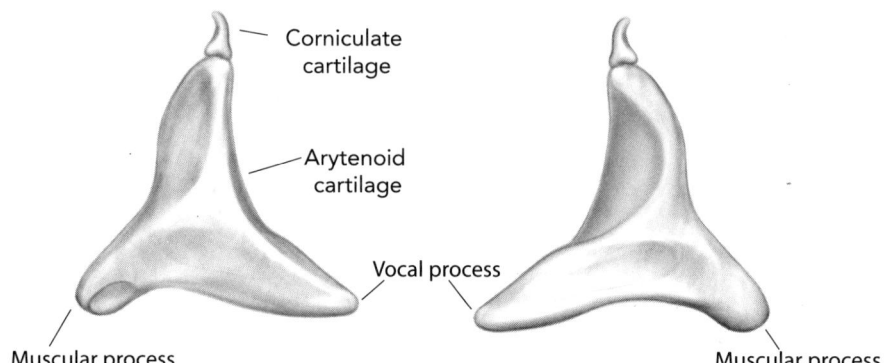

Corniculate cartilage

Arytenoid cartilage

Vocal process

Muscular process

Muscular process

Arytenoid and corniculate cartilages - lateral views
(shown in a larger scale than cricoid cartilage below)

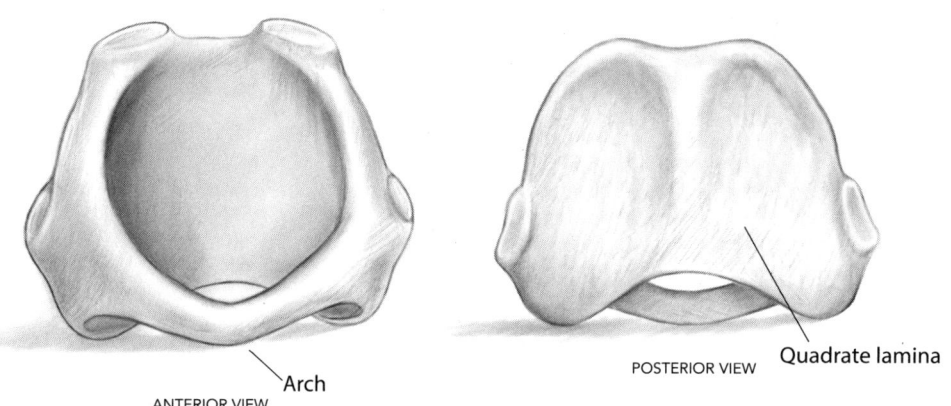

Arch

ANTERIOR VIEW

POSTERIOR VIEW

Quadrate lamina

Four views of the cricoid cartilage

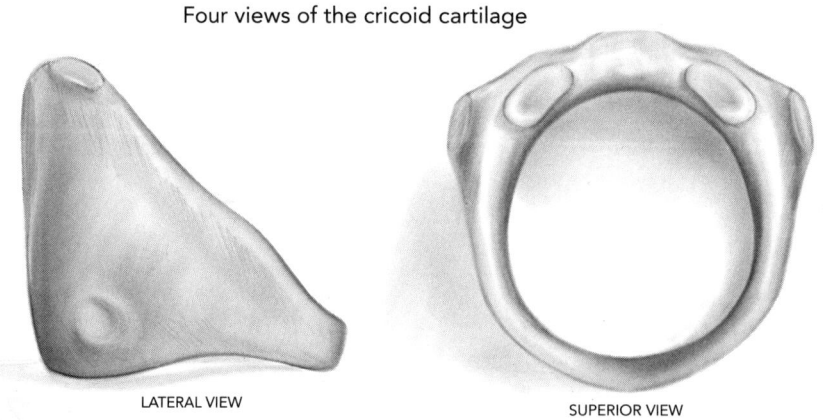

LATERAL VIEW

SUPERIOR VIEW

Corniculate, arytenoid, and cricoid cartilages

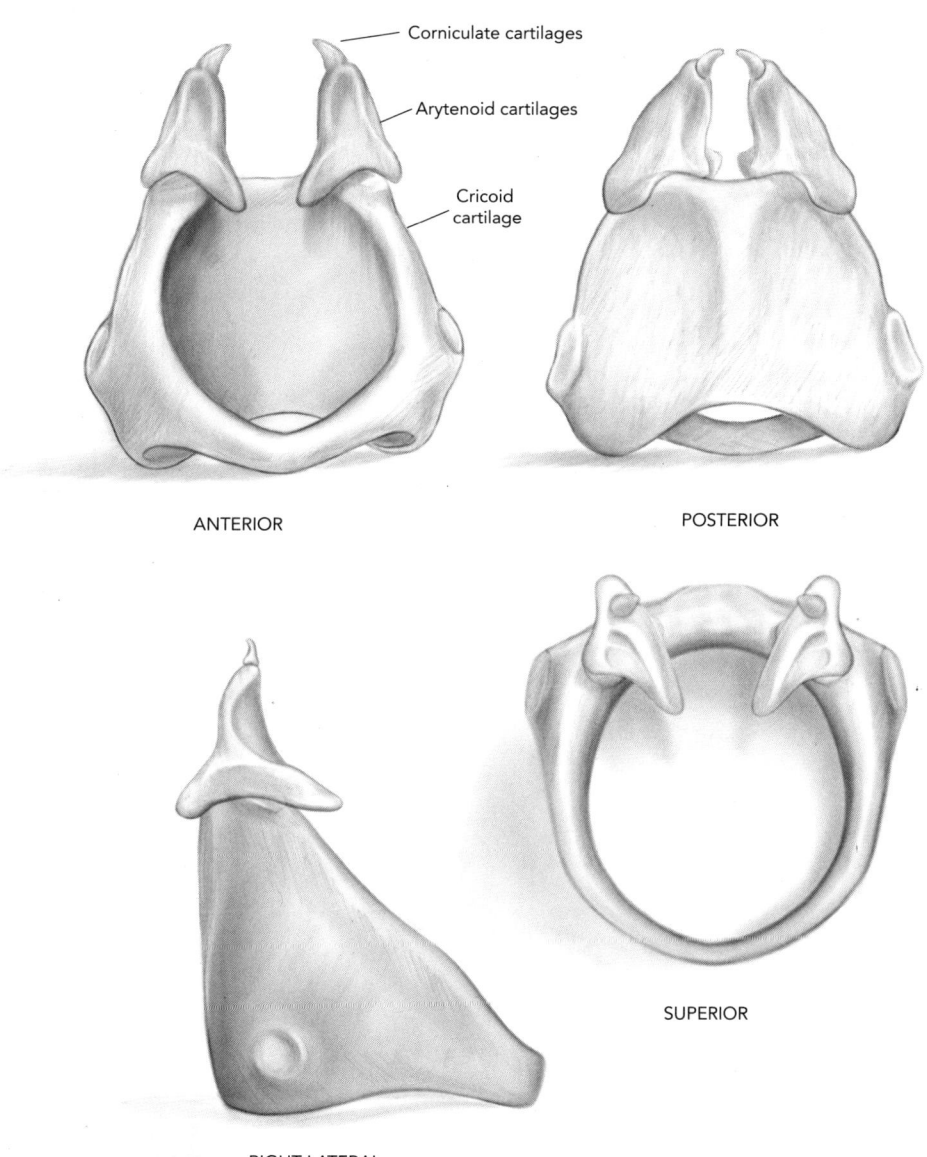

Corniculate cartilages

Arytenoid cartilages

Cricoid cartilage

ANTERIOR

POSTERIOR

SUPERIOR

RIGHT LATERAL

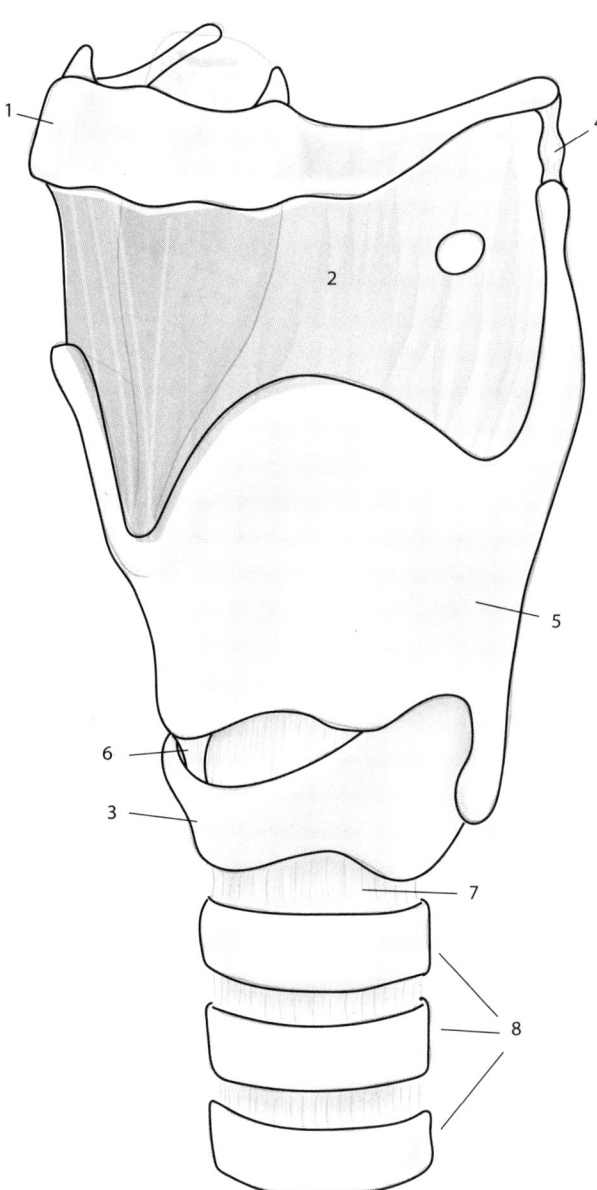

COLOR KEY

☐ 1 Hyoid bone
☐ 2 Thyrohyoid membrane
☐ 3 Cricoid cartilage
☐ 4 Triticeal cartilages
☐ 5 Thyroid cartilage
☐ 6 Median cricothyroid ligament
☐ 7 Cricotracheal membrane
☐ 8 Tracheal cartilage rings

Label:
A Major and minor horns
   of the hyoid bone
B Superior and inferior horns
   of the thyroid cartilage
C Superior thyroid notch

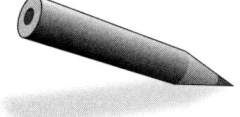

COLOR KEY

☐ 1 Corniculate cartilages
☐ 2 Arytenoid cartilages
☐ 3 Cricoid cartilage
☐ 4 Thyroid cartilage
☐ 5 Hyoid bone

Label:

A Articular facets of
   the cricoid cartilage
B Superior and inferior horns
   of the thyroid cartilage
C Thyroid notch
D Oblique line of the
   thyroid cartilage
E Vocal process of
   arytenoid cartilages
F Muscular process of
   arytenoid cartilages
G Major and minor horns
   of the hyoid bone

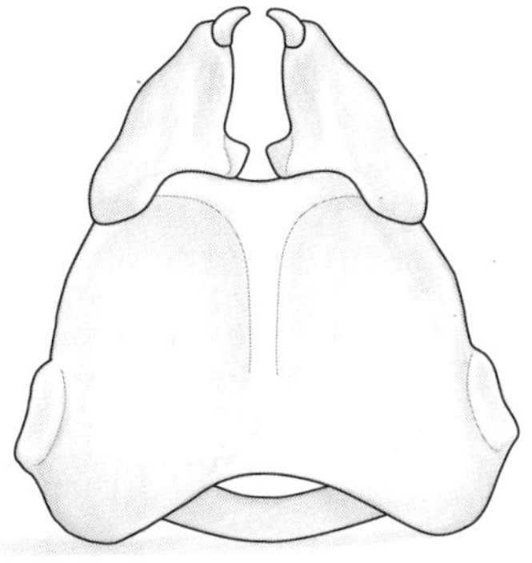

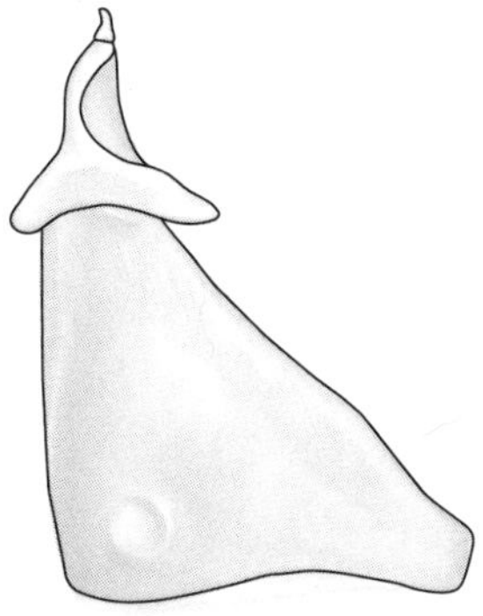

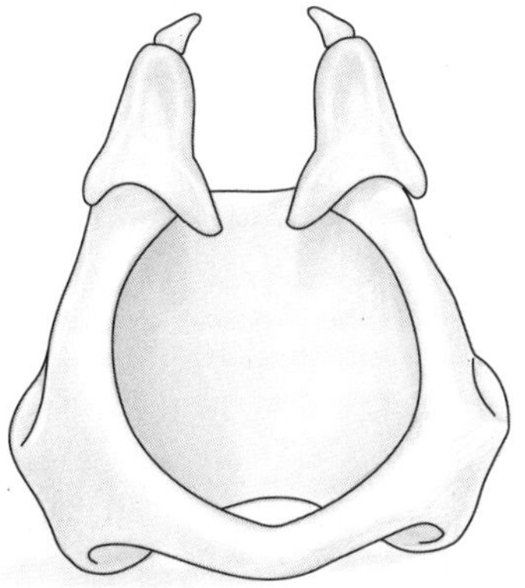

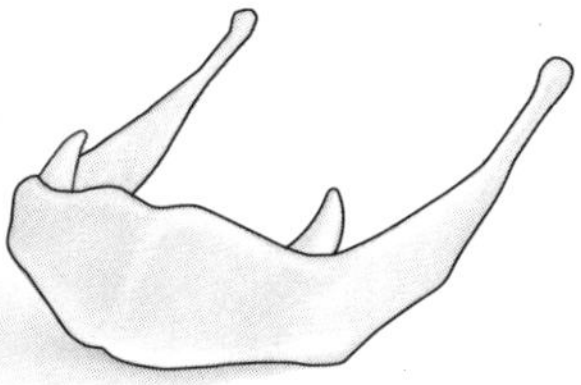

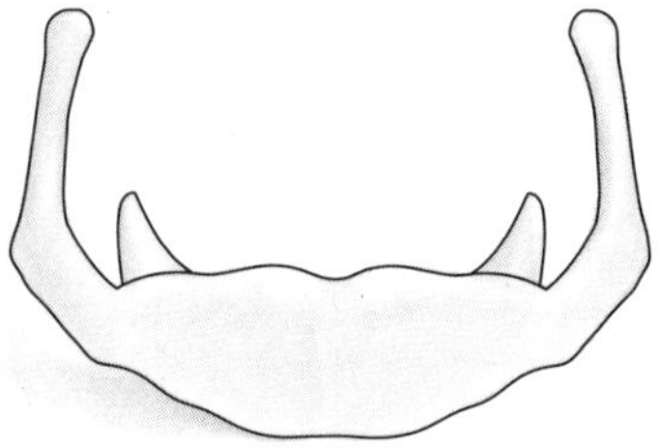

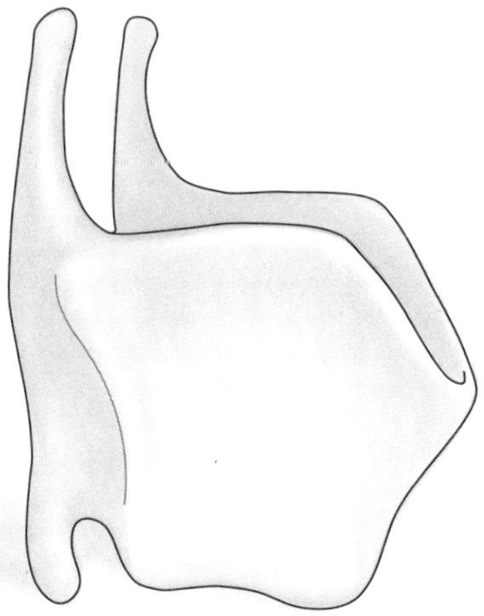

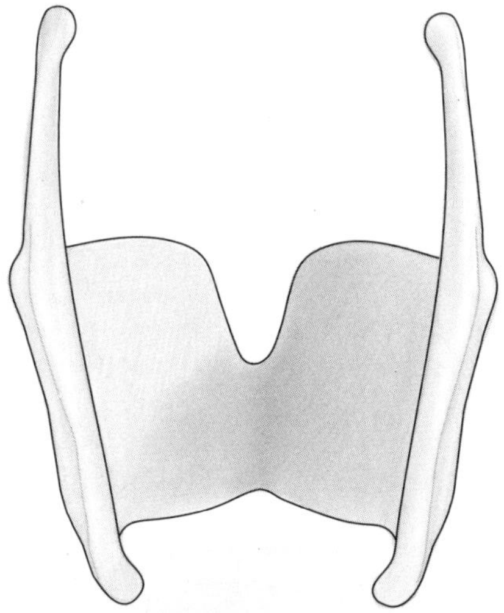

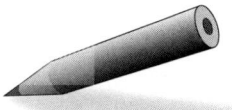

COLOR KEY
- 1 Hyoid bone
- 2 Cuneiform cartilages
- 3 Corniculate cartilages
- 4 Arytenoid cartilages
- 5 Triticeal cartilages
- 6 Thyroid cartilage
- 7 Cricoid cartilage
- 8 Tracheal cartilage rings

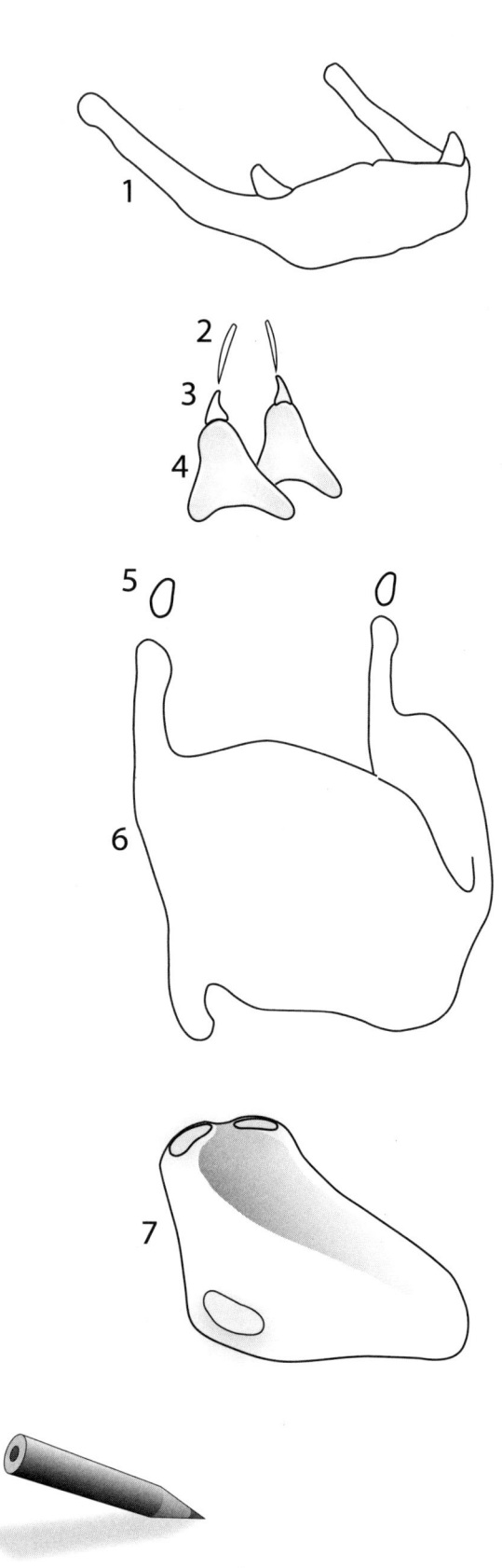

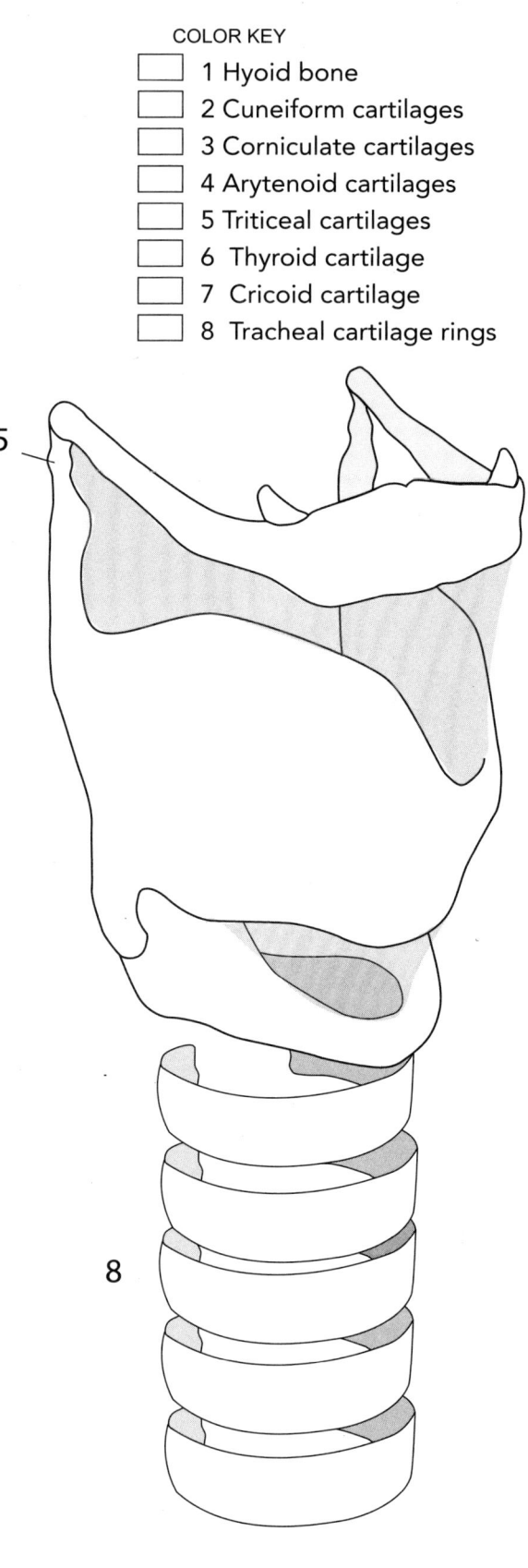

Posterior views of laryngeal cartilages

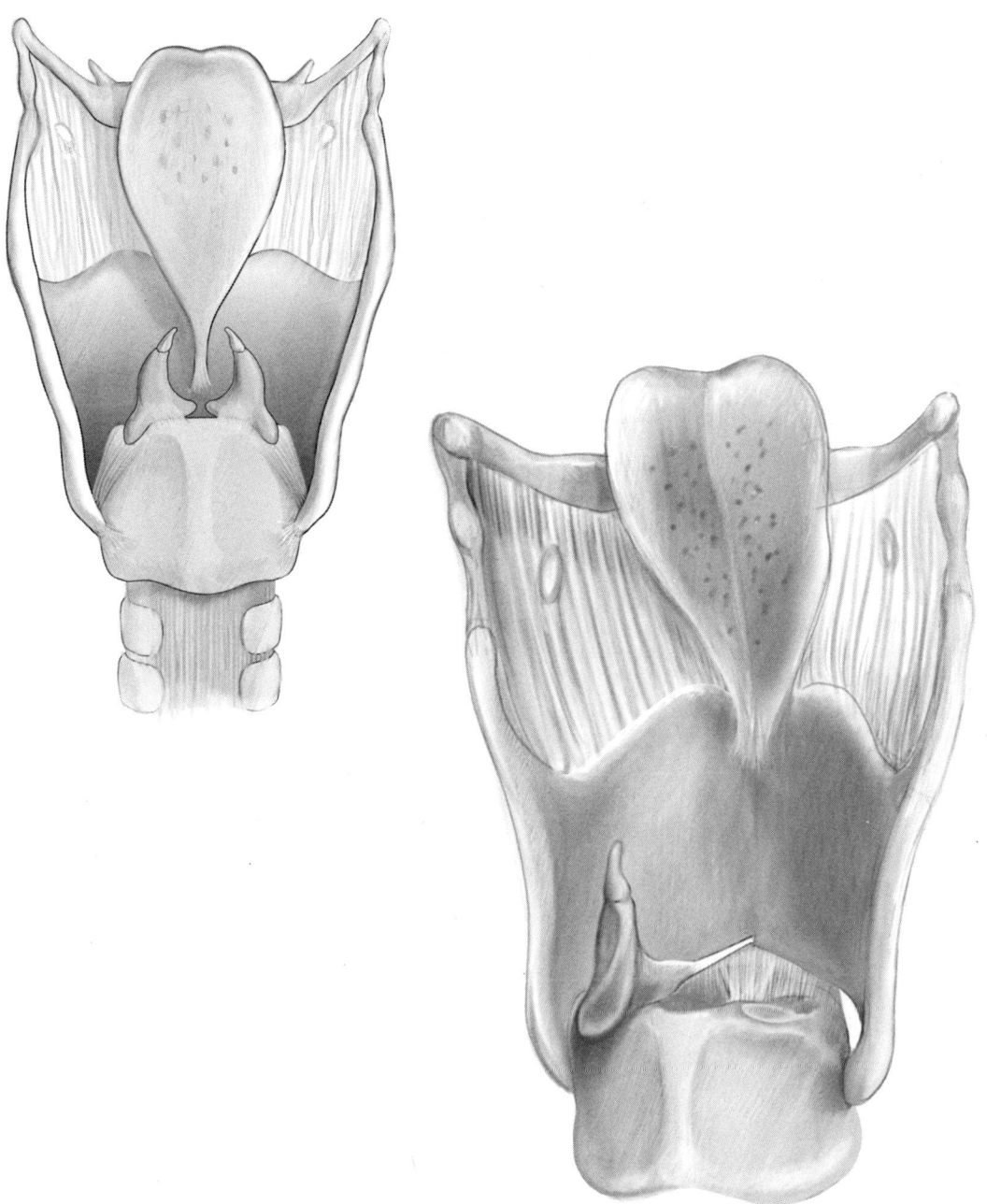

In this illustration, the right arytenoid
and corniculate cartilages have been removed
in order to reveal the right articular facet
of the cricoid cartilage.

The epiglottic cartilage

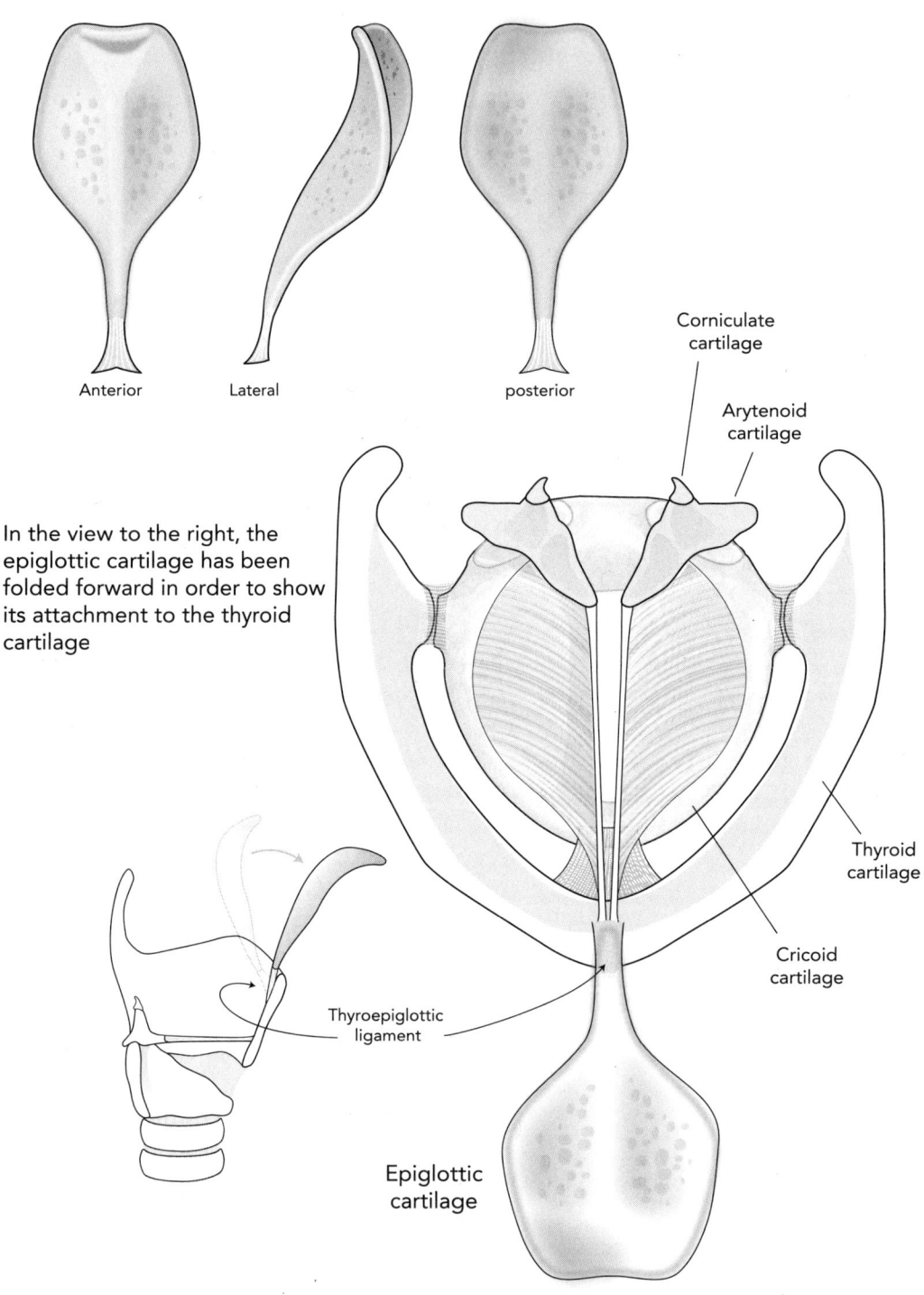

Anterior   Lateral   posterior

In the view to the right, the
epiglottic cartilage has been
folded forward in order to show
its attachment to the thyroid
cartilage

Corniculate
cartilage

Arytenoid
cartilage

Thyroid
cartilage

Cricoid
cartilage

Thyroepiglottic
ligament

Epiglottic
cartilage

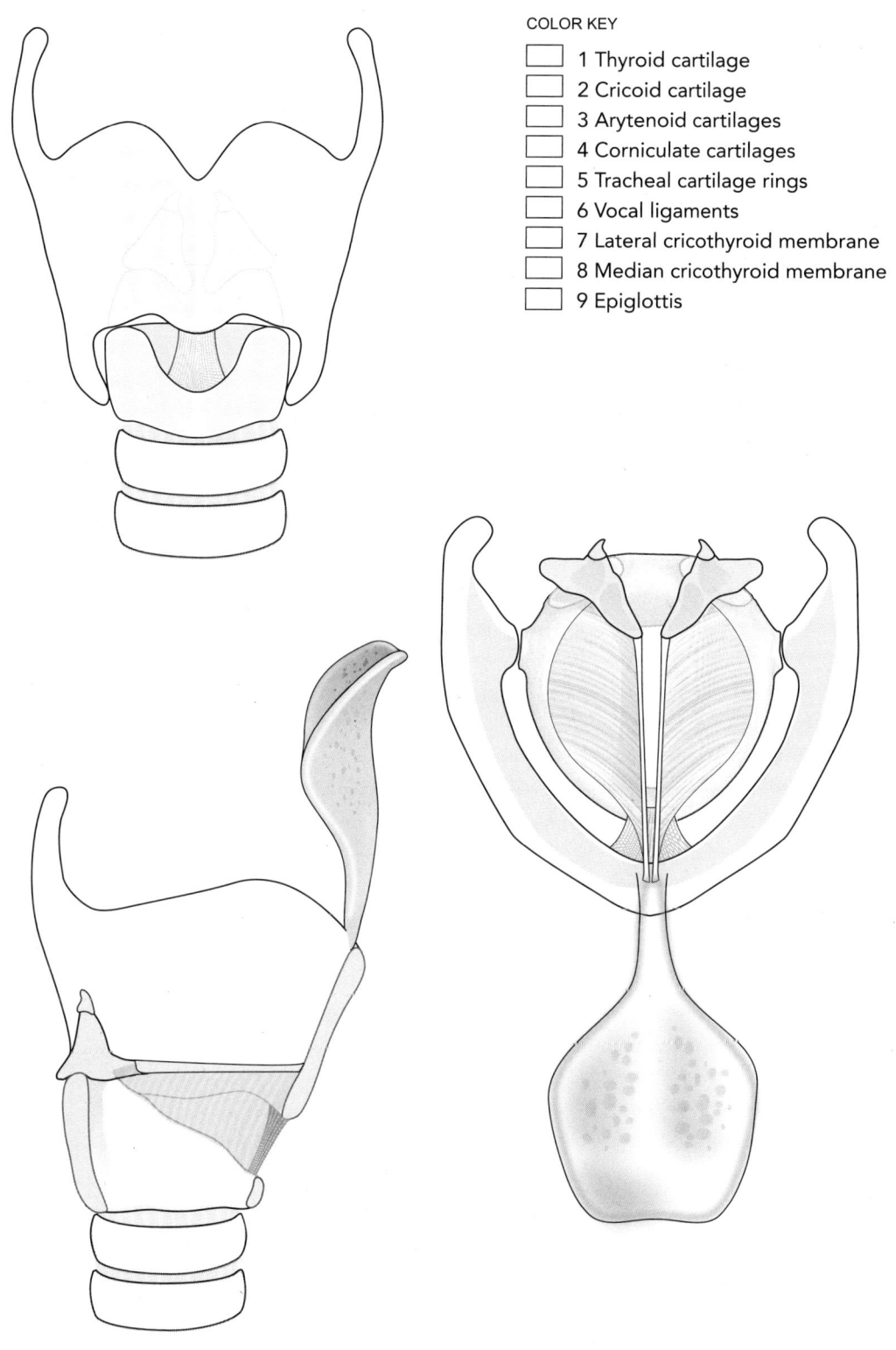

COLOR KEY

- ☐ 1 Thyroid cartilage
- ☐ 2 Cricoid cartilage
- ☐ 3 Arytenoid cartilages
- ☐ 4 Corniculate cartilages
- ☐ 5 Tracheal cartilage rings
- ☐ 6 Vocal ligaments
- ☐ 7 Lateral cricothyroid membrane
- ☐ 8 Median cricothyroid membrane
- ☐ 9 Epiglottis

Laryngeal cartilages, membranes and ligaments

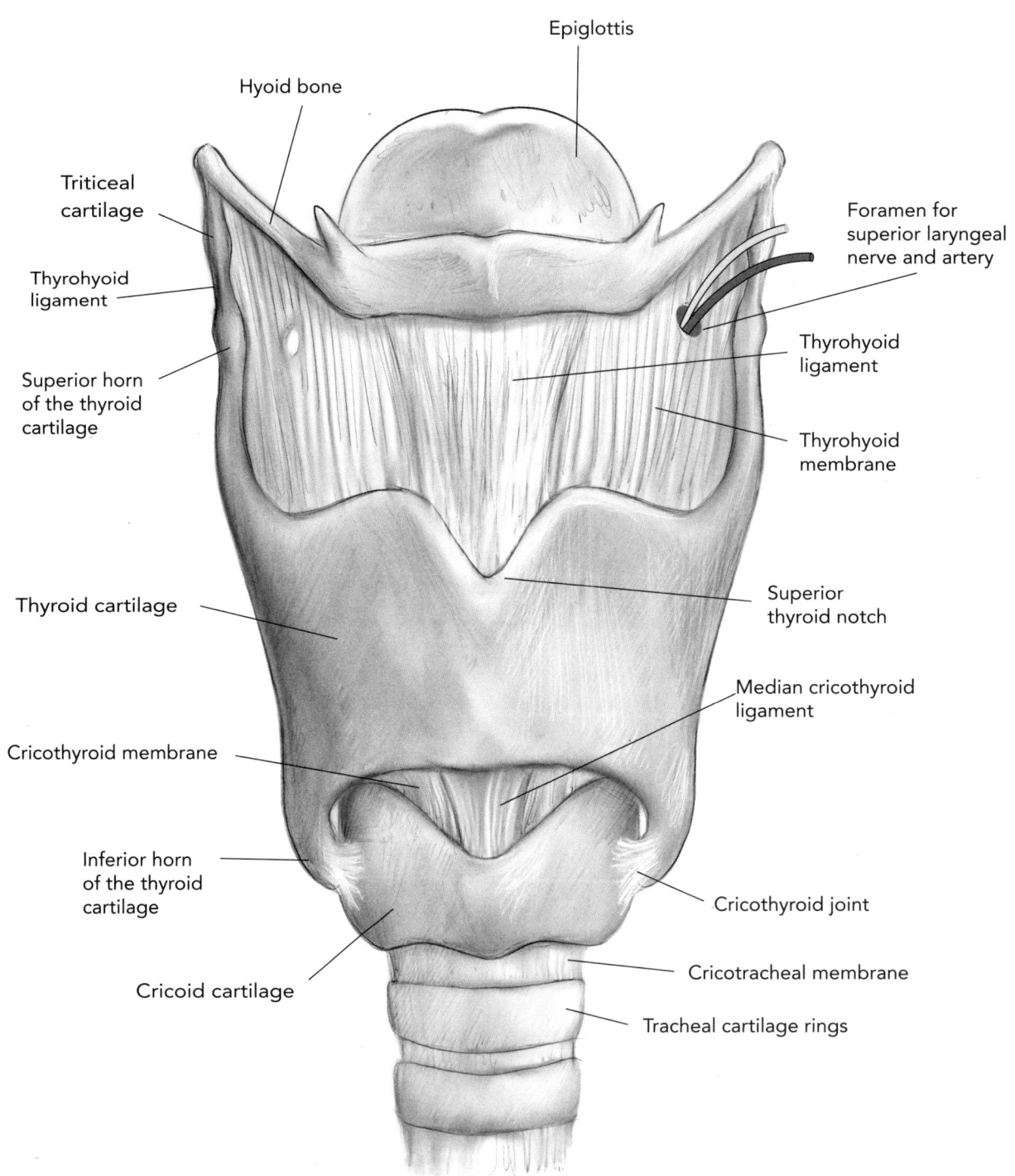

Epiglottis

Hyoid bone

Triticeal cartilage

Foramen for superior laryngeal nerve and artery

Thyrohyoid ligament

Thyrohyoid ligament

Superior horn of the thyroid cartilage

Thyrohyoid membrane

Thyroid cartilage

Superior thyroid notch

Median cricothyroid ligament

Cricothyroid membrane

Inferior horn of the thyroid cartilage

Cricothyroid joint

Cricotracheal membrane

Cricoid cartilage

Tracheal cartilage rings

Arytenoid cartilages location

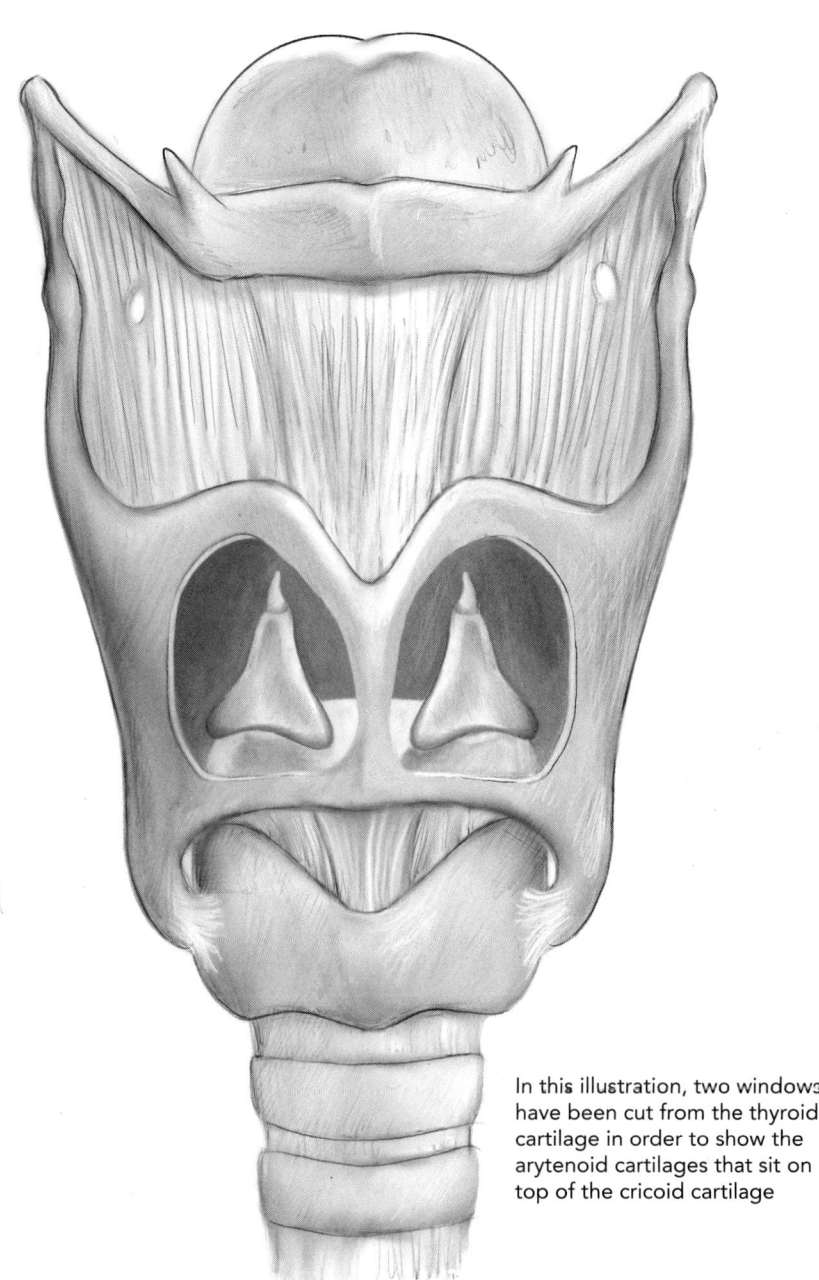

In this illustration, two windows have been cut from the thyroid cartilage in order to show the arytenoid cartilages that sit on top of the cricoid cartilage

Refer to the previous illustrations to locate and color the structures

COLOR KEY

- ☐ 1 Epiglottis
- ☐ 2 Hyoid bone
- ☐ 3 Triticeal cartilage
- ☐ 4 Thyroid cartilage
- ☐ 5 Thyrohyoid membrane
- ☐ 6 Thyrohyoid ligament

- ☐ 7 Corniculate cartilages
- ☐ 8 Arytenoid cartilages
- ☐ 9 Median cricothyroid ligament
- ☐ 10 Cricotracheal membrane
- ☐ 11 Corniculate cartilages
- ☐ 12 Tracheal cartilage rings

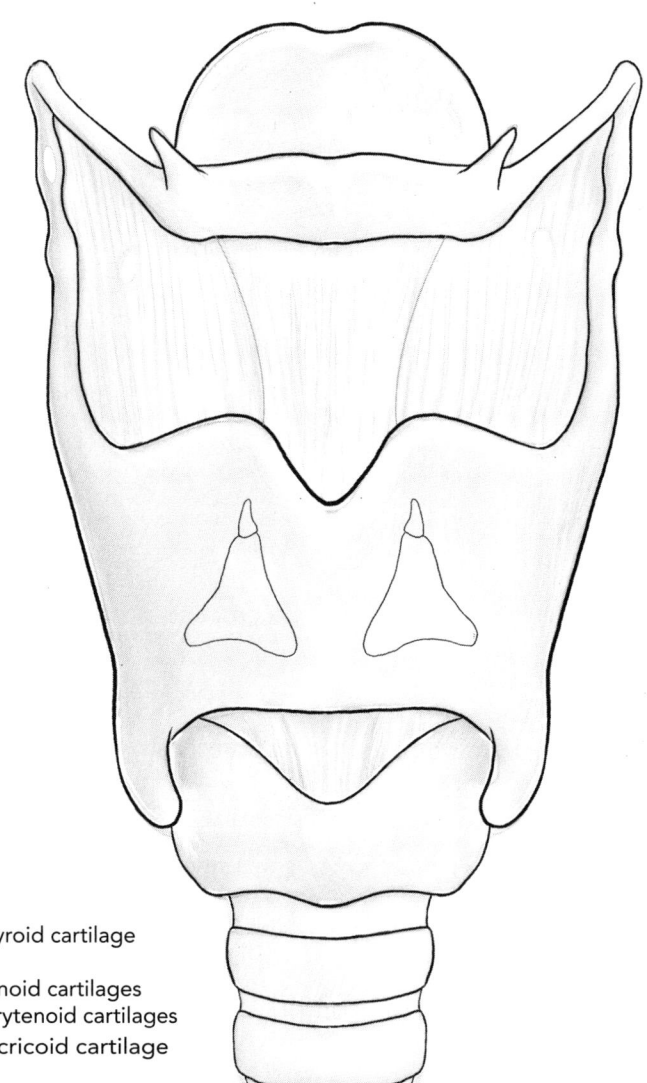

Label:
Superior horns of the thyroid cartilage
Cricothyroid joints
Vocal processes of arytenoid cartilages
Muscular processes of arytenoid cartilages
Articular facets of the cricoid cartilage

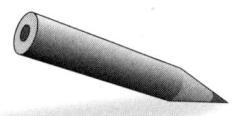

COLOR KEY

☐ 1 Hyoid bone
☐ 2 Epiglottis
☐ 3 Thyroid cartilage
☐ 4 Arytenoid cartilages
☐ 5 Corniculate cartilages
☐ 6 Cricoid cartilage
☐ 7 Triticeal cartilages
☐ 8 Tracheal cartilage rings

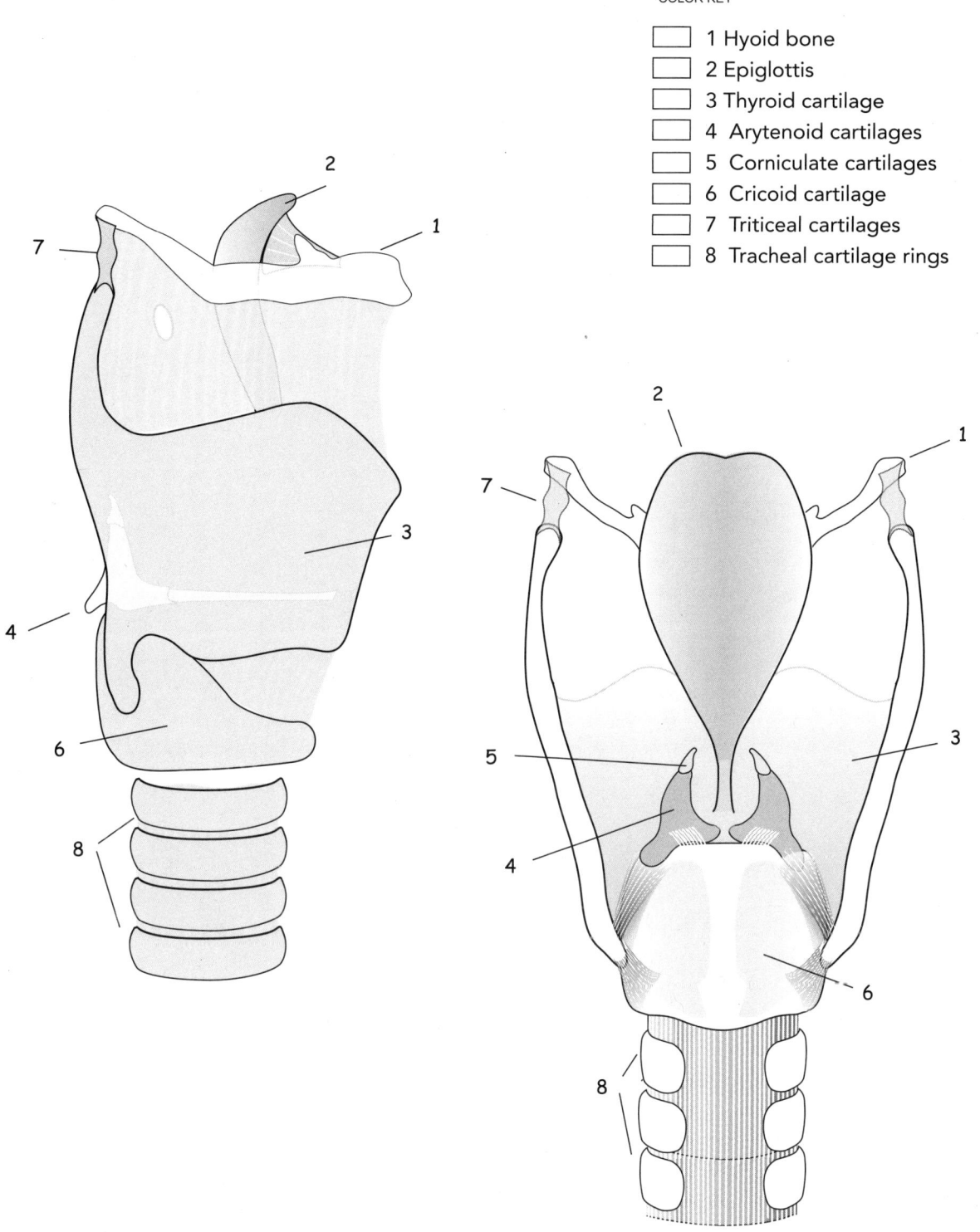

Superior view of laryngeal cartilages

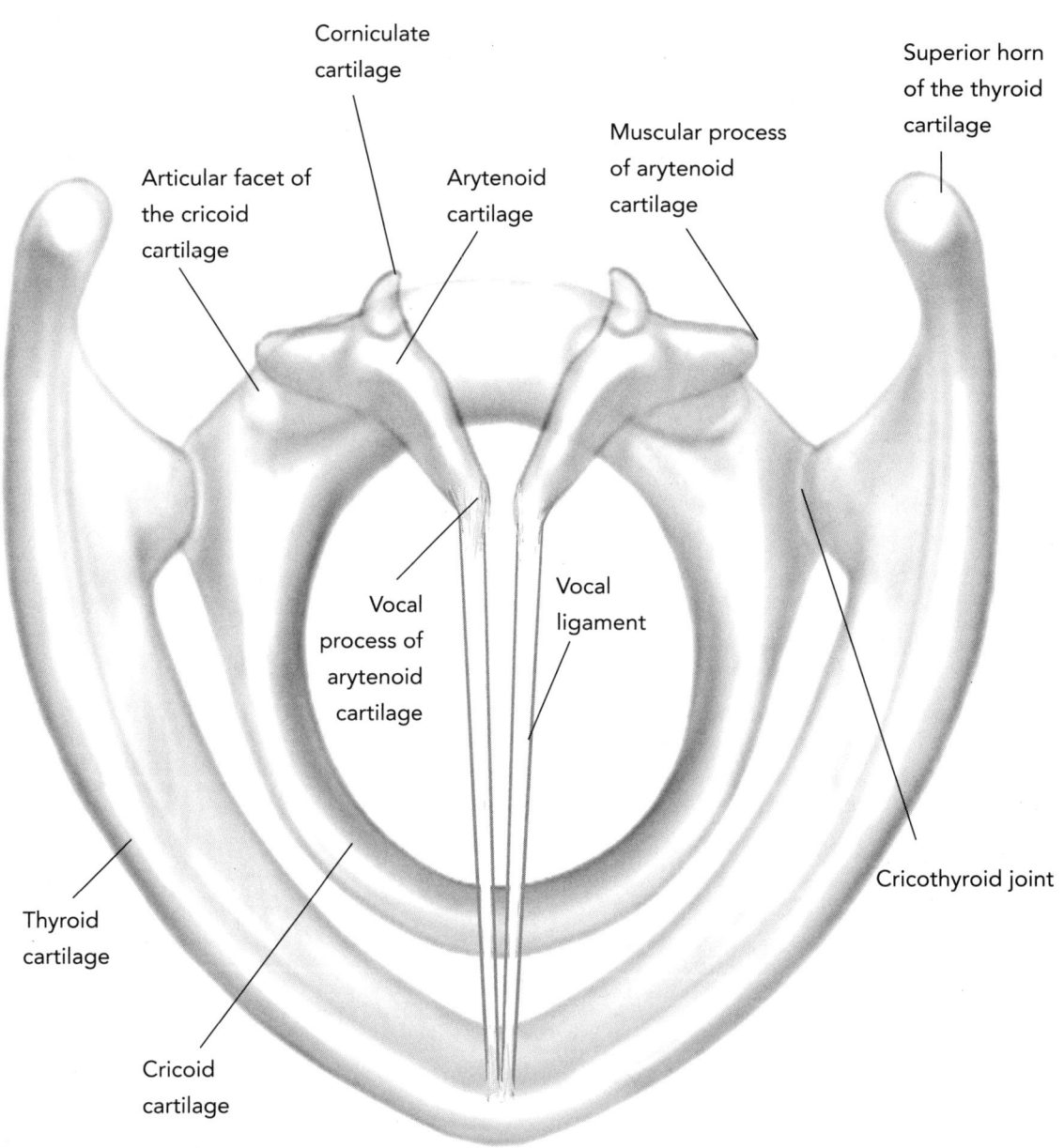

Corniculate cartilage

Articular facet of the cricoid cartilage

Arytenoid cartilage

Muscular process of arytenoid cartilage

Superior horn of the thyroid cartilage

Vocal process of arytenoid cartilage

Vocal ligament

Cricothyroid joint

Thyroid cartilage

Cricoid cartilage

COLOR KEY

☐ 1 Thyroid cartilage
☐ 2 Cricoid cartilage
☐ 3 Vocal ligaments
☐ 4 Arytenoid cartilages
☐ 5 Corniculate cartilages

Label:
Superior horns of the thyroid cartilage
Cricothyroid joints
Vocal processes of arytenoid cartilages
Muscular processes of arytenoid cartilages
Articular facets of the cricoid cartilage

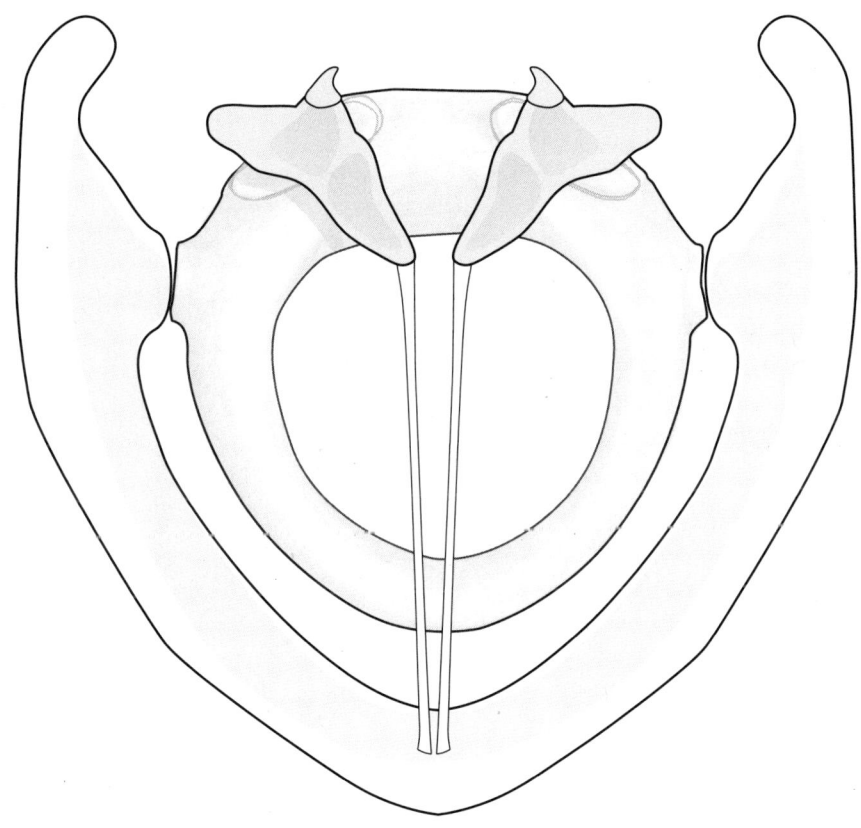

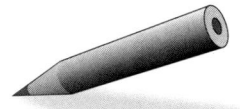

Sectional views of the larynx

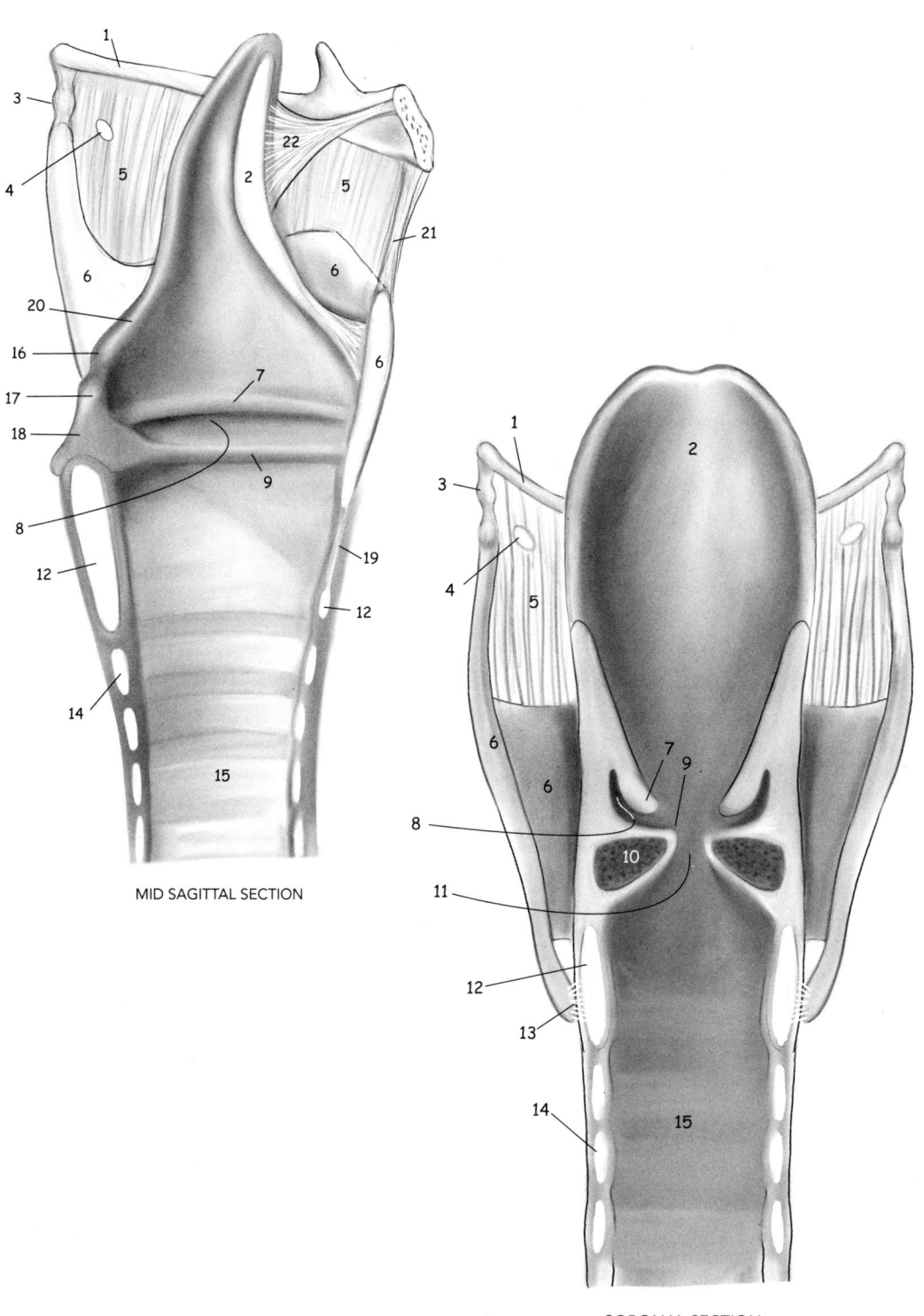

MID SAGITTAL SECTION

CORONAL SECTION

Color or label items 1 through 22

1 Hyoid bone
2 Epiglottis
3 Triticeal cartilage
4 Foramen
5 Thyrohyoid membrane
6 Thyroid cartilage
7 Vestibular fold (false vocal fold)
8 Ventricle
9 True vocal fold
10 Vocalis muscle

MID SAGITTAL SECTION

11 Opening of the glottis
12 Cricoid cartilage
13 Cricothyroid joint
14 Tracheal cartilage rings
15 Trachea
16 Cuneiform cartilage (beneath flesh)
17 Corniculate cartilages (beneath flesh)
18 Arytenoid cartilage (beneath flesh)
19 Middle cricothyroid ligament
20 Aryepiglottic fold
21 Middle thyrohyoid ligament
22 Hyoepiglottic ligament

CORONAL SECTION

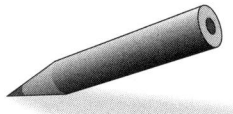

Posterior view of larynx

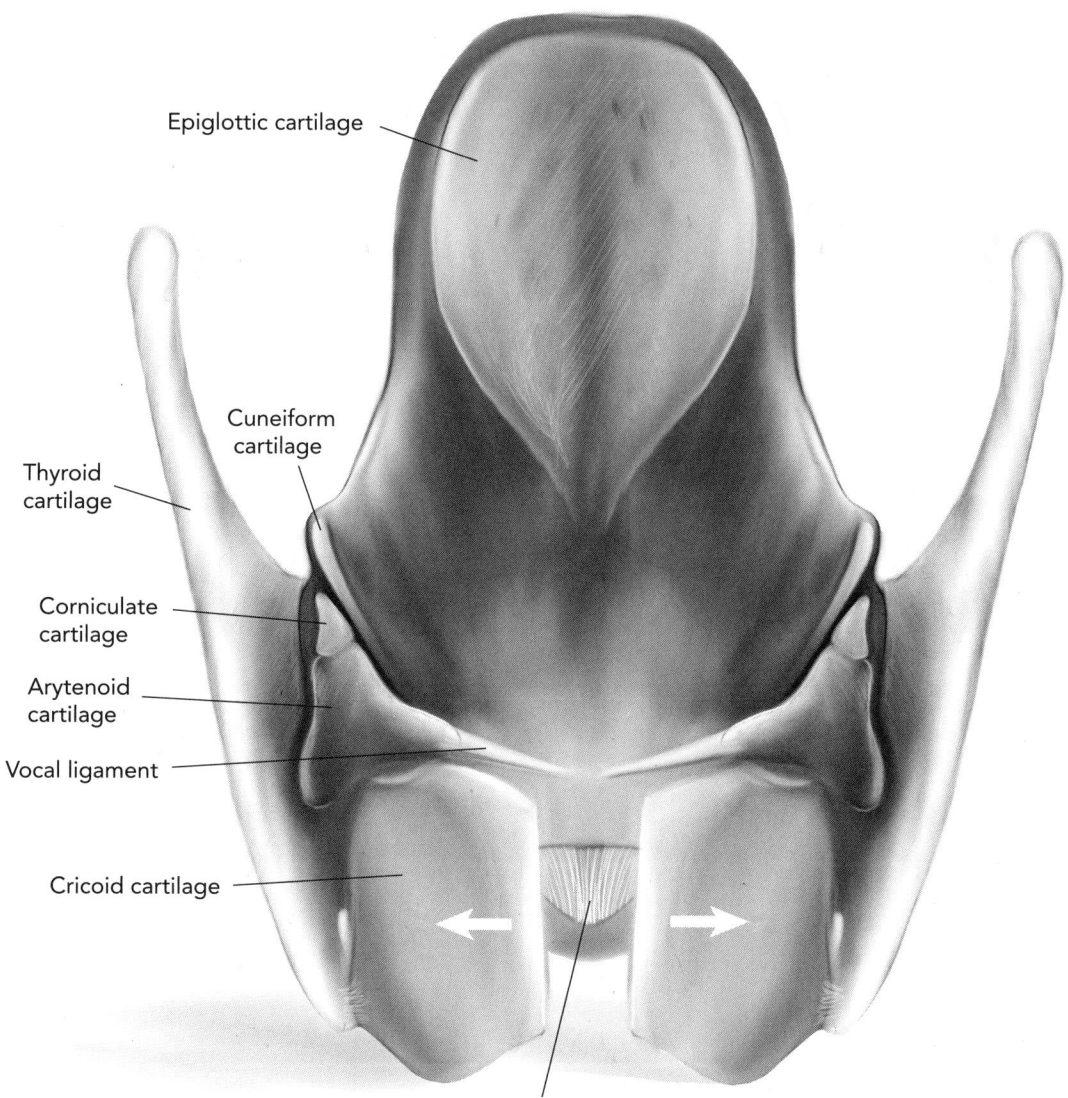

Epiglottic cartilage

Cuneiform cartilage

Thyroid cartilage

Corniculate cartilage

Arytenoid cartilage

Vocal ligament

Cricoid cartilage

Cricothyroid ligament.

In this posterior view, the back of the cricoid cartilage has been split and pulled apart to reveal the front of the cricoid and the cricothyroid ligament.

The flesh has been rendered as if it is transparent to reveal the arytenoid, corniculate, cuneiform and epiglottic cartilages.

Posterior view of larynx in relation to superior structures

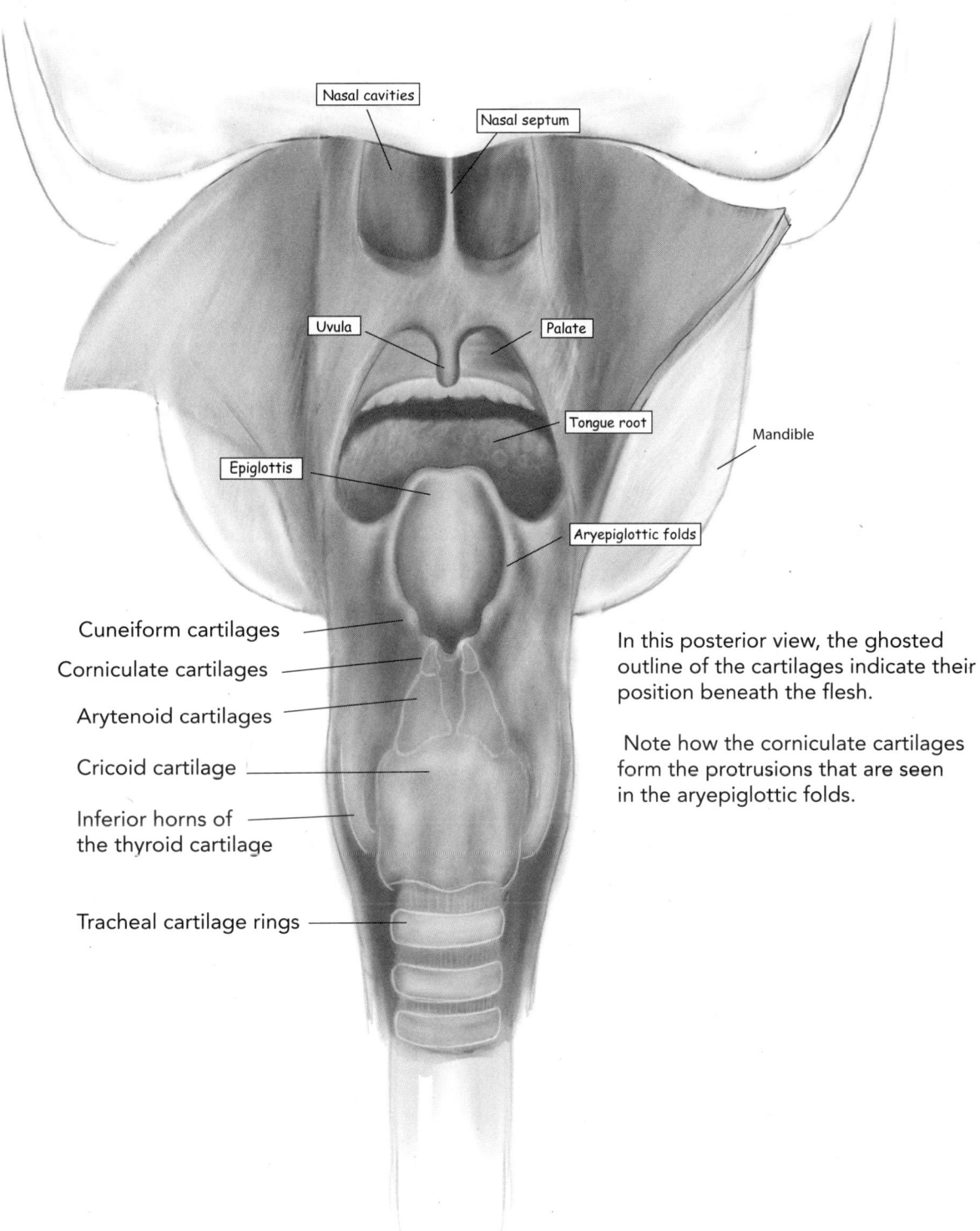

Nasal cavities

Nasal septum

Uvula

Palate

Tongue root

Epiglottis

Mandible

Aryepiglottic folds

Cuneiform cartilages

Corniculate cartilages

Arytenoid cartilages

Cricoid cartilage

Inferior horns of
the thyroid cartilage

Tracheal cartilage rings

In this posterior view, the ghosted outline of the cartilages indicate their position beneath the flesh.

Note how the corniculate cartilages form the protrusions that are seen in the aryepiglottic folds.

JOINTS OF THE LARYNX

Cricoarytenoid joint: connects the base of each arytenoid cartilage and the superior surface of the quadrate lamina of the cricoid. The CA is a synovial joint that allows for a wide range of movements of the arytenoid cartilages. When the appropriate muscles contract the arytenoid cartilages undergo a rotational movement. Depending on which muscle is contracted the vocal processes either approximate medially and in a downward closing motion (towards one another), or laterally and in an upward opening motion (away from one another). Because the vocal folds are attached to the vocal processes, they follow the movement, and are either brought toward or away from the midline, to close or open the glottis.

Cricothyroid joint: is located between the inferior horns of the thyroid cartilage and the sides of the cricoid cartilage. Like the CA joints, the CT joints are synovial. They allow the thyroid cartilage to tilt superiorly and inferiorly and the cricoid cartilage to be tilted upward and backward. These movements increase the distance between the anterior commissure of the thyroid cartilage and the arytenoid cartilages. Increasing the distance has the effect of stretching and tensing the vocal folds, which increases their frequency and pitch. Decreasing the distance between the anterior commissure and the vocal processes shortens the vocal folds, decreasing frequency and pitch.

Various ligaments hold the joints in place and limit the amount and type of movements allowed.

Cricothyroid joint

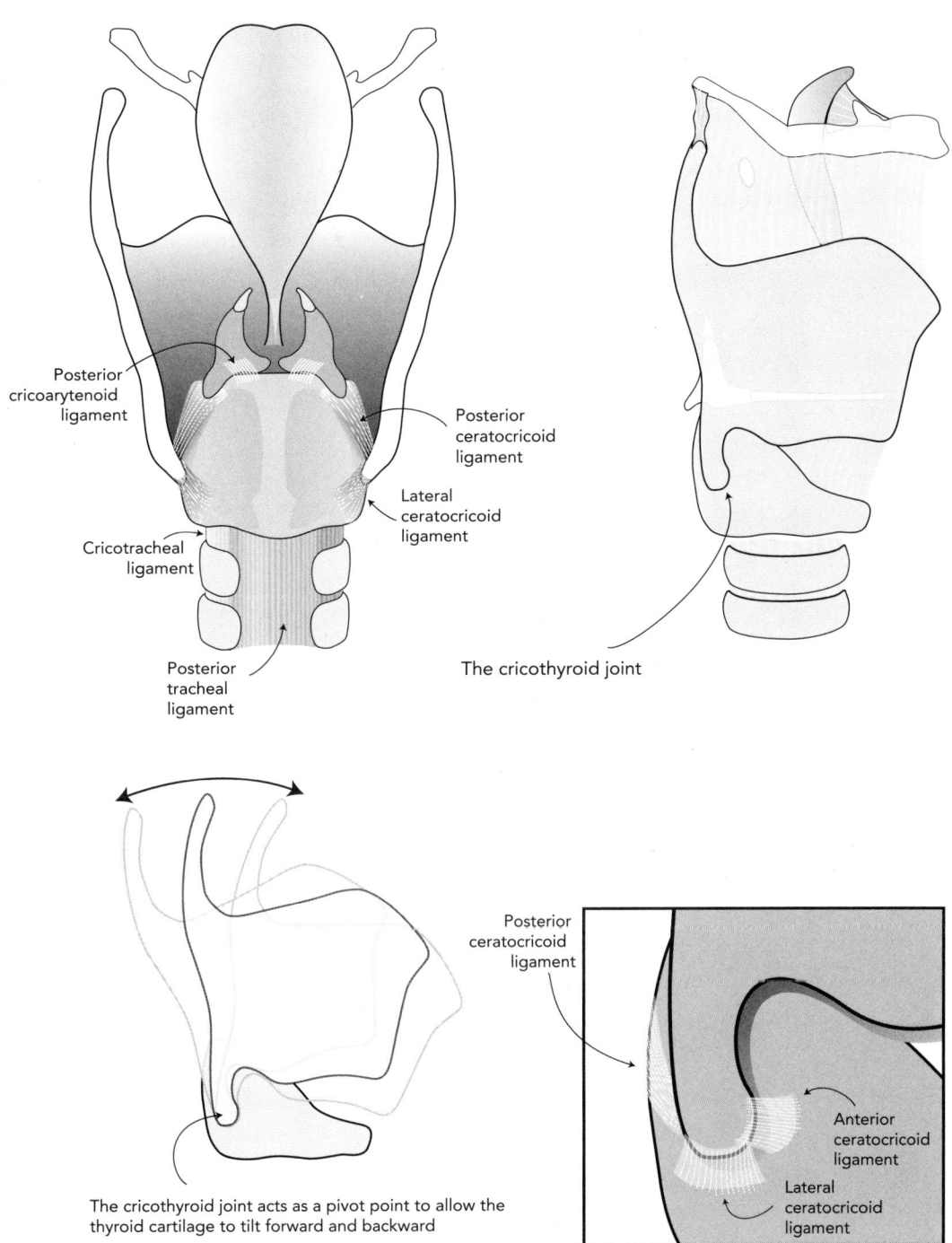

Posterior cricoarytenoid ligament

Posterior ceratocricoid ligament

Lateral ceratocricoid ligament

Cricotracheal ligament

Posterior tracheal ligament

The cricothyroid joint

The cricothyroid joint acts as a pivot point to allow the thyroid cartilage to tilt forward and backward

Posterior ceratocricoid ligament

Anterior ceratocricoid ligament

Lateral ceratocricoid ligament

Movement of the arytenoid cartilages

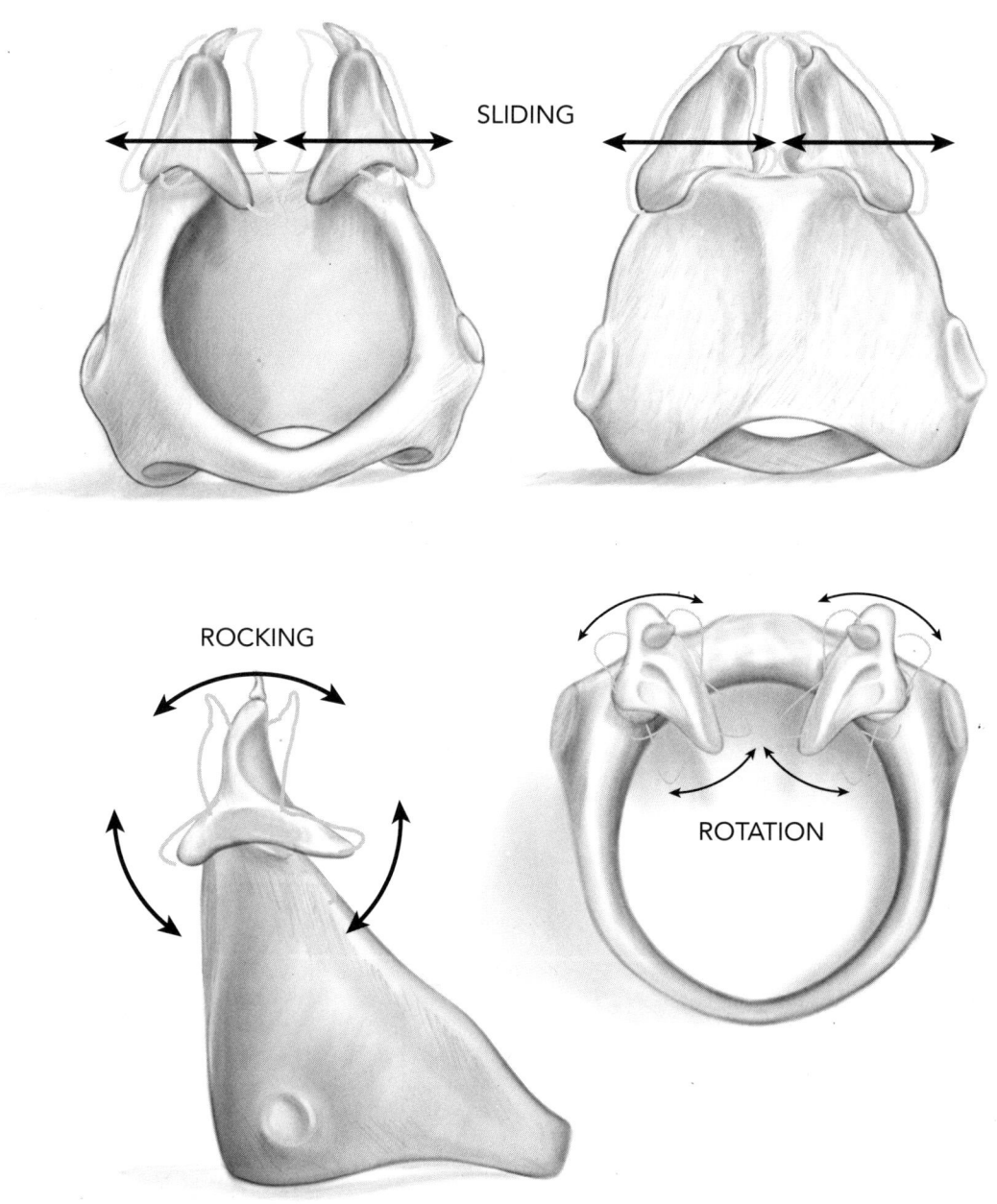

Schematic: types of movement of arytenoid cartilages

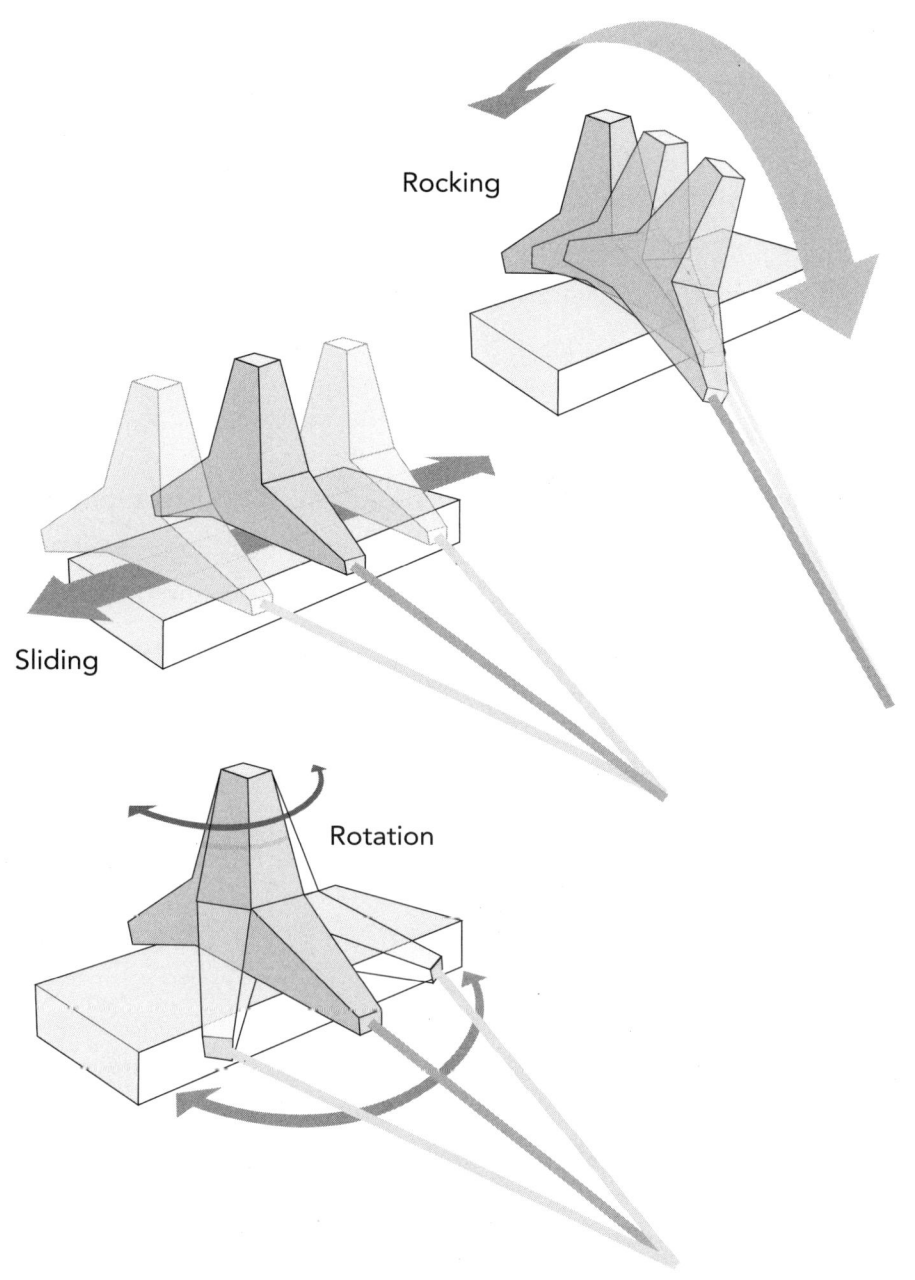

LARYNGEAL VALVES

There are three sets of valves within the laryngeal lumen. From superior to inferior they are:

Aryepiglottic folds

The aryepiglottic folds are bundles of connective tissue and muscle that run from the superior and lateral margins of the epiglottis to the apex of each arytenoid. This forms a roughly oval-shaped sphincter. The elastic cuneiform cartilages are located within these tissues. The function of the cuneiform cartilages is to provide some firmness that helps the aryepiglottic folds to withstand the negative pressures of inhalation. When the aryepiglottic muscle contracts, the epiglottis is pulled backwards to cover the entrance to the larynx during swallowing.

False (ventricular) folds

The false vocal folds are located inferior to the aryepiglottic folds and superior to the true folds but do not extend as far to the midline. They run roughly run parallel to the true folds. The false vocal folds are composed primarily of connective and some muscle tissue and contain numerous mucous glands and goblet cells that help to lubricate the true vocal folds beneath them.

Laryngeal ventricle

The laryngeal ventricle is the space between the false and true vocal folds containing numerous glands.

True vocal folds

The true vocal folds attach anteriorly at the anterior commissure of the thyroid cartilage, and posteriorly to the vocal process of each arytenoid. The true vocal folds are composed of five layers, each with a different cellular make-up and different biomechanical properties. From superficial to deep, the layers are the epithelium, superficial layer of the lamina propria (SLLP), intermediate layer of the lamina propria (ILLP), deep layer of the lamina propria (DLLP), and muscle.

Layers of the vocal folds

Epithelium

The epithelium is the outermost surface of the true vocal folds composed of non-keratinizing stratified squamous cell epithelium. This type of epithelium is found mainly in wet cavities such as the oral and nasal cavities and protects against abrasion and other forms of damage.

Lamina propria

The lamina propria is a three-part layer of mucous membrane that lies deep to the epithelium. Each layer of the lamina propria is composed of different types of connective tissue.

Superficial layer (also called Reinke's space): consists mostly of loosely organized elastin fibers as well as small amounts of collagen. This allows the superficial layer a great deal of compliance.

Intermediate layer: is composed of densely organized elastin fibers. This layer is still compliant, but less so than the superficial layer.

Deep layer: consists mostly of collagen fibers. Collagen fibers are less flexible and compliant than elastin fibers.

Thyroarytenoid muscle

The thyroarytenoid muscle is the innermost layer of the vocal folds. Because muscle fibers are denser than connective tissues this layer is less compliant than the other layers.

Cover-body model

The cover-body model describes the vibratory characteristics of the vocal folds in terms of the compliance of the layers.

Cover: comprises the flexible epithelium and superficial layer of the lamina propria and is the most compliant layer.

Vocal ligament: formed by the intermediate and deep layers of the lamina propria. This layer is less compliant than the cover.

Body: made up of the thyroarytenoid (vocalis) muscle. It is the least compliant layer.

Vocal fold layers

COLOR KEY

- ☐ 1 Squamous epithelium
- ☐ 2 Lamina propria superficial layer
- ☐ 3 Lamina propria intermediate layer
- ☐ 4 Lamina propria deep layer
- ☐ 5 Vocalis muscle

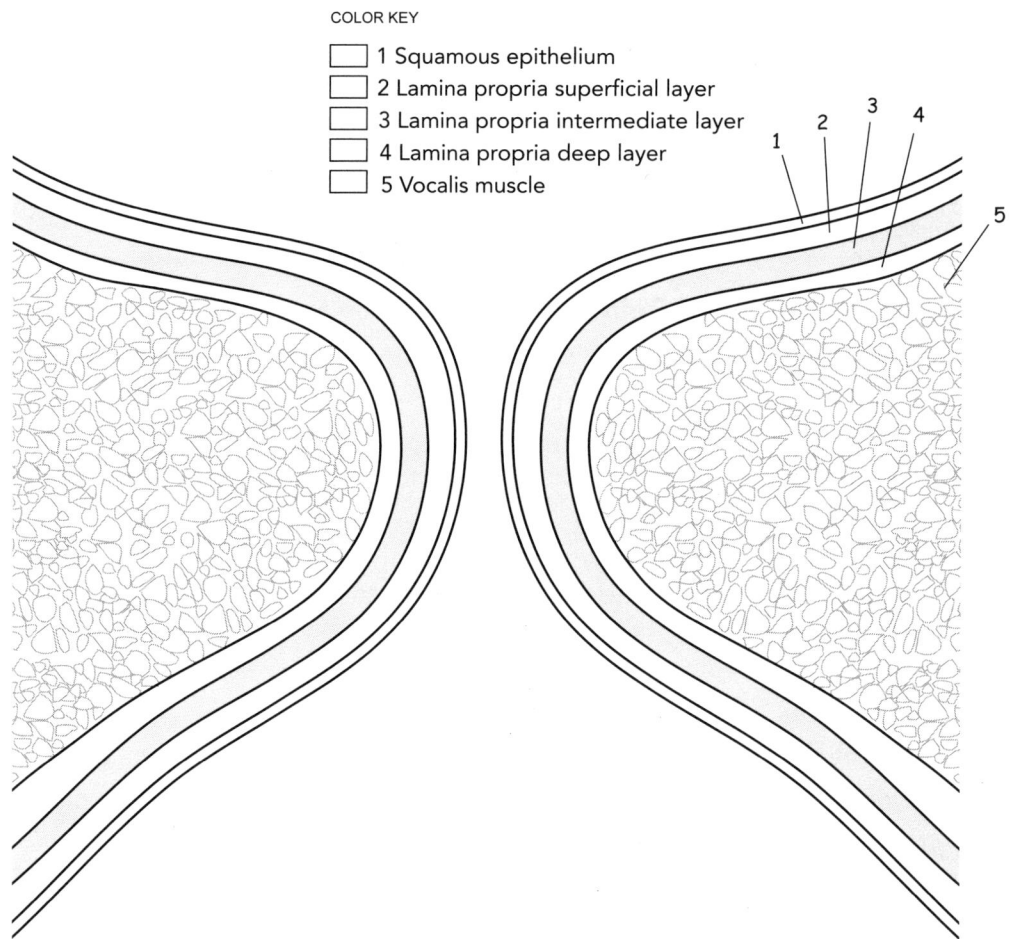

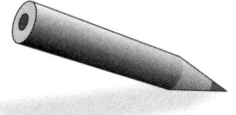

GLOTTIS

The glottis is the space between the vocal folds. The anterior three fifths of the glottis is bounded by ligament and is called the membranous glottis. The posterior two fifths is bounded by cartilage and is called the cartilaginous glottis.

The glottis changes shape depending on the positioning of the vocal folds at any time.

For phonation of a voiced sound, the glottis is closed with the folds in a median position. Normal quiet breathing is associated with a somewhat open glottis. When large amounts of air are needed the glottis is very widely open with the folds in a position called forced abduction. Whispering is associated with a glottis that is closed along most of its length, but with a small posterior opening.

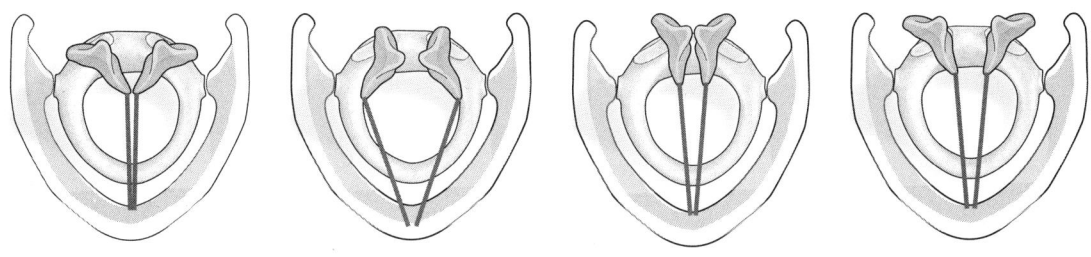

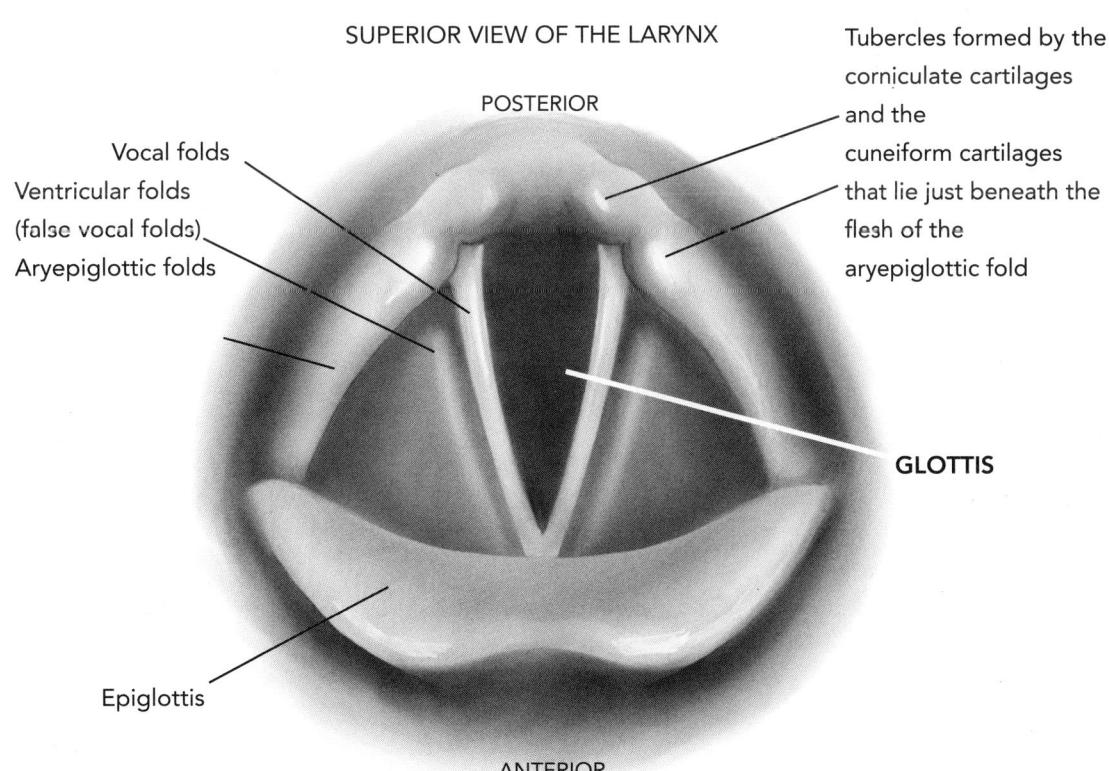

SUPERIOR VIEW OF THE LARYNX

POSTERIOR

Vocal folds

Ventricular folds
(false vocal folds)

Aryepiglottic folds

Tubercles formed by the corniculate cartilages and the cuneiform cartilages that lie just beneath the flesh of the aryepiglottic fold

GLOTTIS

Epiglottis

ANTERIOR

MUSCLES OF THE LARYNX

The muscles of the larynx are divided into extrinsic and intrinsic groups. Extrinsic muscles are those which have one attachment to the cartilages of the larynx or hyoid bone, and the other to some structure external to the larynx. Intrinsic muscles have both their attachments to or within the larynx.

Extrinsic muscles of the larynx

There are two groups of extrinsic muscles that attach to the hyoid bone and to structures above and below the hyoid (sternum, scapula, mandible, and temporal bone). The groups of muscles attaching below the hyoid are known as the infrahyoids. This group of muscles lower the larynx. Those attaching above the level of the hyoid are the suprahyoids. The suprahyoids raise the larynx. The muscles are named according to their attachments.

Infrahyoid muscles

Sternohyoid: runs from the clavicle and sternum to the body of the hyoid. This muscle depresses the hyoid bone and larynx.

Sternothyroid: runs from the first costal (rib)cartilage and sternum to the oblique line of thyroid lamina. It lowers the hyoid bone and larynx.

Omohyoid: courses from the scapula to the inferior border of the hyoid. This muscle depresses and retracts the hyoid bone.

Thyrohyoid: runs from the oblique line of the thyroid lamina to the major horn of the hyoid. The thyrohyoid muscle draws the hyoid bone and thyroid cartilage closer to each other.

Suprahyoid muscles

Digastric: consists of two portions (bellies), the anterior and posterior bellies. Both bellies elevate the hyoid bone.

Stylohyoid: runs between the styloid process of the temporal bone to the body of the hyoid bone. The stylohyoid muscle elevates and retracts the hyoid bone.

Mylohyoid: courses between the body of the mandible and the hyoid bone. It elevates the hyoid bone.

Geniohyoid: runs from the mandible to the body of the hyoid bone. The geniohyoid muscle pulls the hyoid bone anteriorly and superiorly.

Extrinsic muscles of the larynx

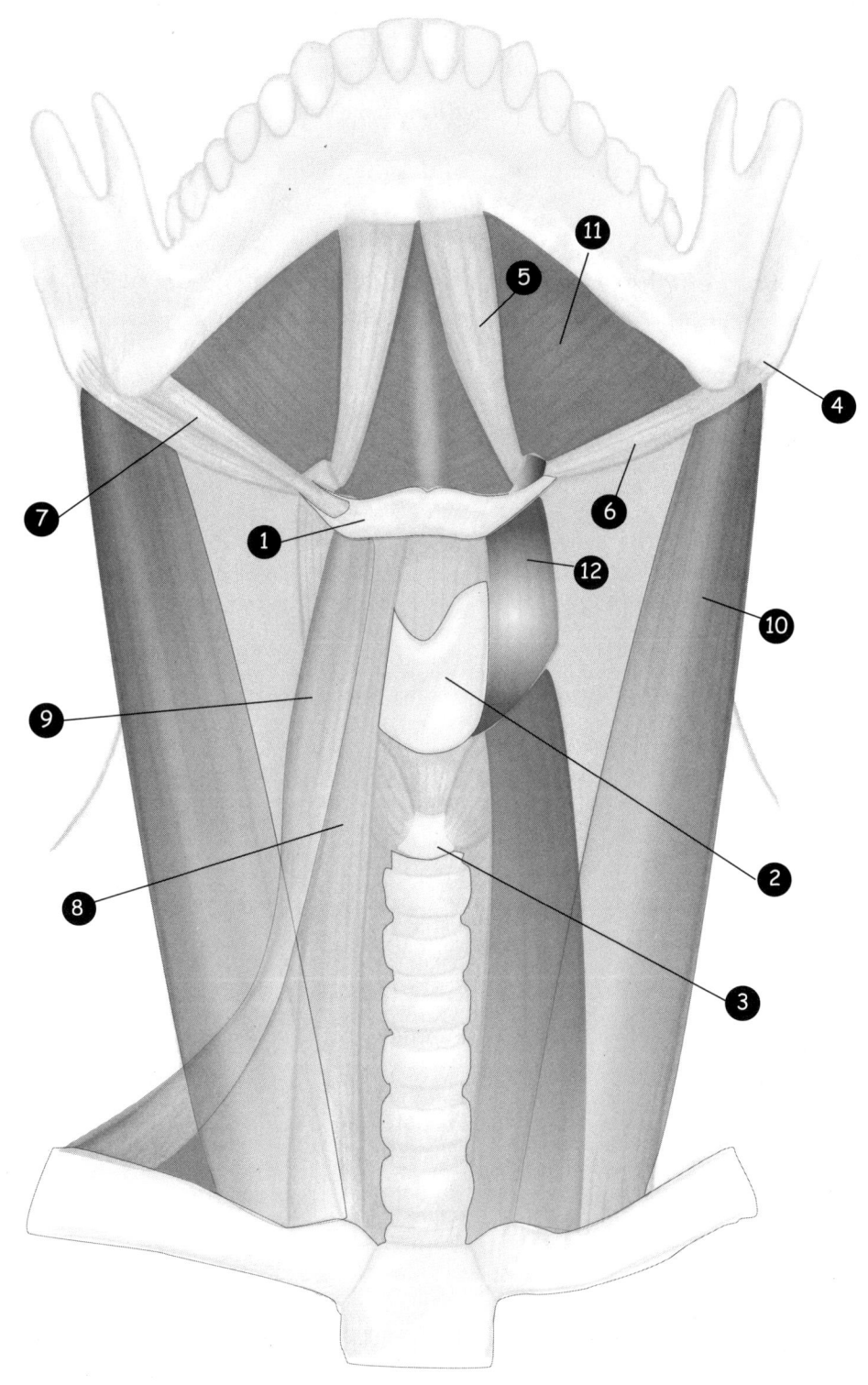

Refer to the illustration on the facing page to locate and color the structures

COLOR KEY
☐ 1 Hyoid bone
☐ 2 Thyroid cartilage
☐ 3 Cricoid cartilage
☐ 4 Mastoid process
☐ 5 Anterior belly of digastric muscle
☐ 6 Posterior belly of digastric muscle
☐ 7 Stylohyoid muscle
☐ 8 Sternohyoid muscle
☐ 9 Omohyoid muscle
☐ 10 Sternocleidomastoid muscle
☐ 11 Mylohyoid muscle
☐ 12 Thyrohyoid muscle

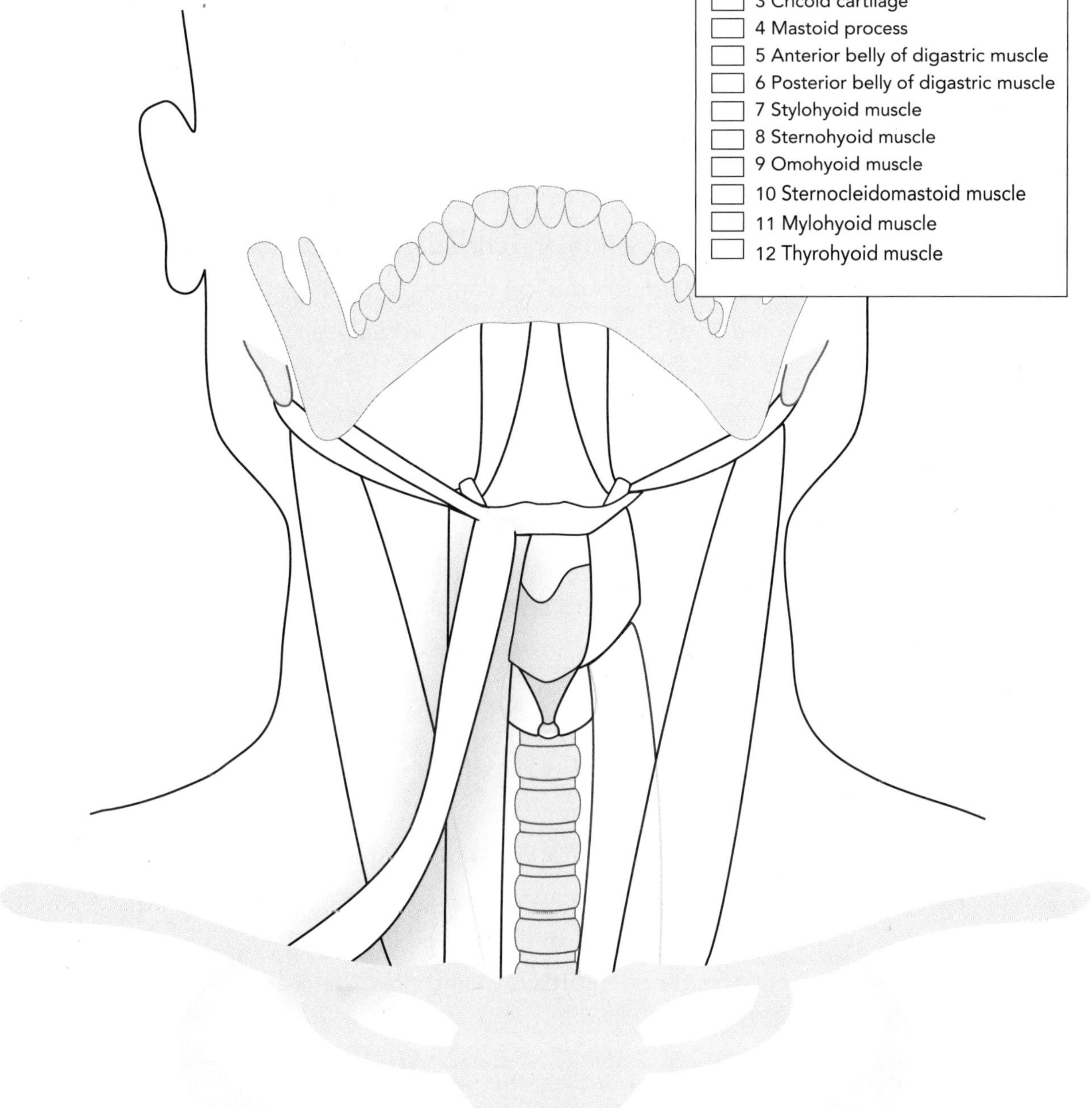

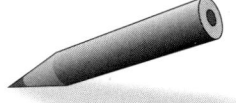

Intrinsic muscles of the larynx

There are five intrinsic muscles of the larynx, which function to adduct, abduct, tense, and relax the vocal folds. One intrinsic muscle forms the body of the vocal folds. The intrinsic muscles are named according to their attachments.

Posterior cricoarytenoid (PCA): originates on the quadrate lamina of the cricoid cartilage. Fibers course upward and attach to the muscular process of each arytenoid. This pattern gives the PCA muscle a leaf shaped appearance. Contraction rotates the vocal processes of the arytenoid cartilages laterally and upwards, abducting the vocal folds and opening the glottis.

Lateral cricoarytenoid (LCA): fibers course from the cricoid cartilage to the muscular process of each arytenoid cartilage. When the muscle contracts it swings the vocal processes medially and downward to adduct the vocal folds and close the membranous glottis.

Interarytenoid (IA): only unpaired muscle of the larynx. It is composed of two bundles of muscle fibers. Each bundle runs in different directions across and between the posterior surfaces of the arytenoid cartilages. Contraction pulls the arytenoid cartilages medially toward each other, adducting the vocal folds to close the cartilaginous glottis.

>   **Transverse Interarytenoid:** attaches at the side and back of each arytenoid and courses across the backs of the arytenoids in a broad horizontal sheet.

>   **Oblique Interarytenoid:** originates at the base of each arytenoid and attaches at the apex of the opposite arytenoid, resulting in a crossing pattern of the fibers. Some of the oblique IA fibers continue laterally around the apex of the arytenoid and insert into the lateral margins of the epiglottis. These fibers form the aryepiglottic muscle. When the aryepiglottic muscle contracts the epiglottis is pulled downward and backward to cover the entrance to the larynx.

Cricothyroid (CT): consists of two muscle bundles, the pars recta and the pars oblique. Both bundles originate on the sides of the cricoid arch and attach to the inferior surface of the thyroid cartilage. The fibers of the pars recta run in a relatively vertical direction. The oblique fibers run at a more oblique angle. Contraction tilts the thyroid cartilage downward toward the cricoid cartilage or tilts the cricoid cartilage upward toward the thyroid cartilage. Either motion results in an increased distance between the thyroid and arytenoid cartilages. Because the vocal folds are attached anteriorly and posteriorly to these cartilages, they are stretched and tensed. This causes an increase in their rate of vibration which is perceived as a higher pitch.

Thyroarytenoid (TA): consists of two sections. The more medial fibers extend from the anterior commissure to the vocal processes of the arytenoid cartilages. These fibers are called the thyrovocalis muscle. The thyrovocalis fibers make fine tension adjustments along the vocal fold edge. The more lateral fibers extend from the anterior commissure to the muscular processes of the arytenoids and are called the thyromuscularis. The muscularis portion works to rapidly shorten the vocal folds. The TA muscle forms the body of the vocal folds and is thereby acted upon indirectly by the functioning of the other intrinsic muscles.

Refer to the narrative to locate and color the numbered structures

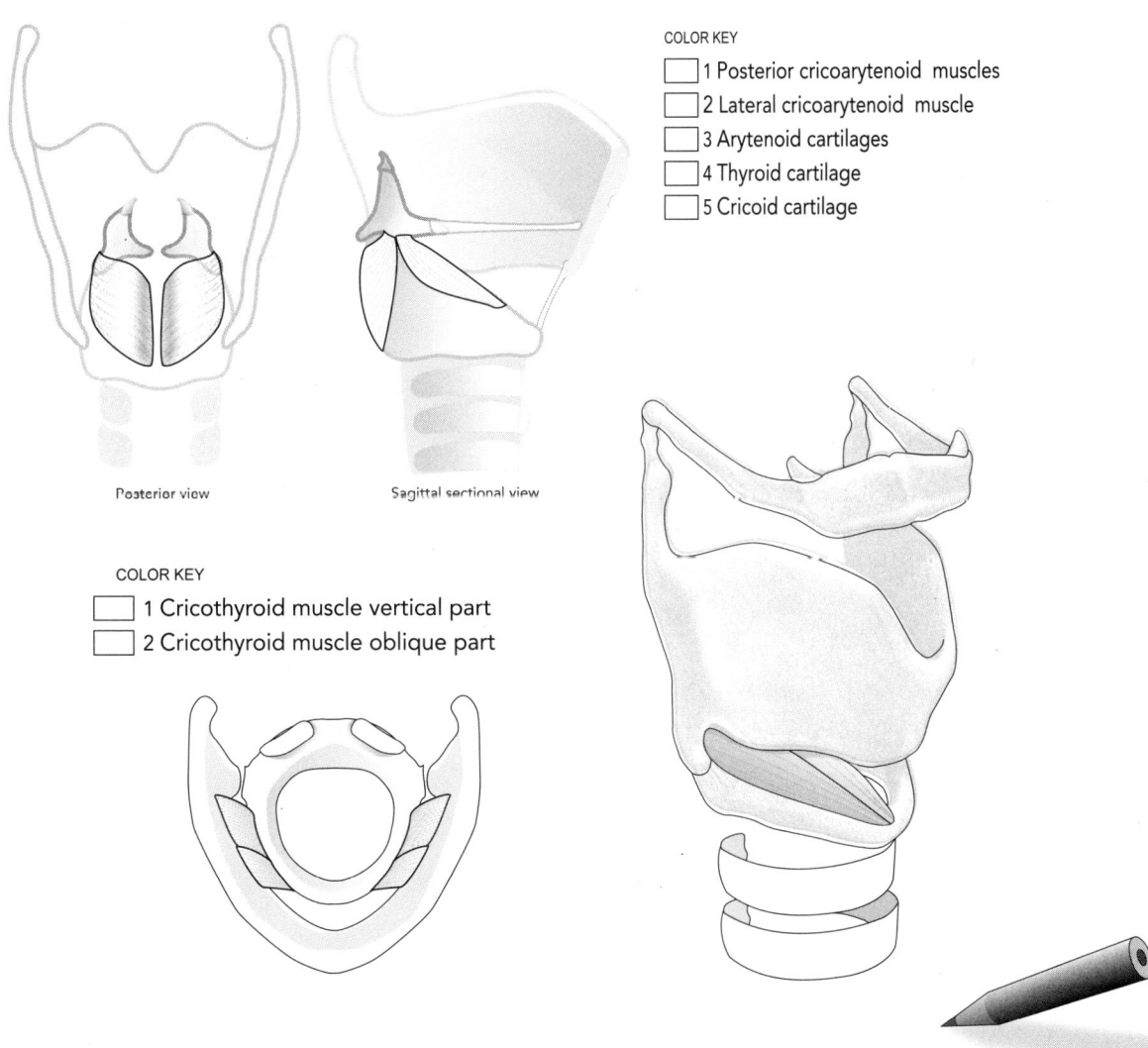

COLOR KEY
☐ 1 Posterior cricoarytenoid muscles
☐ 2 Lateral cricoarytenoid muscle
☐ 3 Arytenoid cartilages
☐ 4 Thyroid cartilage
☐ 5 Cricoid cartilage

Posterior view   Sagittal sectional view

COLOR KEY
☐ 1 Cricothyroid muscle vertical part
☐ 2 Cricothyroid muscle oblique part

Superior view of intrinsic laryngeal cartilages and muscles

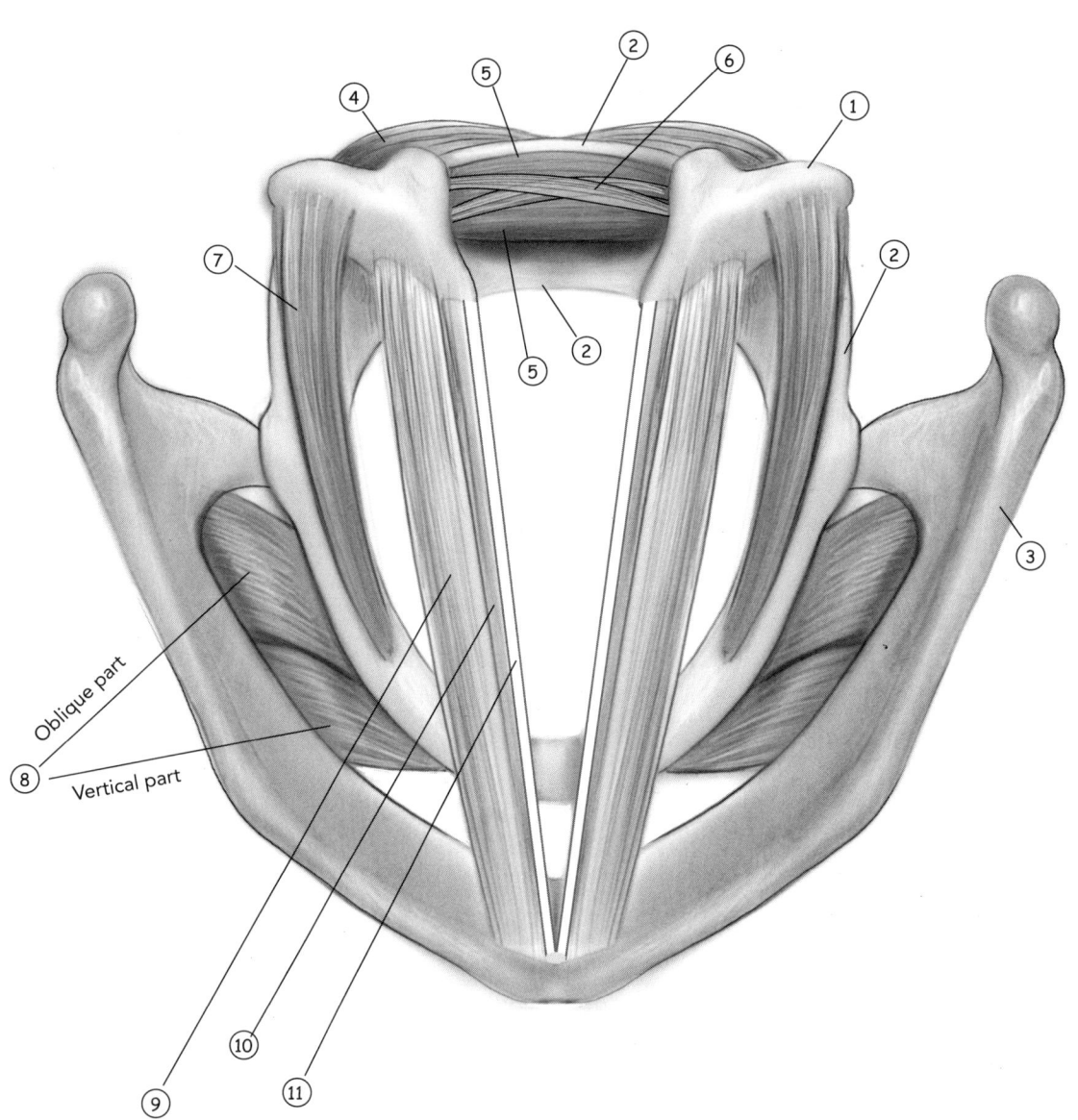

Oblique part

Vertical part

COLOR KEY

☐ 1 Arytenoid cartilage
☐ 2 Cricoid cartilage
☐ 3 Thyroid cartilage
☐ 4 Posterior cricoarytenoid m
☐ 5 Transverse arytenoid m
☐ 6 Oblique arytenoid m
☐ 7 Lateral cricoarytenoid m

8 Cricothyroid m
☐ A Oblique part
☐ B Vertical part

☐ 9 Thyroarytenoid m
☐ 10 Vocalis m
☐ 11 Vocal ligament

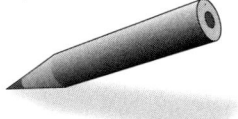

Posterior view of laryngeal muscles

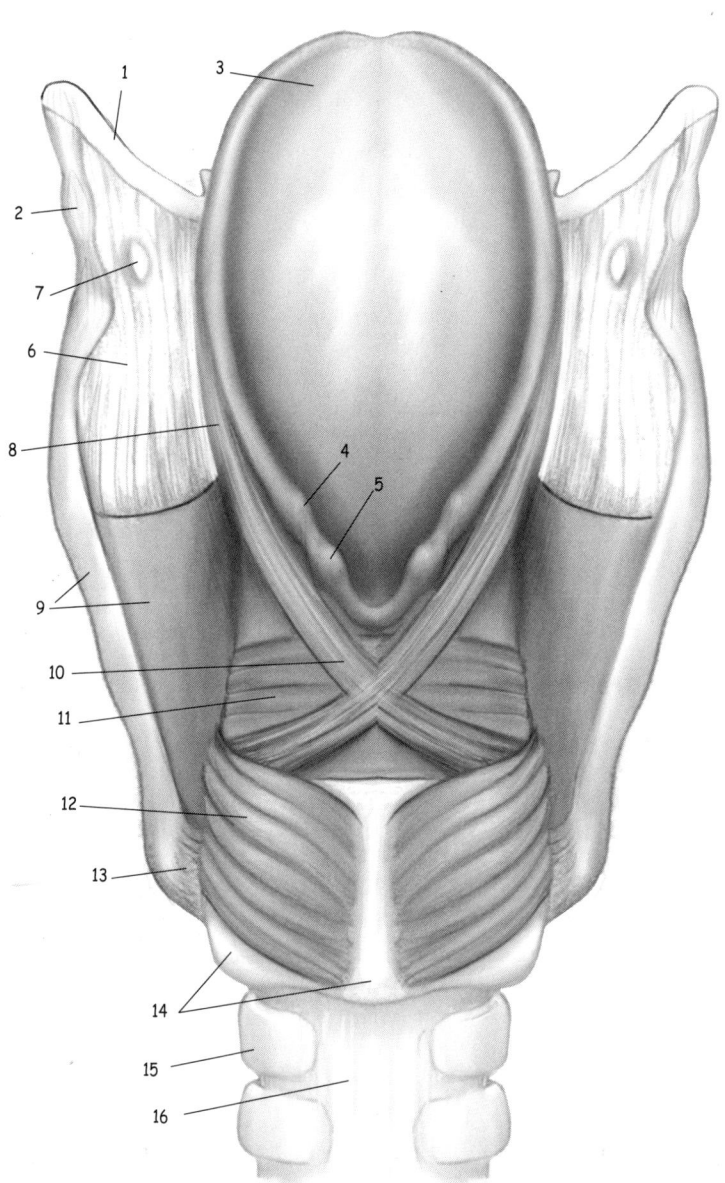

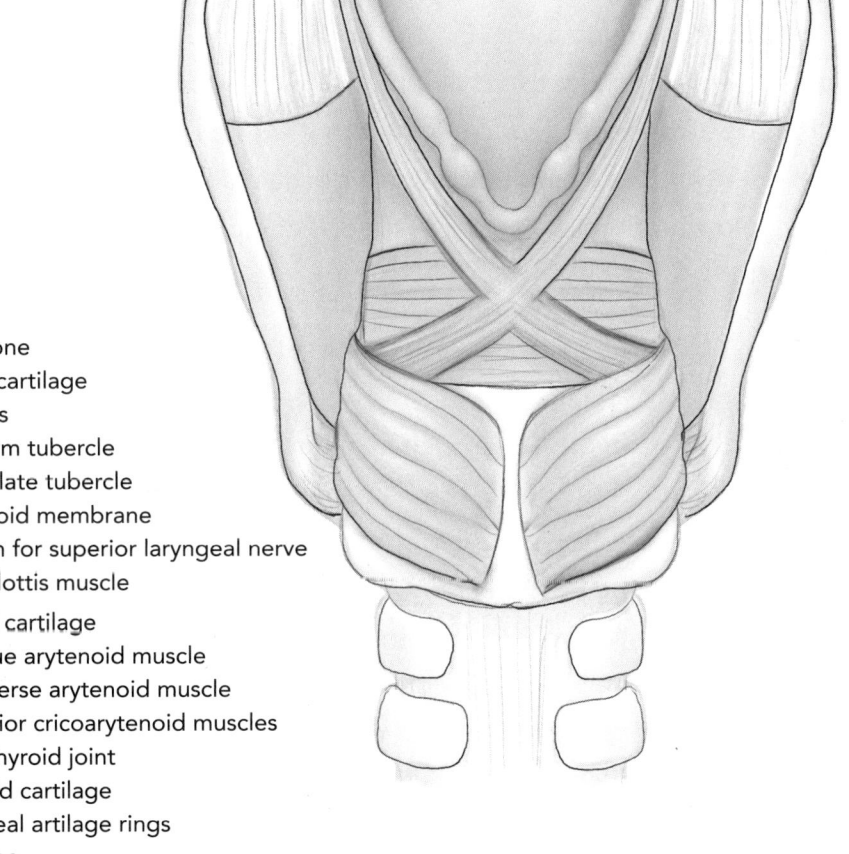

COLOR KEY

- 1 Hyoid bone
- 2 Triticeal cartilage
- 3 Epiglottis
- 4 Cuneiform tubercle
- 5 Corniculate tubercle
- 6 Thyrohyoid membrane
- 7 Foramen for superior laryngeal nerve
- 8 Aryepiglottis muscle
- 9 Thyroid cartilage
- 10 Oblique arytenoid muscle
- 11 Transverse arytenoid muscle
- 12 Posterior cricoarytenoid muscles
- 13 Cricothyroid joint
- 14 Cricoid cartilage
- 15 Tracheal artilage rings
- 16 Trachea

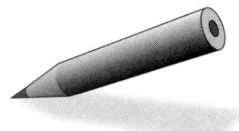

MYOELASTIC-AERODYNAMIC THEORY

The myoelastic-aerodynamic theory describes one cycle of vocal fold vibration. This theory proposes that vocal fold vibration occurs as an interaction of muscle forces, elastic recoil forces, and aerodynamic forces. The cycle of vocal fold vibration begins as the lateral cricoarytenoid and interarytenoid muscles adduct the vocal folds, a process called medial compression. Voice is produced on the exhalation of air, so when the vocal folds initially adduct, air is still flowing through the bronchi and trachea. This air is prevented from passing through the glottis by the adducted vocal folds. The air pressure underneath the vocal folds (subglottal pressure) increases, until it overcomes the medial compression. The positive subglottal pressure forces the glottis open, and a puff of air travels through the glottis and into the vocal tract. Once separated, the vocal folds close very quickly again due to the forces of elasticity and negative pressure. Elastic recoil of the vocal folds begins to return them to the midline, creating a negative pressure within the glottis. The negative pressure traveling through the glottis exerts a suction effect that draws the vocal folds together. The cycle then repeats itself. It is the interplay between positive and negative pressures that maintains the vocal fold vibration for as long as medial compression continues to be exerted.

Mucosal wave

Vocal fold vibration is highly complex, due to the layered structure and different biomechanical characteristics of the cover, vocal ligament, and body. The vocal folds open and close in a rippling wave-like fashion called the mucosal wave. This occurs because of changes in pressure between the bottom and top edges of the vocal folds. As subglottal pressure (positive pressure) builds up underneath the closed glottis, the vocal folds begin to separate at their bottom edges. The positive pressure continues to separate the folds in an upward direction. However, by the time the superior portion of the glottis is open, the inferior margins of the vocal folds are already closing due to the negative pressure generated within the glottis. The glottal closing also proceeds from inferior to superior margins of the vocal folds. The slight time lag between the closing and opening of the lower and upper edges of the vocal folds gives rise to a vertical phase difference. The vocal folds also open and close the glottis horizontally from anterior to posterior and posterior to anterior.

In this case, in a motion rather like that of a zipper, the glottis opens first from the posterior portion at the vocal processes, and the opening travels toward the anterior commissure. Glottal closing occurs in the opposite direction, from anterior to posterior. This creates a slight time lag called the longitudinal phase difference. It is this complex vibration with the resulting mucosal wave that generates the rich, resonant sound of the human voice. Anything that interferes with the mucosal wave can result in dysphonia.

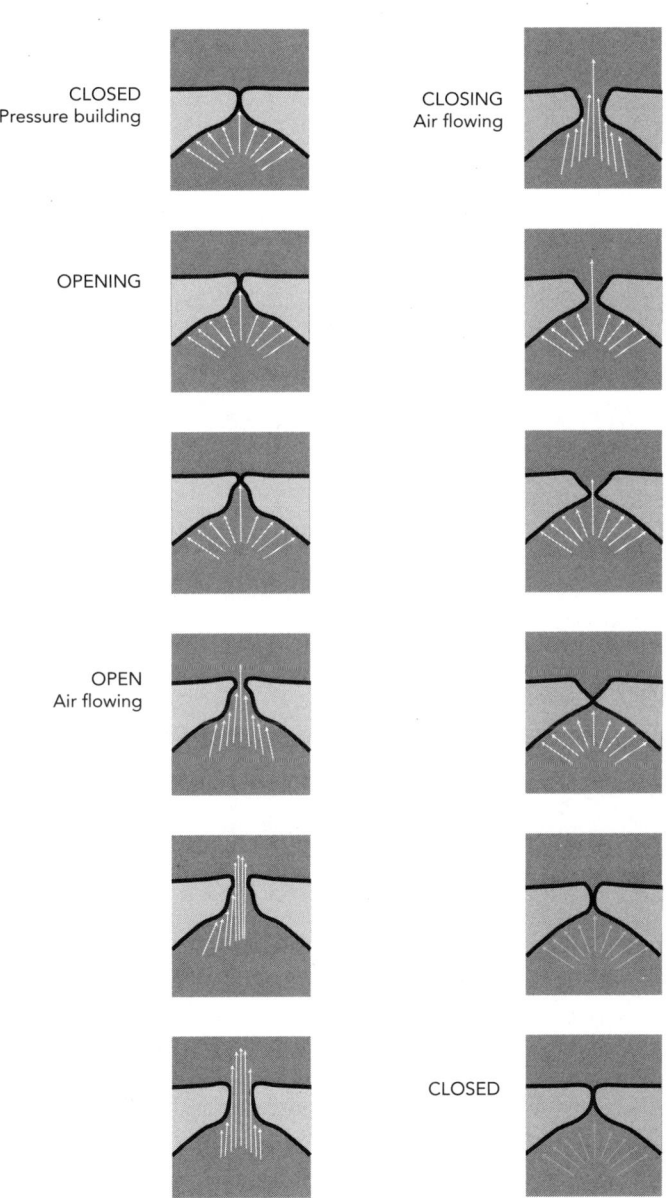

CLOSED
Pressure building

CLOSING
Air flowing

OPENING

OPEN
Air flowing

CLOSED

TEST YOURSELF: THE PHONATORY SYSTEM

MULTIPLE CHOICE LARYNGEAL FRAMEWORK

1 _____   Which of the following statements If any) is NOT true of the hyoid bone?

    a. It consists of a body, major horns, and minor horns

    b. The larynx is suspended from it by means of the hyothyroid membrane

    c. It is formed by two sheets of cartilage

    d. All the above statements are true

2 _____   Which of the following cartilages contains superior and inferior horns?

    a. Cricoid

    b. Arytenoid

    c. Epiglottis

    d. None of the above

3 _____   The epiglottis

    a. Is located on the apex of each arytenoid cartilage

    b. Is a leaf shaped cartilage attached to the thyroid cartilage and hyoid bone

    c. Is a complete ring of cartilage inferior to the thyroid cartilage

    d. Is embedded within the aryepiglottic folds

4 _____ The thyroid cartilage

    a. Formed by two sheets of cartilage which are fused in the front and open in the back

    b. Contains the thyroid notch and anterior commissure

    c. Contains an oblique line to which muscles attach

    d. All the above

5 _____   The true vocal folds attach to the

    a. Anterior commissure

    b. Posterior commissure

    c. Cricoid cartilage

    d. Oblique line

6 _____   Which cartilage is located immediately superior to the trachea?

    a. Cricoid

    b. Thyroid

    c. Corniculate

    d. Epiglottis

7 _____   Which of the following statements is NOT true of the arytenoid cartilages?

    a. They are located on the inferior surface of the cricoid cartilage

    b. The vocal and muscular processes extend from the base of the arytenoid cartilages

    c. They form a joint with the cricoid cartilage

    d. Several muscles attach to the arytenoids, allowing the vocal folds to

       adduct and abduct

8 ____   The arch and quadrate lamina form part of which cartilage?
   a. Thyroid
   b. Arytenoid
   c. Cricoid
   d. Epiglottis

9 ____   Which cartilages are located on the apex of each arytenoid cartilage?
   a. Cuneiform
   b. Corniculate
   c. Epiglottis
   d. None of the above

10 ____   The cricoarytenoid joints are
   a. Synovial
   b. Capable of a wide range of movements
   c. Involved in vocal fold adduction and abduction
   d. All the above

11 ____   The cricothyroid joints
   a. Regulate pitch by increasing the distance between the thyroid and epiglottis
   b. Regulate pitch by changing the distance between the thyroid and arytenoid cartilages
   c. Regulate pitch by increasing the distance between the cricoid and epiglottis
   d. None of the above

12 ____   The petiole is part of which cartilage?
   a. Cuneiform
   b. Corniculate
   c. Epiglottis
   d. None of the above

TRUE OR FALSE LARYNGEAL FRAMEWORK

1 ____   The most important role of the larynx is voice production.

2 ____   The larynx is continuous with both the pharynx and the nasal cavities.

3 ____   The hyoid bone is formed by two sheets of hyaline cartilage.

4 ____   The thyroid cartilage is connected to the hyoid bone by means of the thyrohyoid ligament.

5 ____   The inferior horns of the thyroid cartilage project downward and form a joint
             with the cricoid cartilage.

6 ____   The cricoid cartilage is broad in the front and narrow in the back.

7 ____   The cricothyroid membrane attaches the cricoid cartilage to the trachea.

8 ____   The space between the base of the tongue and the epiglottis forms the vallecula.

9 ____   The petiole is located at the tip of the arytenoid cartilage.

10 ____ The arytenoid cartilages each have a vocal process and a muscular process.

11 ____ The vocal folds attach anteriorly to the arytenoid cartilages and posteriorly

to the thyroid cartilage.

12 ____ The cuneiform cartilages are embedded within the aryepiglottic folds.

13 ____ The joint that is involved in pitch regulation is the cricoarytenoid.

14 ____ The cricothyroid joint allows the distance between the

arytenoid and thyroid cartilages to be increased and decreased.

MATCHING LARYNGEAL FRAMEWORK

	Epiglottis	1 Form the sides of the hyoid bone
	Cricoarytenoid joint	2 Embedded within the aryepiglottic folds
	Quadrate lamina	3 Point at which the vocal folds attach anteriorly
	Cuneiform cartilages	4 Leaf shaped attached to the hyoid bone and thyroid cartilage
	Oblique line	5 Extensions of thyroid cartilage attached to the hyoid bone
	Vocal process	6 Located on the apex of each arytenoid cartilage
	Cricothyroid joint	7 Joint involved in vocal fold adduction and abduction
	Superior horns	8 On thyroid lamina where extrinsic muscles attach
	Major horns	9 Projects posterolaterally from base of the arytenoid cartilage
	Muscular process	10 Joint involved in pitch regulation
	Anterior commissure	11 Posterior portion of the cricoid cartilage
	Corniculate cartilages	12 Projects anteriorly from the base of each arytenoid cartilage

FILL IN THE BLANK LARYNGEAL FRAMEWORK

1.   The _____ cartilage is formed by two sheets which are

fused in the front and open in the back.

2.   The larynx is suspended from the _____.

3.   The major and minor horns are part of the _____.

4.   The superior and inferior horns are part of the _____.

5.   The true vocal folds attach to the thyroid cartilage at the _____.

6   The posterior portion of the cricoid cartilage is called the _____.

7   The _____ membrane attaches the cricoid cartilage to the

        thyroid cartilage.

8   The _____ is the narrowest part of the epiglottis.

9   The space between the base of the tongue and the epiglottis forms the _____.

10   The _____ of the arytenoids projects anteriorly and

        attaches to the vocal folds .

11   Several muscles attach to the _____ of the thyroid cartilage.

12   The _____ cartilages are located on the apex of each arytenoid cartilage.

13   The _____ cartilages are embedded within the aryepiglottic folds.

14   Vocal fold abduction and adduction are permitted by the _____ joints.

15   The _____ joints allow the vocal folds to be elongated and shortened.

MULTIPLE CHOICE   FOLDS AND MUSCLES

1 ____   Which of the following statements best characterizes the aryepiglottic folds?
        a. Attach anteriorly at the anterior commissure of the thyroid cartilage, and
            posteriorly to the vocal process of each arytenoid
        b. Located inferior to the false vocal folds
        c. Composed of five layers with differing biomechanical properties
        d. Form a roughly oval shaped sphincter superior to the false vocal folds

2 ____   Which of the following statements (if any) is NOT true of the false vocal folds?
        a. Located inferiorly to the true vocal folds
        b. Composed mainly of connective tissue with some muscle tissue
        c. Contain mucous glands and goblet cells
        d. All the above are true

3 ____   The true vocal folds
        a. Are composed of five layers
        b. Have differing biomechanical properties in each layer
        c. Attach anteriorly at the anterior commissure of the thyroid cartilage, and
            posteriorly to the vocal process of each arytenoid
        d. All the above

4 _____   The outermost layer of the vocal folds is the
    a. Superficial layer of the lamina propria
    b. Epithelium
    c. Muscle
    d. None of the above

5 _____   The type of epithelium covering the true vocal folds is
    a. Keratinizing simple squamous
    b. Non-keratinizing simple squamous
    c. Keratinizing stratified squamous
    d. Non-keratinizing stratified squamous

6 _____   The layer of the lamina propria that is composed mostly of collagen fibers is the
    a. Superficial
    b. Intermediate
    c. Deep
    d. Muscle

7 _____   The layer of the lamina propria that is composed mostly of loosely organized elastin fibers is the
    a. Superficial
    b. Intermediate
    c. Deep
    d. Muscle

8 _____   Which of the following statements (if any) is NOT true of the cover-body model?
    a. Describes the vibratory characteristics of the vocal folds in terms of stiffness
    b. From most to least superficial, goes from most to least stiff
    c. Consists of the cover, vocal ligament, and body
    d. All the above are true

9 _____   For phonation, the glottis is
    a. Open
    b. Closed
    c. Partially open
    d. None of the above

10 _____   The extrinsic muscles of the larynx
    a. Control fine movements of the vocal fold edge
    b. Raise and lower the larynx in the neck
    c. Are composed of medial and lateral bundles
    d. None of the above

11 _____ The infrahyoid muscles
        a. Depress the hyoid bone
        b. Raise the hyoid bone
        c. Lower the pitch of the voice
        d. Raise the pitch of the voice

12 _____ The glottis is closed by which muscle?
        a. Cricothyroid
        b. Thyroarytenoid
        c. Lateral cricoarytenoid
        d. Posterior cricoarytenoid

13 _____ The glottis is opened by which muscle?
        a. Cricothyroid
        b. Thyroarytenoid
        c. Lateral cricoarytenoid
        d. Posterior cricoarytenoid

14 _____ The Interarytenoid muscle
        a. Consists of the pars recta and pars oblique
        b. Stretches and tenses the vocal folds
        c. Opens the vocal folds
        d. None of the above

15 _____ Which muscle contains transverse and oblique bundles?
        a. Cricothyroid
        b. Interarytenoid
        c. Thyroarytenoid
        d. Lateral cricoarytenoid

16 _____ Which muscle is made up of lateral and medial bundles?
        a. Cricothyroid
        b. Interarytenoid
        c. Thyroarytenoid
        d. Lateral cricoarytenoid

17 _____ Which muscle stretches and tenses the vocal folds?
        a. Cricothyroid
        b. Interarytenoid
        c. Thyroarytenoid
        d. Lateral cricoarytenoid

18 ____   Which of the following statements (if any) is NOT true of the myoelastic

aerodynamic theory?

a. The vocal folds are closed by medial compression

b. Positive subglottal pressure forces the vocal folds apart

c. Negative pressure causes the vocal folds to close

d. All the above are true

19 ____   Which of the following statements best describes the mucosal wave?

a. Bottom to top opening and closing of the vocal folds

b. The four phases of vocal fold movement: opening, open, closing, and closed

c. Top to bottom opening and closing of the vocal folds

d. Vocal folds recoil to midline due to their natural elasticity

TRUE/FALSE   FOLDS AND MUSCLES

1 ____   The aryepiglottic folds are located superior to the false vocal folds.

2 ____   The false vocal folds contain mucous glands and goblet cells that help to

lubricate the true vocal folds.

3 ____   The true vocal folds are composed primarily of dense connective tissue.

4 ____   The outermost surface of the true vocal folds is composed of non-keratinizing

stratified squamous cell epithelium.

5 ____   Both the superficial and intermediate layers of the lamina propria are composed

of densely organized elastin fibers.

6 ____   The thyroarytenoid muscle is the least compliant layer of the true vocal folds.

7 ____   The cover comprises the epithelium and superficial layers and is the most compliant.

8 ____   The vocal ligament is formed by the superficial and intermediate layers of the lamina propria.

9 ____   The glottis is divided into the membranous and cartilaginous portions of equal length.

10 ____   Phonation occurs when the glottis is partly open.

11 ____   The extrinsic muscles raise and lower the larynx within the neck.

12 ____   The digastric is a suprahyoid muscle that elevates the hyoid bone.

13 ____   The posterior cricoarytenoid and the interarytenoids are both vocal fold adductors.

14 ____   The interarytenoids are made up of transverse and oblique fibers.

15 ____   The aryepiglottic muscle is formed by the continuation of cricoarytenoid fibers.

16 ____   Contraction of the posterior cricoarytenoid muscle rotates the vocal processes.

of the arytenoid cartilages laterally and upwards, opening the glottis.

17 ____   The cricothyroid muscle is formed by the pars recta and the pars oblique.

18 ____   The cricothyroid muscle acts to open and close the glottis.

19 ____   The muscularis portion of the thyroarytenoid works to rapidly shorten the

vocal folds and the vocalis fibers make fine tension adjustments along the vocal fold edge.

20 ____The myoelastic aerodynamic theory combines muscular, elastic, and aerodynamic forces.

MATCHING   FOLDS AND MUSCLES

	Omohyoid	1 Base of one arytenoid cartilage to apex of the opposite arytenoid cartilage
	Cricothyroid	2 Side of cricoid to muscular process of arytenoid
	Sternothyroid	3 Anterior commissure to vocal processes
	Sternohyoid	4 Clavicle and sternum to body of hyoid
	Lateral cricoarytenoid	5 Posterior portion of cricoid cartilage to muscular processes of arytenoid cartilages
	Thyrohyoid	6 Body of mandible to hyoid bone
	Digastric	7 First costal cartilage and sternum to oblique line of thyroid lamina
	Oblique interarytenoid	8 Scapula to inferior border of hyoid
	Posterior cricoarytenoid	9 Oblique line of thyroid lamina to major horn of hyoid
	Mylohyoid	10 Lateral portion of cricoid cartilage to inferior portion of thyroid cartilage
	Transverse interarytenoid	11 Consists of anterior and posterior bellies
	Stylohyoid	12 One side of an arytenoid cartilage to the other side of the other arytenoid cartilage
	Thyroarytenoid	13 Styloid process of temporal bone to body of hyoid bone

FILL IN THE BLANK   FOLDS AND MUSCLES

1.   The cuneiform cartilages are located within the _____ '_____.

2.   The _____ _____ are composed of connective tissue and some muscle tissue and

contain numerous mucous glands and goblet cells.

3.   The _____ attach anteriorly at the anterior commissure of the thyroid

cartilage and posteriorly to the vocal process of each arytenoid.

4.   The outermost surface of the true vocal folds is composed of _____.

5.   The _____ layer of the lamina propria consists mostly of collagen fibers.

6   The _____ layer of the lamina propria consists mostly of loosely organized elastin fibers.

7   The intermediate layer of the lamina propria consists mainly of _____.

8   The least flexible layer in the cover-body model is the _____.

9   The _____ is the most flexible layer of the cover-body model.

10   The vocal ligament is formed by the _____

   and _____ layers of the lamina propria.

11.   The cover is formed by the _____ and _____.

12   Normal quiet breathing is associated with a _____ vocal fold position.

13   The _____ glottis comprises the anterior three fifths, and the

   _____ glottis comprises the posterior two fifths.

14   The _____ attach at the lateral posterior margins of each arytenoid

   and course across the backs of the arytenoids in a sheet of muscle .

15   The muscle that abducts the vocal folds is the _____.

16   The _____ muscle regulates pitch.

17   The muscle that pulls the epiglottis downward and backward to cover the entrance to

   the larynx is the _____.

18   The _____ muscle closes the membranous glottis.

19   The cartilaginous glottis is closed by the _____ muscle.

20   The _____ fibers of the thyroarytenoid muscle make fine tension

   adjustments along the vocal fold edge .

21   Medial compression is exerted by the _____

   and _____ muscles.

22   During a cycle of vibration, the vocal folds are closed by _____

   and _____.

23   The vibratory motion of the vocal folds is known as the _____.

24.   The _____ refers to the slight time lag between the

   approximation and separation of the lower and upper edges of the vocal folds.

Fill in the names of these structures of the larynx

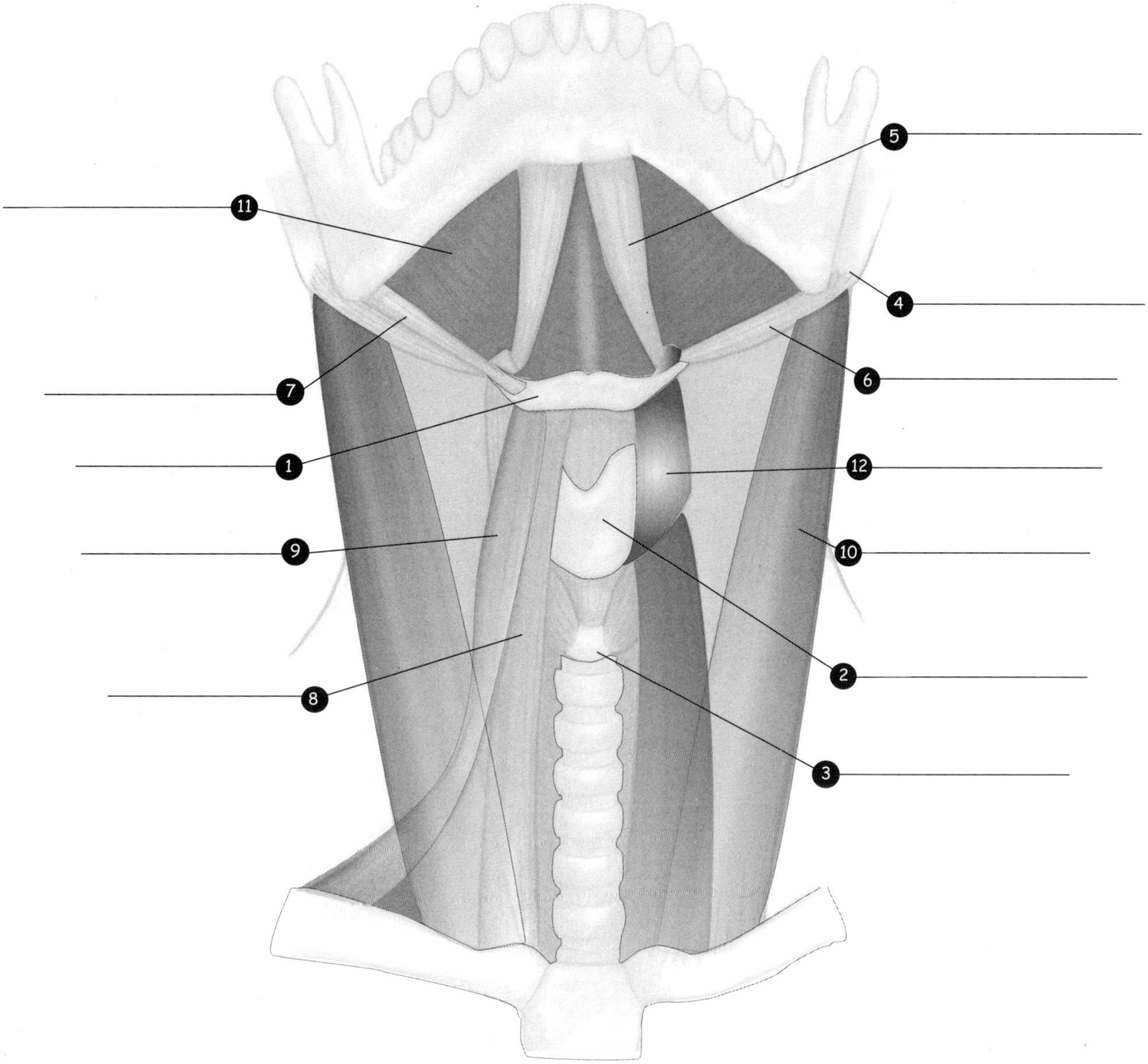

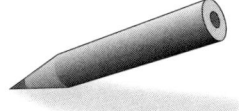

1

2

4

3

5

6

8

7

11

12

9

10

14

15

13

s

Laryngeal Jumble
Identify theses structures
and fill in the names.
Some may appear more than once
and they are not shown to scale.

1_____

2_____

3_____

4_____

5_____

6_____

7_____

8_____

9_____

10_____

11_____

12_____

13_____

14_____

15_____

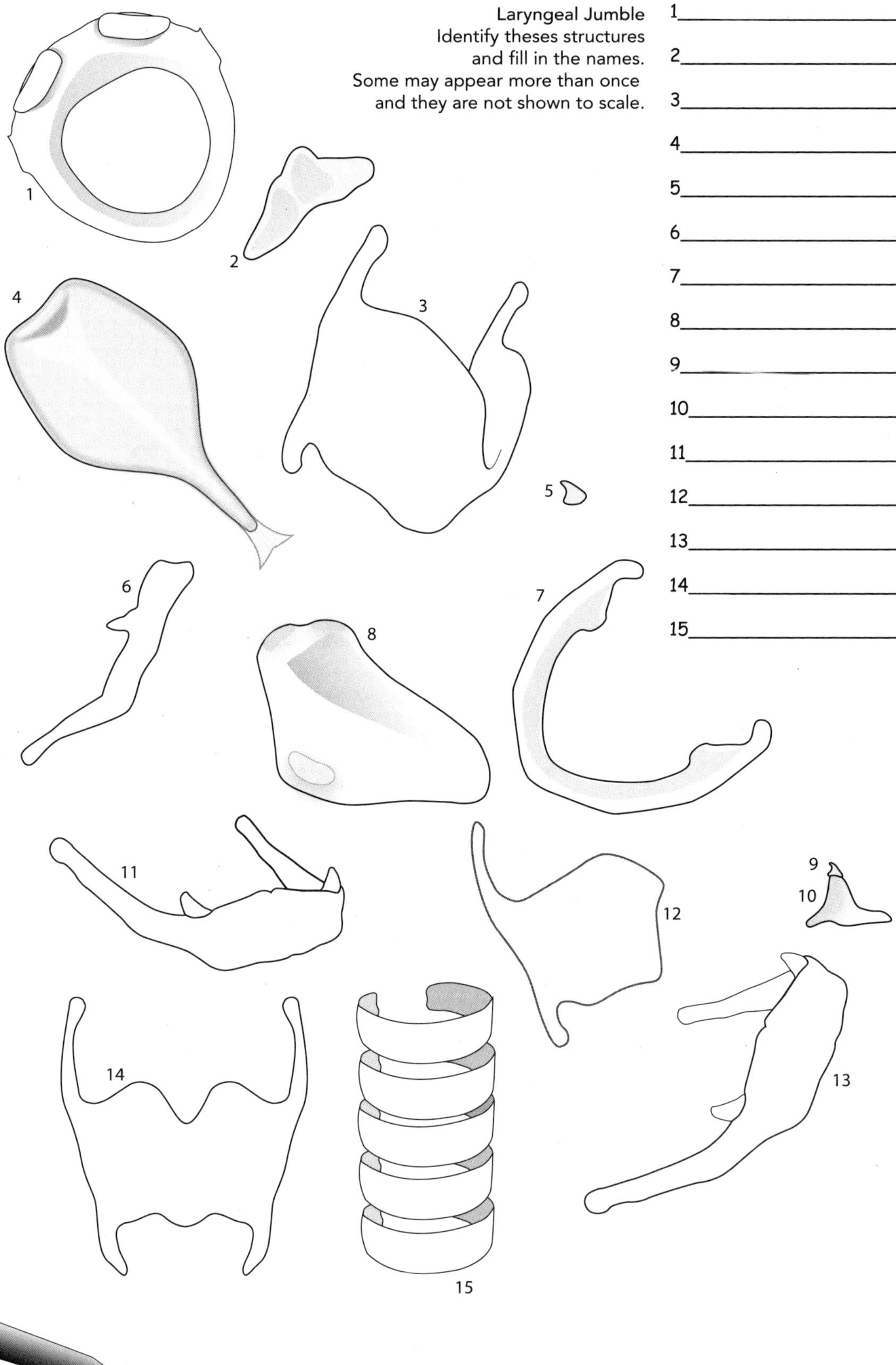

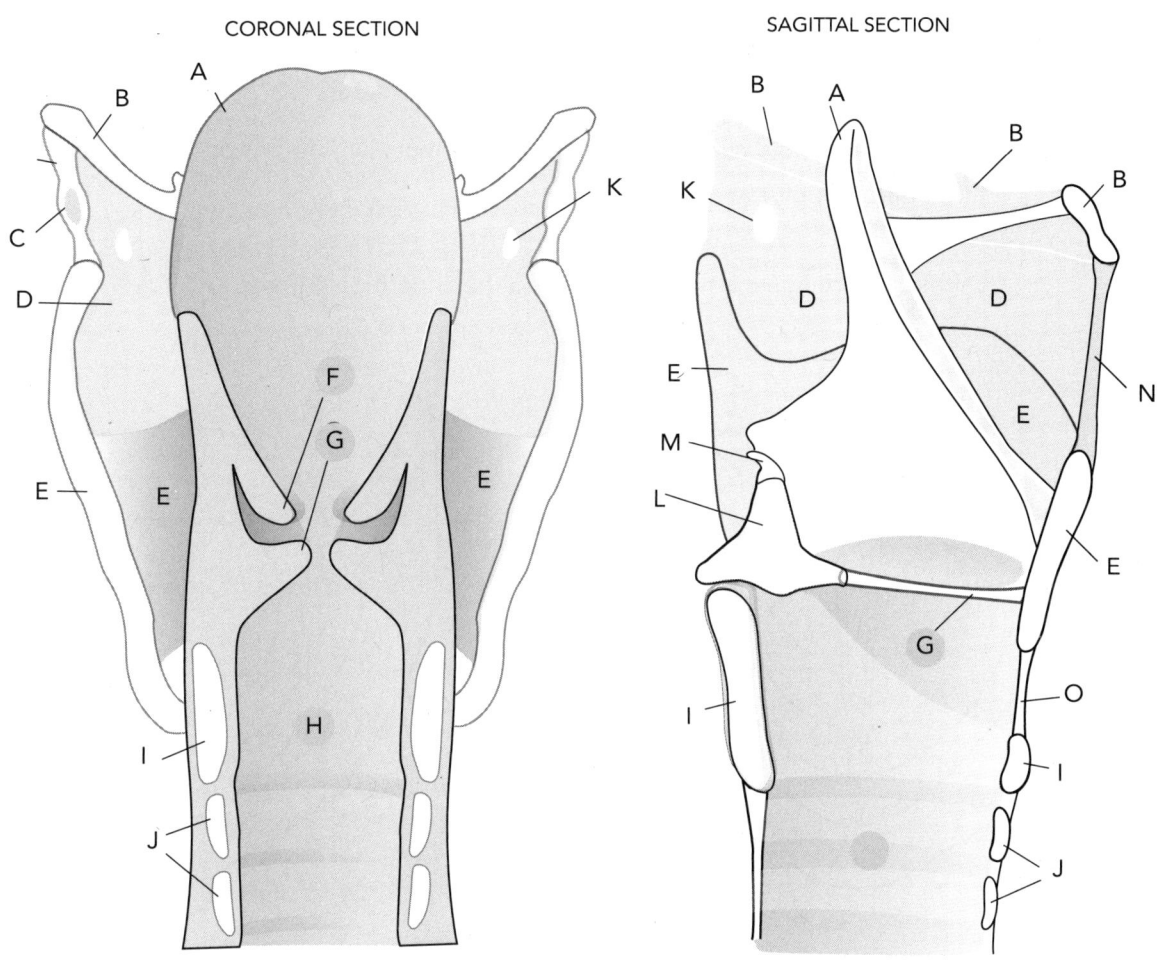

CORONAL SECTION

SAGITTAL SECTION

Fill in the names of the structures labeled in the two sectional views of the larynx

A_____

B_____

C_____

D_____

E_____

F_____

G_____

H_____

I_____

J_____

K_____

L_____

M_____

N_____

O_____

Based on the upper left drawing, complete the three other
superior views of the laryngeal cartilages by drawing in the arytenoid cartilages
and the vocal ligaments.

Show the arytenoid cartilages and vocal ligaments in different positions creating
three different glottal shapes.

Label the cartilages, articular facets and the cricothyroid joints.

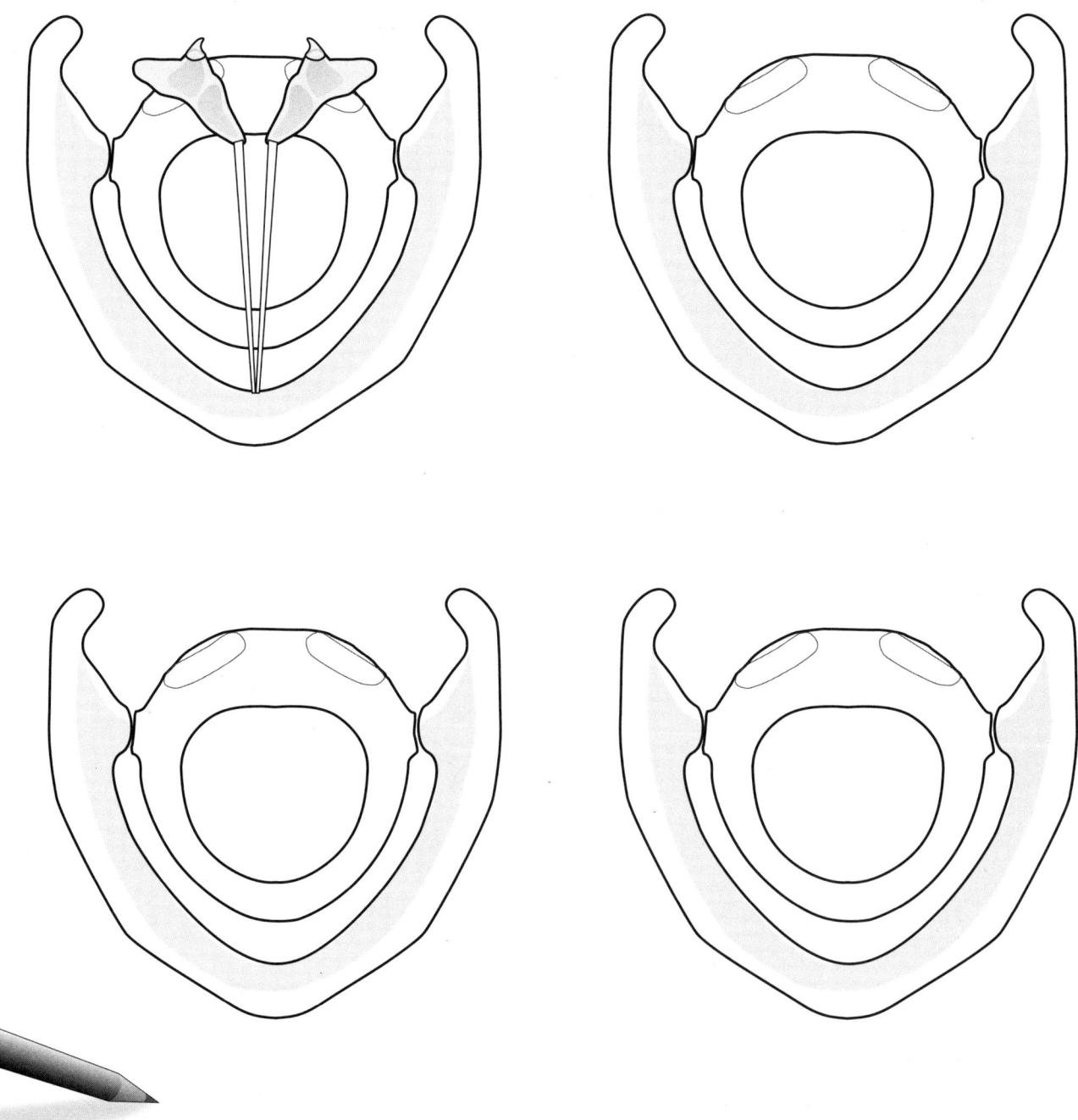

Across

4. Muscle that has transverse and oblique portions

5. During vibration the vocal folds are opened by ___ pressure

7. Runs from the mandible to the hyoid bone

9. Medial portion of the thyroarytenoid muscle

Muscles of the Larynx

Down

1. Consists of anterior and posterior bellies and elevates the hyoid bone

2. Runs from the sternum to the thyroid cartilage

3. These muscles lower the larynx

6. Muscle that closes the membranous glottis

8. Vocal fold opener

Cartilages and Membranes of the Larynx

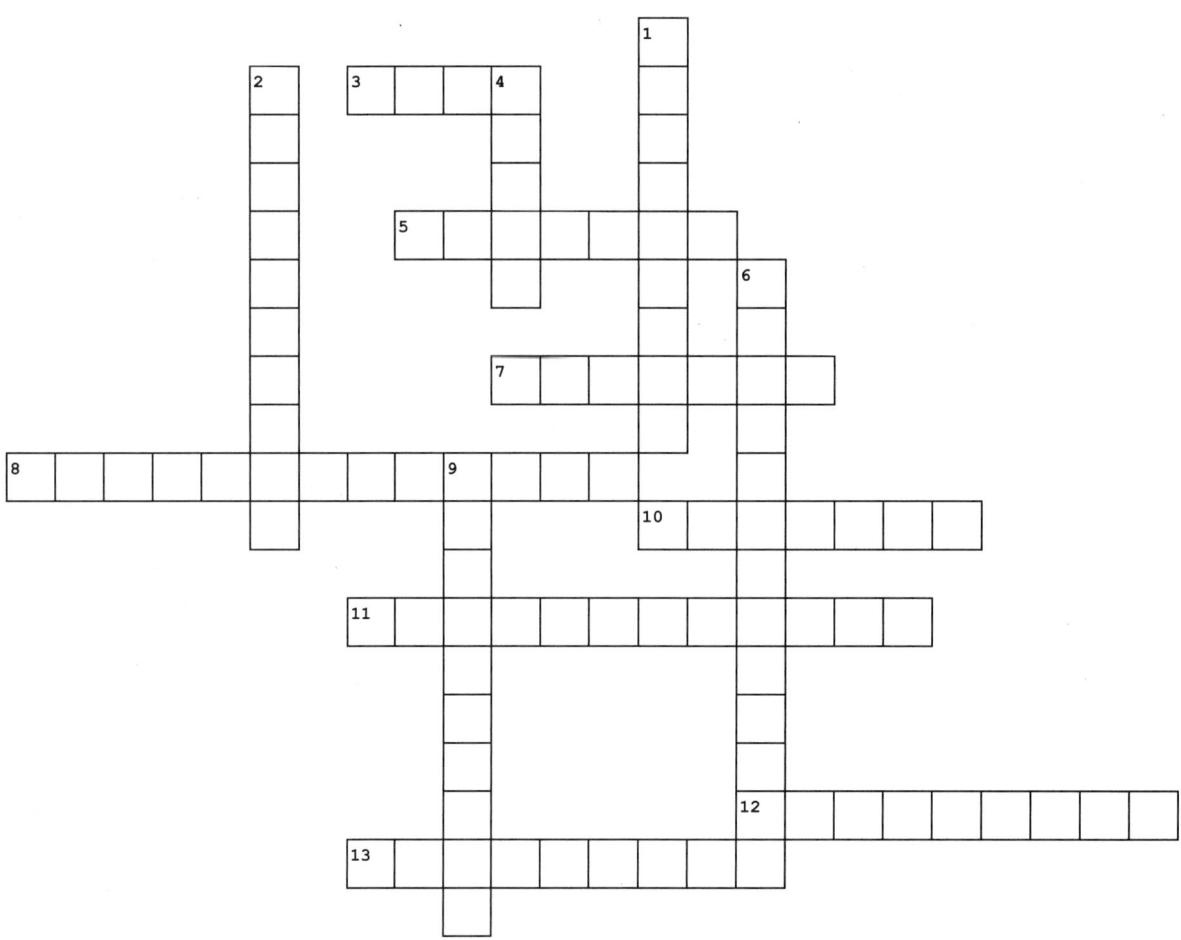

Across

3. Front portion of the cricoid cartilage
5. Most inferior of the laryngeal cartilages
7. Cartilage that forms the "Adam's Apple"
8. Folds: arytenoids to epiglottis
10. Narrowest portion of the epiglottis
11. These cartilages sit on top of the arytenoids
12. Contain vocal and muscular processes
13. Some people have these small cartilages within the thyrohyoid membrane

Down

1. Cartilage embedded in the aryepiglottic folds
2. Covers the larynx during swallowing
4. Has a body, major horns, and minor horns
6. Membrane that connects the cricoid cartilage and trachea
9. Membrane that connects the thyroid cartilage and hyoid bone

Joints and Folds
of the Larynx

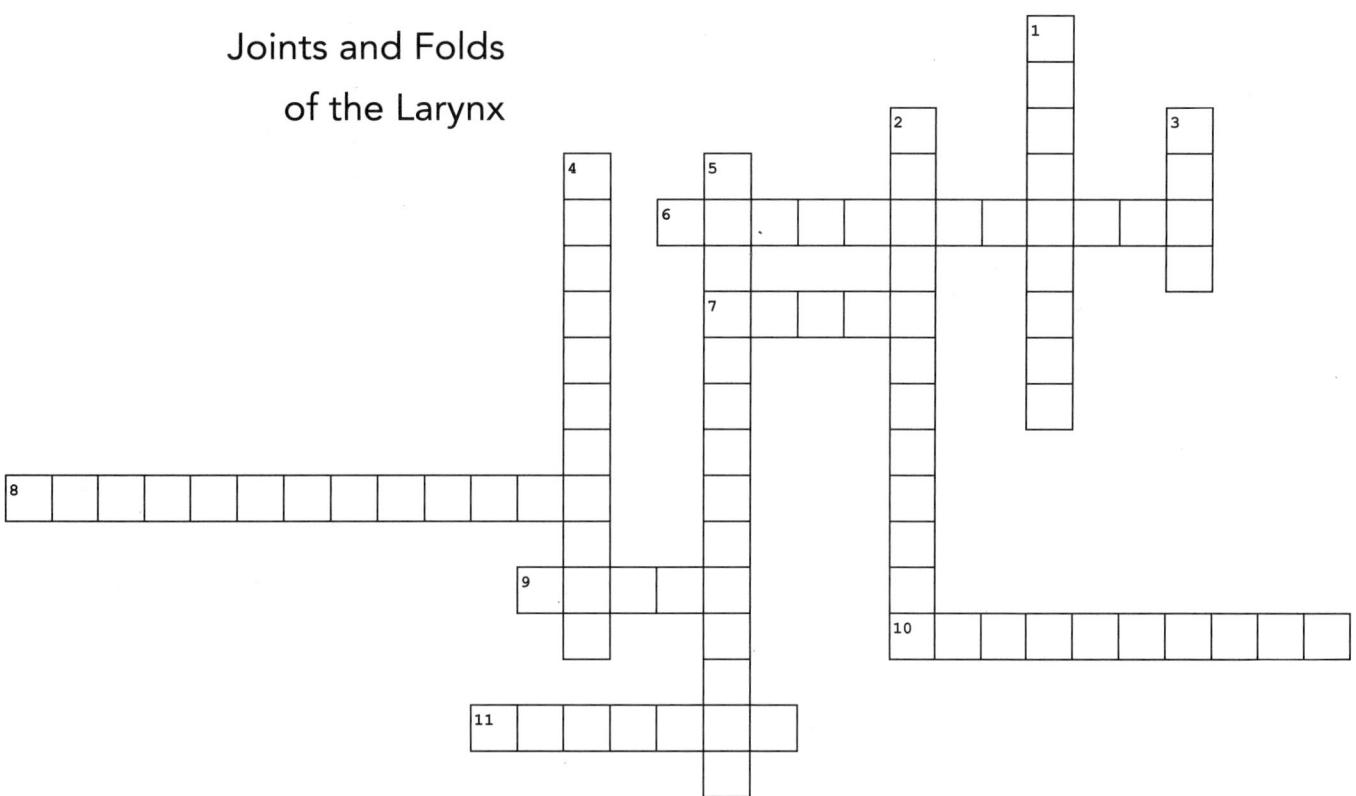

Across

6. This joint helps to regulate pitch changes
7. Comprising the epithelium and superficial layer of the lamina propria
8. Most superior folds in the larynx
9. These folds contain mucous glands
10. Outermost layer of the true vocal folds
11. Space between the vocal folds

Down

1. Space between the true and false vocal folds
2. Layer of the lamina propria composed of densely packed elastin fibers
3. Least compliant layer of the vocal folds
4. Layer of the lamina propria composed of loosely organized elastin fibers
5. The joint is involved in adducting and abducting the vocal folds

Section Four

The Articulatory System

Articulation is the process whereby the
structures of the vocal tract
such as the lips, tongue, mandible,
and velum, modify exhaled air
to shape specific speech sounds (phonemes).

The articulatory system includes the vocal tract and
the structures within and outside of the vocal tract.

The vocal tract is located within the craniofacial skeleton
and many of the muscles involved in articulation have
their attachments to the bones of the skull.

CRANIOFACIAL SKELETON

The craniofacial skeleton is the foundation for the soft tissues of the face and head. The cranium is formed by 8 bones that are held together by synarthrodial (immovable) sutures. The brain is enclosed within a large cavity called the cranial vault. 14 facial bones form the lower front of the skull and provide the framework for most of the face. Together the bones of the cranium and face form cavities that hold the eyes, the internal ear, and the vocal tract.

The 8 Cranial Bones

Frontal bone (1): forms the front portion of the skull above the eyes and includes the forehead, the roof of the nasal cavity, and the roofs of the orbits (bony sockets) of the eyes. Within the frontal bone are two frontal sinuses, one above each eye near the midline.

Parietal bones (2): form the sides and roof of the cranium.

Temporal bones (2): are located at the base and sides of the skull directly inferior to the temple. Each bone consists of five parts: tympanic part, petrous portion, mastoid process, styloid process, and squama temporalis. The petrous portion is the hardest piece of the bone and protects the inner ear.

Occipital bone (1): is situated at the back and lower part of the cranium. The bone is trapezoid in shape and curved on itself. The foramen magnum is a large hole at the base of the bone. This hole allows the spinal cord to pass through.
On either side of the foramen magnum are the occipital condyles, which are the points of articulation between the skull and the atlas vertebra at the top of the vertebral column.

Ethmoid bone (1): separates the nasal cavity from the brain. The bone makes up the roof of the nasal cavity, part of the walls of the nasal cavity, part of the bony orbits around the eyes, and part of the floor of the cranium. The ethmoid bone consists of four main parts. The perpendicular plate forms the septum of the nose. The crista galli is the upper part of the perpendicular plate. The labyrinths (lateral masses) form portions of the bony orbits of the eyes and the nasal cavity structures. The cribriform plate is a horizontal portion of the bone that makes up part of the floor of the cranium.

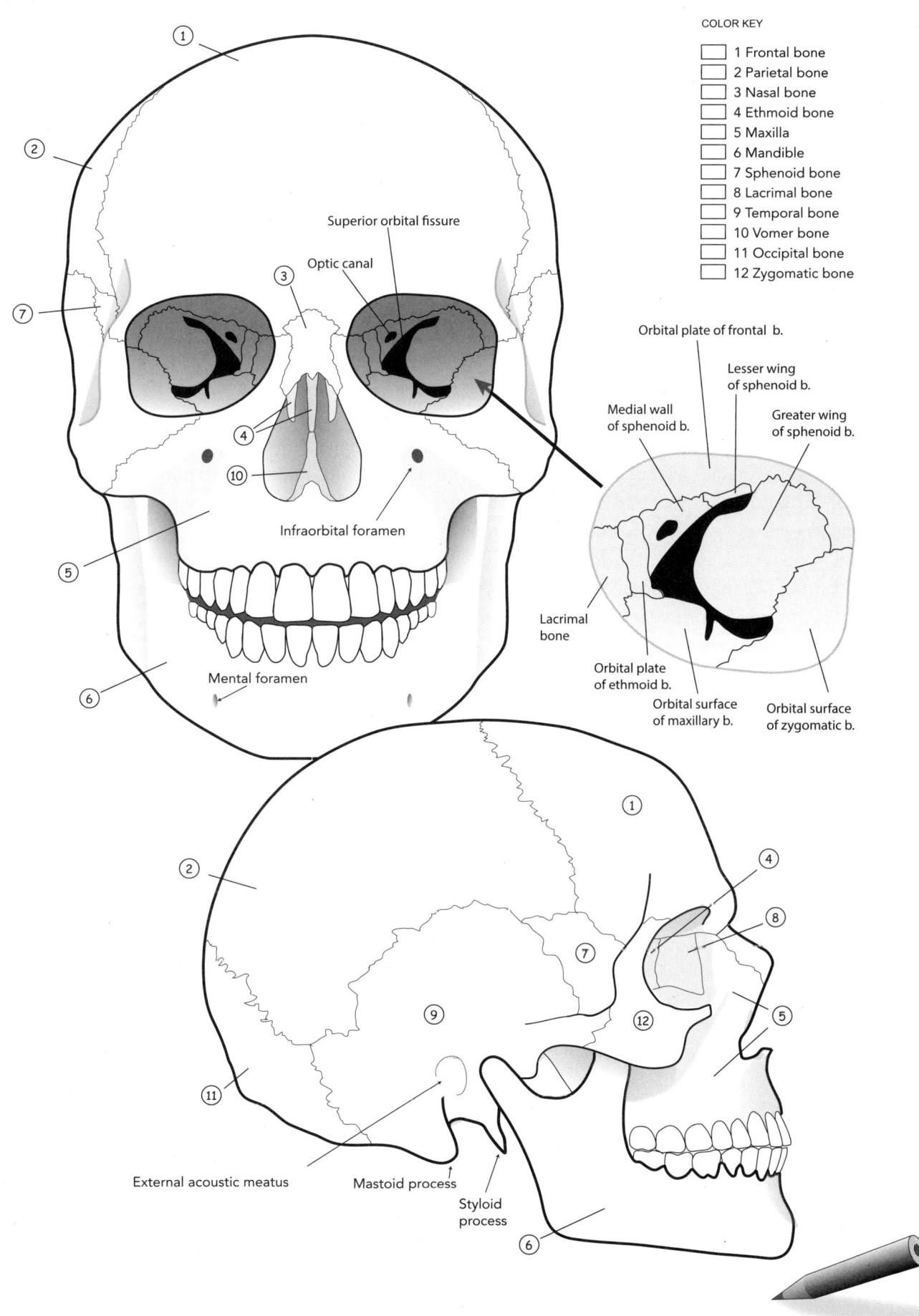

COLOR KEY

- [ ] 1 Frontal bone
- [ ] 2 Parietal bone
- [ ] 3 Nasal bone
- [ ] 4 Ethmoid bone
- [ ] 5 Maxilla
- [ ] 6 Mandible
- [ ] 7 Sphenoid bone
- [ ] 8 Lacrimal bone
- [ ] 9 Temporal bone
- [ ] 10 Vomer bone
- [ ] 11 Occipital bone
- [ ] 12 Zygomatic bone

Superior orbital fissure

Optic canal

Infraorbital foramen

Mental foramen

Orbital plate of frontal b.

Lesser wing
of sphenoid b.

Medial wall
of sphenoid b.

Greater wing
of sphenoid b.

Lacrimal
bone

Orbital plate
of ethmoid b.

Orbital surface
of maxillary b.

Orbital surface
of zygomatic b.

External acoustic meatus

Mastoid process

Styloid
process

Sphenoid bone (1): is located at the base of the skull anterior to the temporal bone and basal portion of the occipital bone. It forms part of the orbit of the eye. It resembles a bat or butterfly with its wings extended. The bone is divided into a median portion or body, two great and two small wings extending outward from the sides of the body, and two processes (pterygoid processes) which project inferiorly. Each process consists of a medial and lateral pterygoid plate. The medial pterygoid plate ends in a hook-like process called the hamulus.

The 14 Facial Bones

Vomer (1): is a thin, quadrilateral-shaped bone located midsagittally in the nasal cavity. It forms the posterior part of the nasal septum which separates the right and left nasal cavities.

Nasal conchae (turbinates) (3) : There are three nasal conchae - inferior, middle, and superior, within each nasal cavity. These small bones are long, narrow, and curled like a seashell. They divide the nasal cavity into four groove-like passages and help to direct airflow, as well as humidify, warm, and filter air inhaled through the nose.

Nasal bones (2): are two small oblong bones located in the upper-middle area of the face, between the frontal processes of the maxilla. The bones are fused forming the bridge of the nose. The bones vary in size and form in different individuals.

Zygomatic bones (2): are paired, small, roughly squarish bones situated at the upper and lateral part of the face. The bones form the prominences of the cheek, and part of the lateral wall and floor of the orbit. Each zygomatic bone has four processes: frontosphenoidal, orbital, maxillary, and temporal. The zygomatic bone extends backward to meet the zygomatic process of the temporal bone, forming the zygomatic arch.

Lacrimal bones (2): are the smallest and most fragile bones of the face, making up the anterior portion of the medial wall of the orbit.

Mandible (1): forms the lower jaw and is a large bone that has a distinctive angled shape. It is composed of the body and two rami (perpendicular portions extending superiorly). Each ramus ends in an anterior projection called the coronoid process, and a posterior projection called the condyle. The mandible also contains an alveolar process, which holds the bottom teeth in place. The mandible is attached to the skull by a joint between the condylar process and the temporal bone. Called the temporomandibular joint, it allows the jaw to open and close—a crucial factor in both eating and articulation. The mandible can be protruded, retracted, and move from side to side. This permits the mandible to move in a rotary motion that is important in chewing.

Maxilla (1): forms the upper jaw. It is composed of two irregularly-shaped bones that are fused at the intermaxillary suture. The maxilla forms the anterior three quarters of the hard palate, as well as parts of the eye orbits, and the floor and lateral walls of the nasal cavity. Each half of the fused bones contains four processes: zygomatic, frontal, palatine, and alveolar processes. The alveolar process contains the roots of the upper teeth.

Palatine bones (2): are situated at the posterior edge of the nasal cavity between the maxilla and the pterygoid process of the sphenoid. The palatine bone is shaped somewhat like the letter L and consists of a horizontal plate and a perpendicular plate. The two horizontal plates form the posterior quarter of the hard palate and the floor of the nasal cavity. Anteriorly, the bones are fused with the maxilla at the transverse palatine suture. The two horizontal plates articulate with each other at the median palatine suture.

Sagittal section of the skull

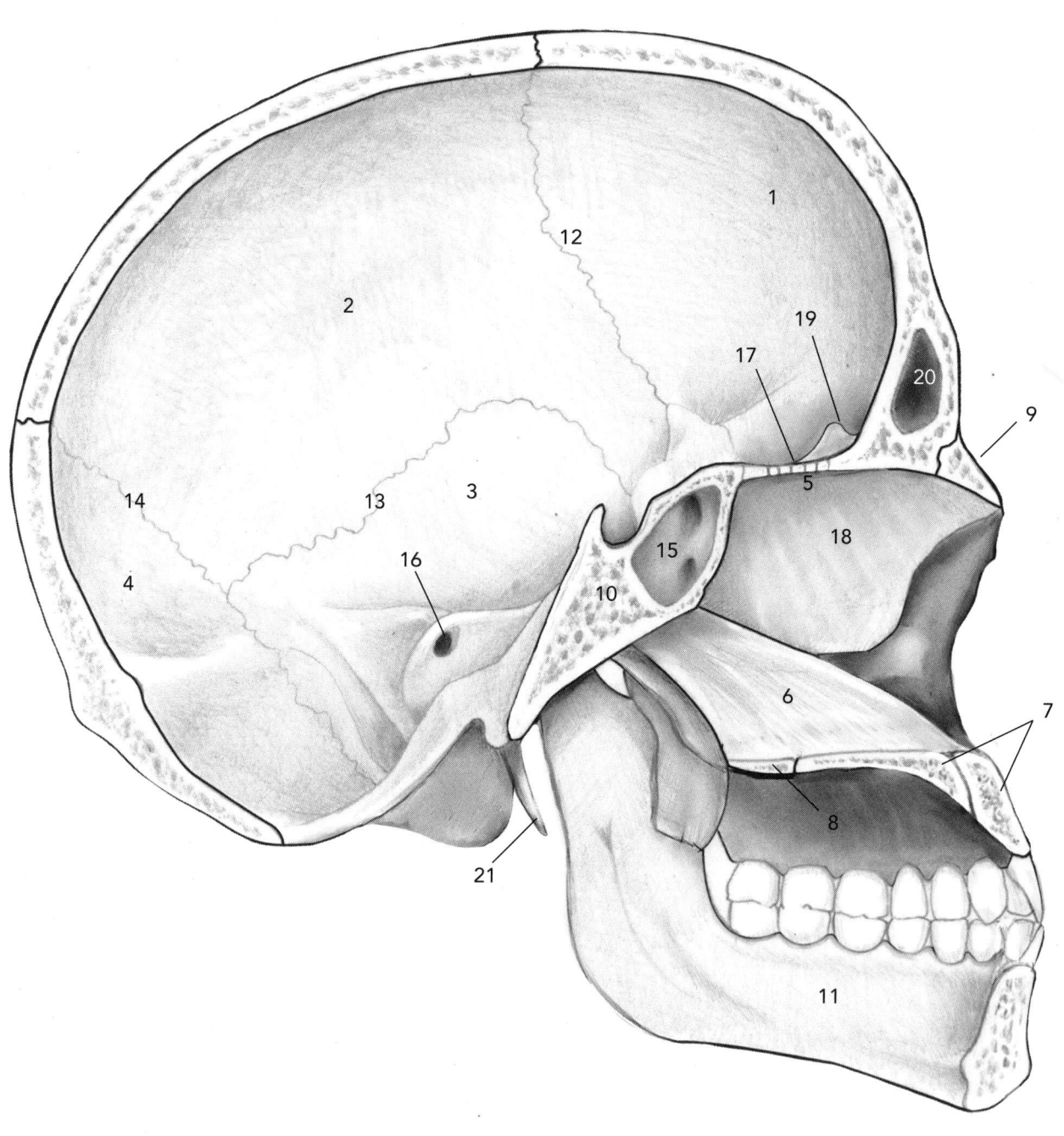

COLOR KEY

- [ ] 1 Frontal bone
- [ ] 2 Parietal bone
- [ ] 3 Temporal bone
- [ ] 4 Occipital bone
- [ ] 5 Ethmoid bone
- [ ] 6 Vomer
- [ ] 7 Maxilla

- [ ] 8 Palatine bone
- [ ] 9 Nasal bone
- [ ] 10 Sphenoid bone
- [ ] 11 Mandible
- [ ] 12 Coronal suture
- [ ] 13 Squamous suture

- [ ] 14 Lambdoidal suture
- [ ] 15 Sphenoid sinus
- [ ] 16 Internal acoustic meatus
- [ ] 17 Cribriform plate of ethmoid bone
- [ ] 18 Perpendicular plate of ethmoid bone
- [ ] 19 Crista galli
- [ ] 20 Frontal sinus
- [ ] 21 Styloid process

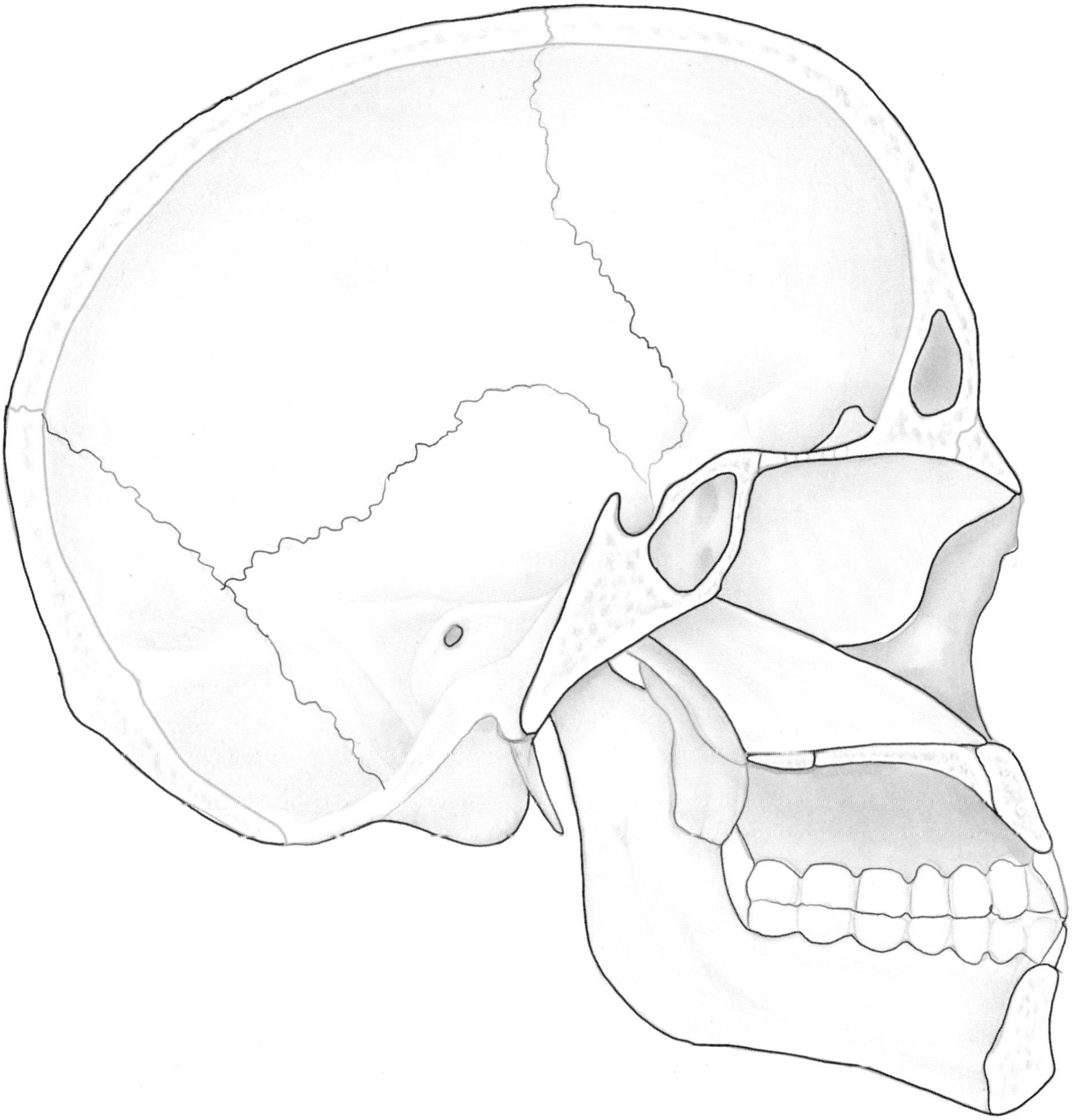

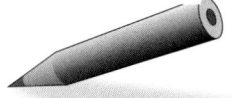

Ethmoid bone

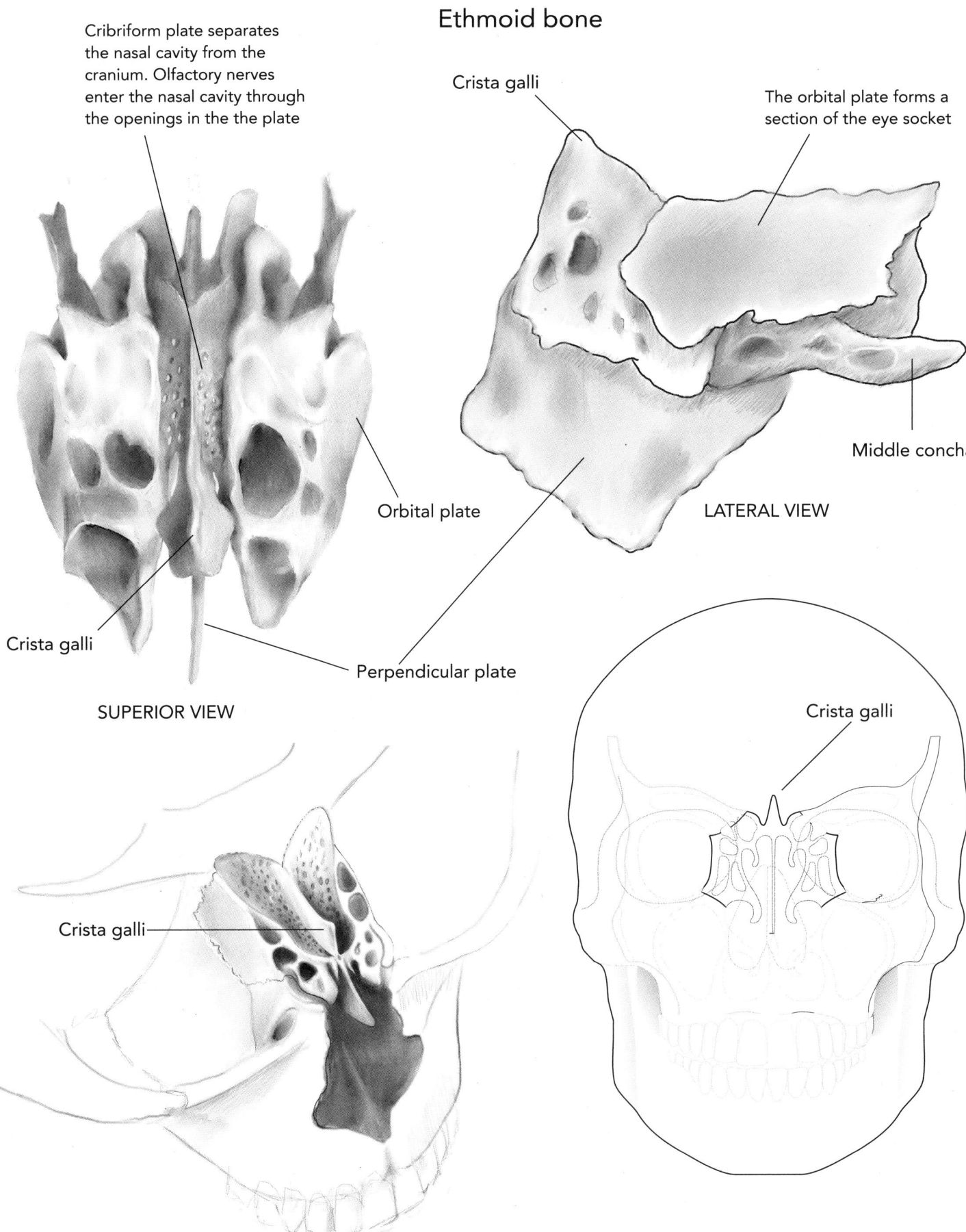

Cribriform plate separates the nasal cavity from the cranium. Olfactory nerves enter the nasal cavity through the openings in the the plate

Crista galli

The orbital plate forms a section of the eye socket

Middle concha

Orbital plate

Crista galli

Perpendicular plate

LATERAL VIEW

SUPERIOR VIEW

Crista galli

Crista galli

Sphenoid bone

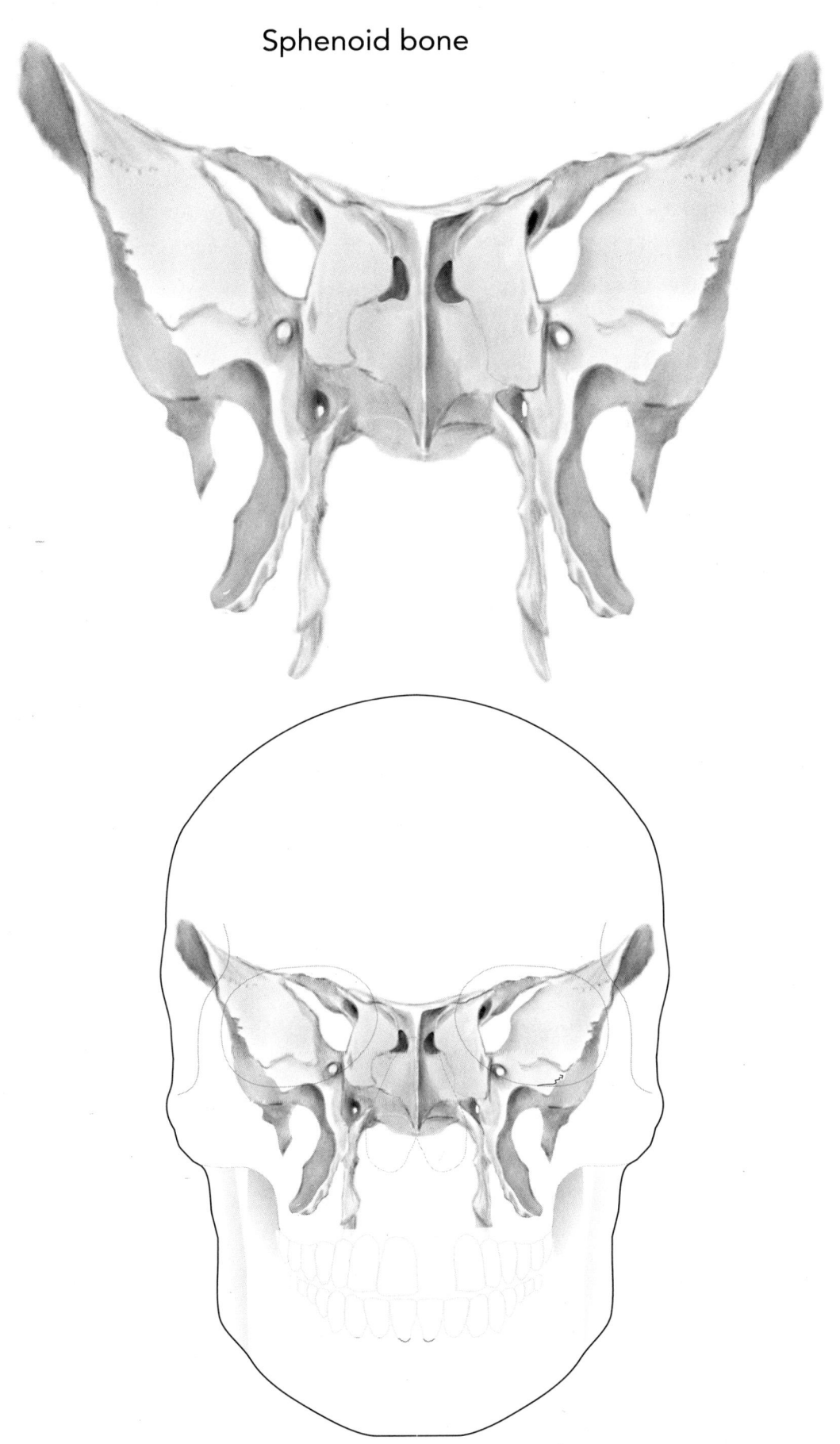

FACIAL MUSCLES

The facial muscles are a group of around 20 flat skeletal muscles that surround the openings of the face (eyes, nose, mouth, ears). The muscles are subcutaneous (lying just underneath the skin). They connect either on to other facial muscles or directly into the connective tissue of the skin. Many originate from the skull. The muscles are divided into muscles of facial expression and muscles of mastication.

Muscles of facial expression

The muscles of expression vary considerably among individuals. The muscles of facial expression can be grouped by region: Forehead, Eyes, Nose, Mouth.

Muscles of the Forehead

Frontalis: elevates the eyebrows and forehead and wrinkles the forehead.

Muscles of the Eyes

Orbicularis oculi: closes the eyelids, and produces winking, blinking, and squinting.

Muscles of the Nose

Procerus: wrinkles the root of the nose.
Nasalis: narrows the nose.
Levator labii superioris alaeque nasi: elevates the upper lip and flares the nostrils.

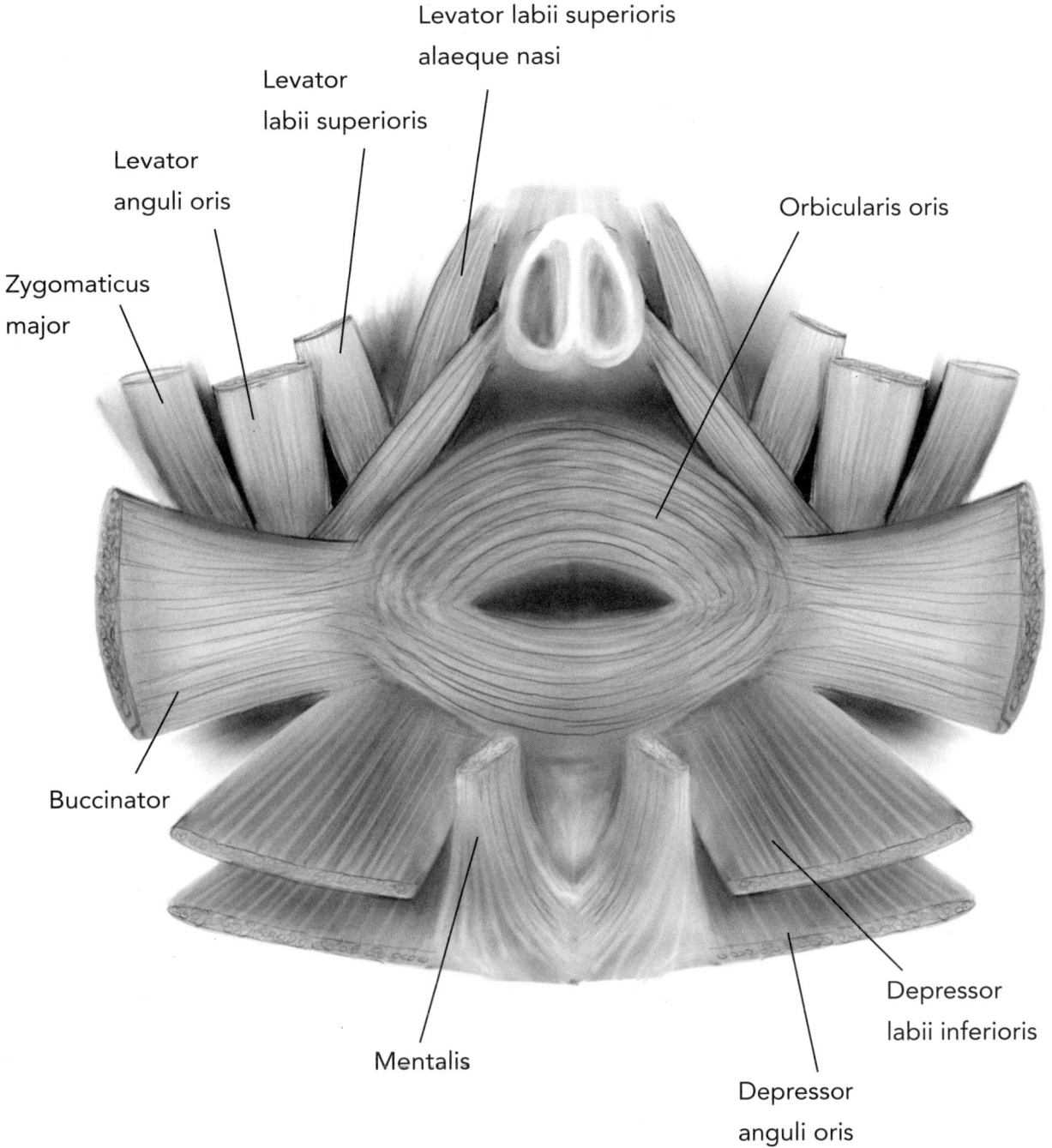

Levator labii superioris
alaeque nasi

Levator
labii superioris

Levator
anguli oris

Orbicularis oris

Zygomaticus
major

Buccinator

Depressor
labii inferioris

Mentalis

Depressor
anguli oris

This is a posterior view of the muscles surrounding the lips.
Think of it as if you were looking at the inside of a mask.

Muscles of the Mouth

Orbicularis oris: is a circular muscle surrounding both the upper and lower lips. Fibers from numerous other facial muscles insert onto the orbicularis oris. These muscles move the skin wherever they insert. A group of muscles (elevators) insert around the upper lip and raise it. The depressors insert around the lower lip and depress it. The orbicularis oris closes and protrudes the lips.

Buccinator: allows the cheeks to draw inwards to keep food between the molars while chewing.

Zygomaticus major: is a large muscle extending from each zygomatic arch to the corners of the mouth. This muscle pulls the angle of the mouth upward and outward, causing the corners of the mouth to rise in a smile.

Zygomaticus minor: is small muscle running from the zygomatic arch to the outer part of the upper lip. Like the zygomaticus major it also creates a smile by moving the upper lip backward, upward, and outward.

Risorius: is located around the mouth area. It stretches the mouth laterally to smile.

Levator labii superioris: elevates the upper lip.

Levator anguli oris: pulls the corner of the mouth upward.

Depressor anguli oris: pulls the corner of the mouth downward.

Depressor labii inferioris: pulls the lower lip downward.

Mentalis: protrudes the lower lip and elevates the skin of the chin.

Platysma: is primarily a muscle of the neck, but many of the muscle fibers blend with the muscles surrounding the angle and lower part of the mouth. This muscle thus contributes to facial expression.

Muscles of the Ears

Auricularis anterior: surrounds the outer ear and draws it forward and upward.

Auricularis superior: surrounds the outer ear and slightly raises it.

Auricularis posterior: surrounds the outer ear and draws it backward.

While these muscles can adjust the direction of the pinna in some animals, they are not very active in humans.

Muscles of mastication

The muscles of mastication are responsible for opening and closing the jaw and moving the jaw laterally.

Temporalis: runs from the temporal bone and inserts into the coronoid process and ramus of the mandible. It elevates the mandible to close the jaw; however, its posterior fibers retract the mandible.

Masseter: runs from the zygomatic arch and inserts into the coronoid process and ramus of mandible. It elevates and protrudes the mandible.

Lateral pterygoid: runs from the sphenoid bone and inserts into the temporomandibular joint and the condylar process of the mandible. Contraction of this muscle can be bilateral or unilateral. Bilateral contraction depresses the chin to open the jaw; unilateral contraction produces side-to-side movements of the jaw.

Medial pterygoid: runs from lateral pterygoid plate and palatine bone and inserts into the ramus of the mandible. It elevates the mandible and produces a grinding motion when fibers act alternately.

Facial muscles

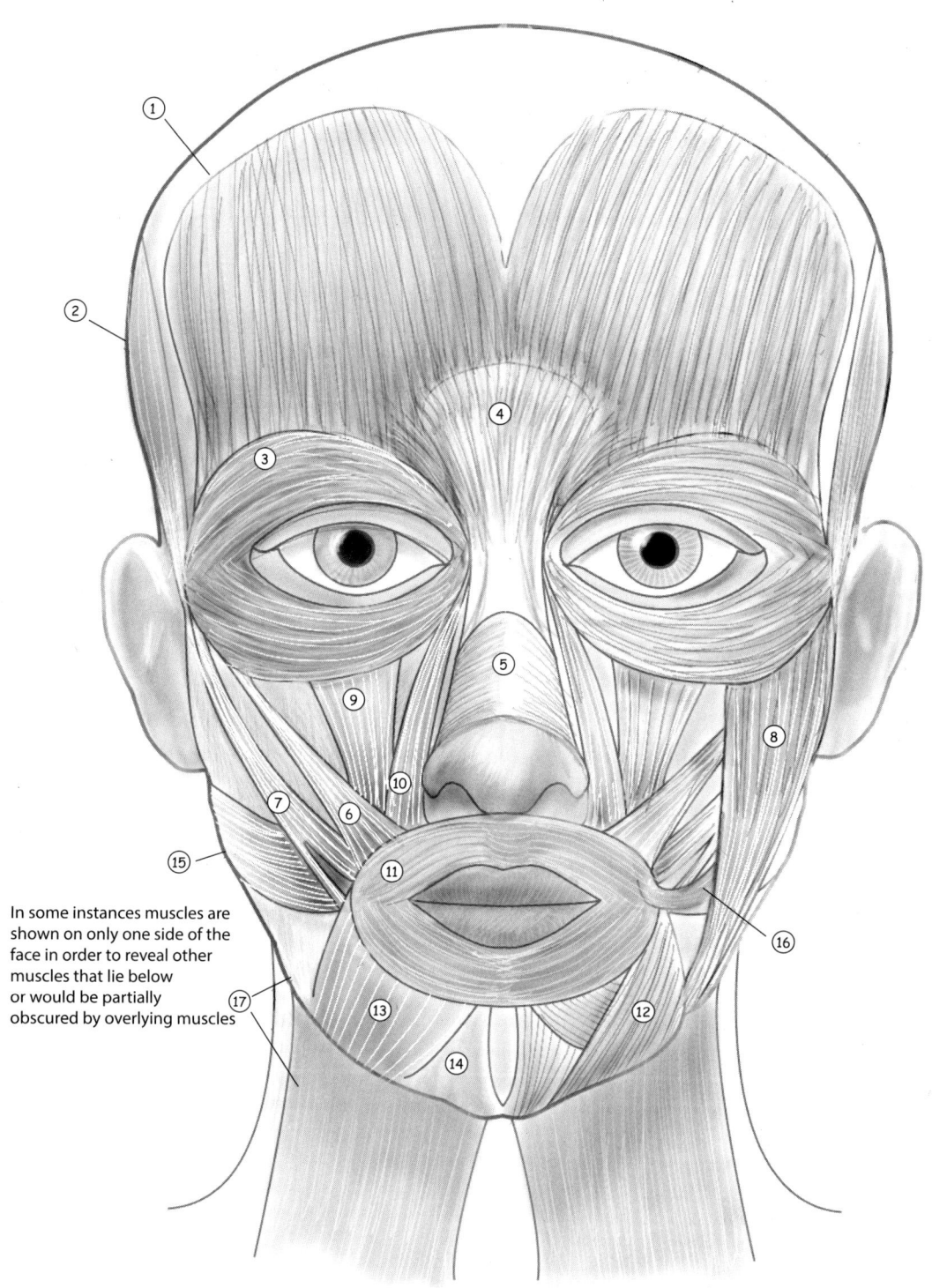

In some instances muscles are
shown on only one side of the
face in order to reveal other
muscles that lie below
or would be partially
obscured by overlying muscles

Facial muscles

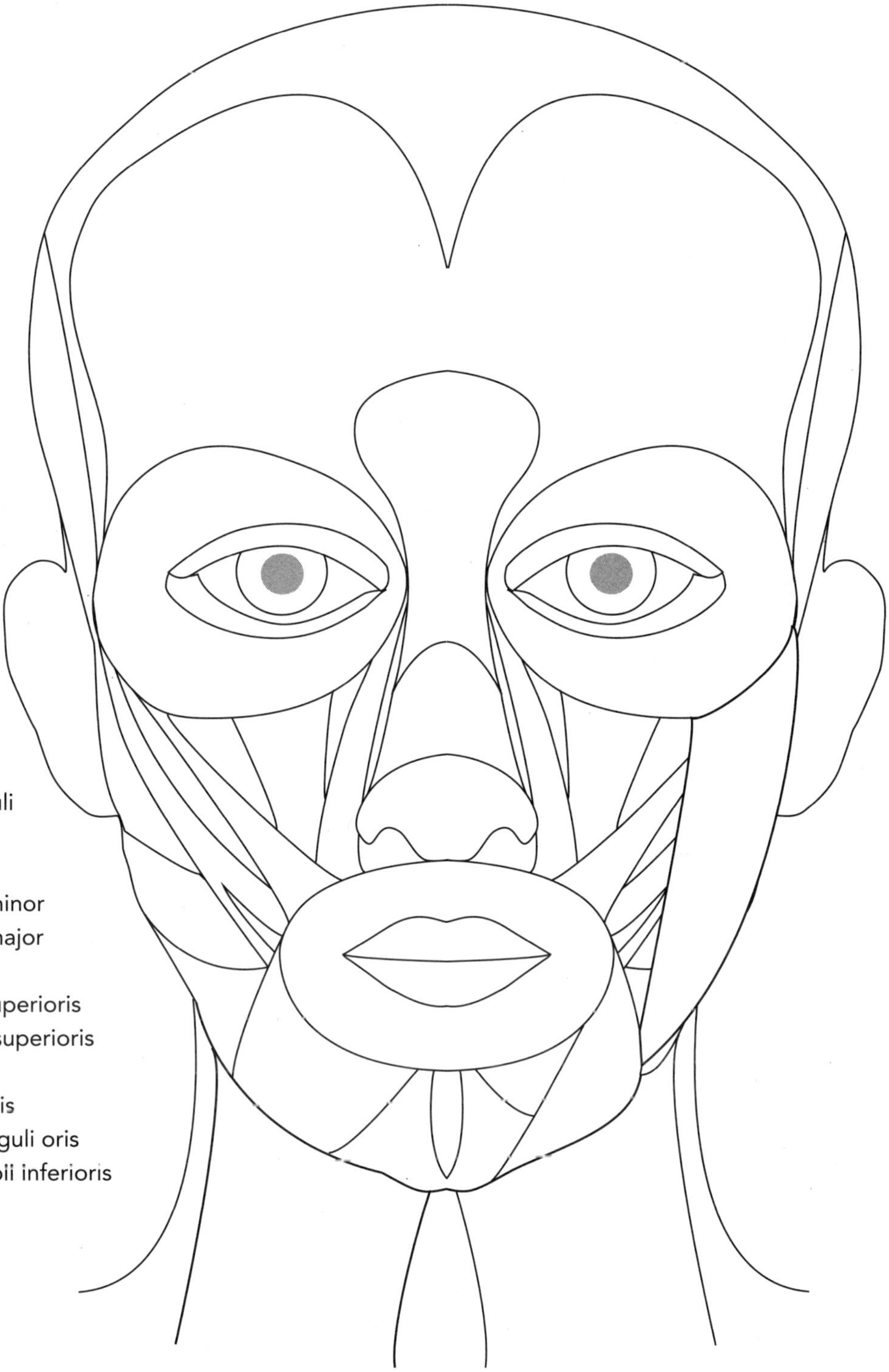

COLOR KEY

- ☐ 1 Frontalis
- ☐ 2 Temporalis
- ☐ 3 Orbicularis oculi
- ☐ 4 Procerus
- ☐ 5 Nasalis
- ☐ 6 Zygomaticus minor
- ☐ 7 Zygomaticus major
- ☐ 8 Masseter
- ☐ 9 Levator labii superioris
- ☐ 10 Levator labii superioris
      allaeque nasi
- ☐ 11 Orbicularis oris
- ☐ 12 Depressor anguli oris
- ☐ 13 Depressor labii inferioris
- ☐ 14 Mentalis
- ☐ 15 Buccinator
- ☐ 16 Risorius
- ☐ 17 Platysma

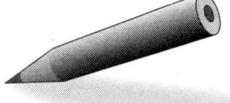

Facial muscles

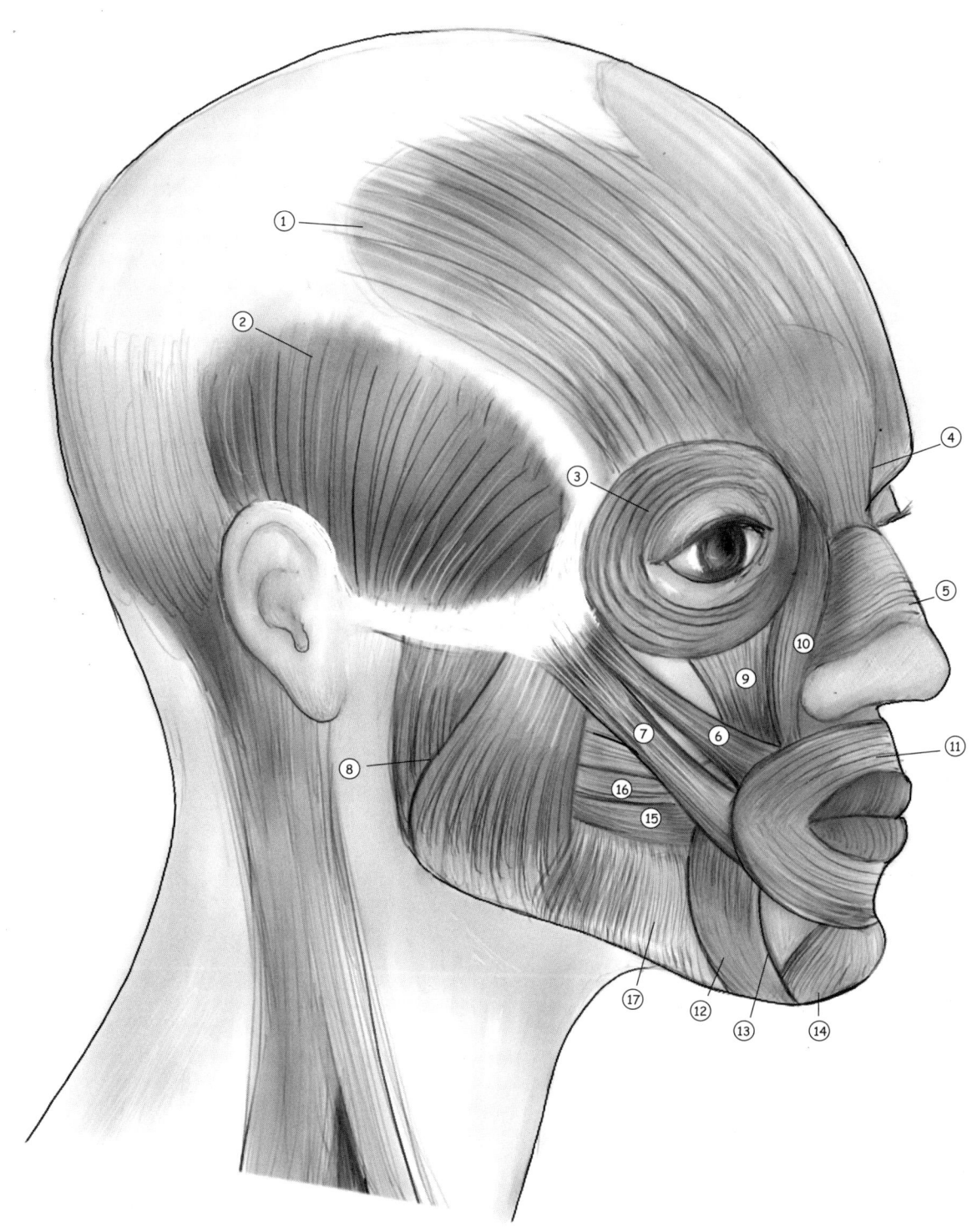

Facial muscles

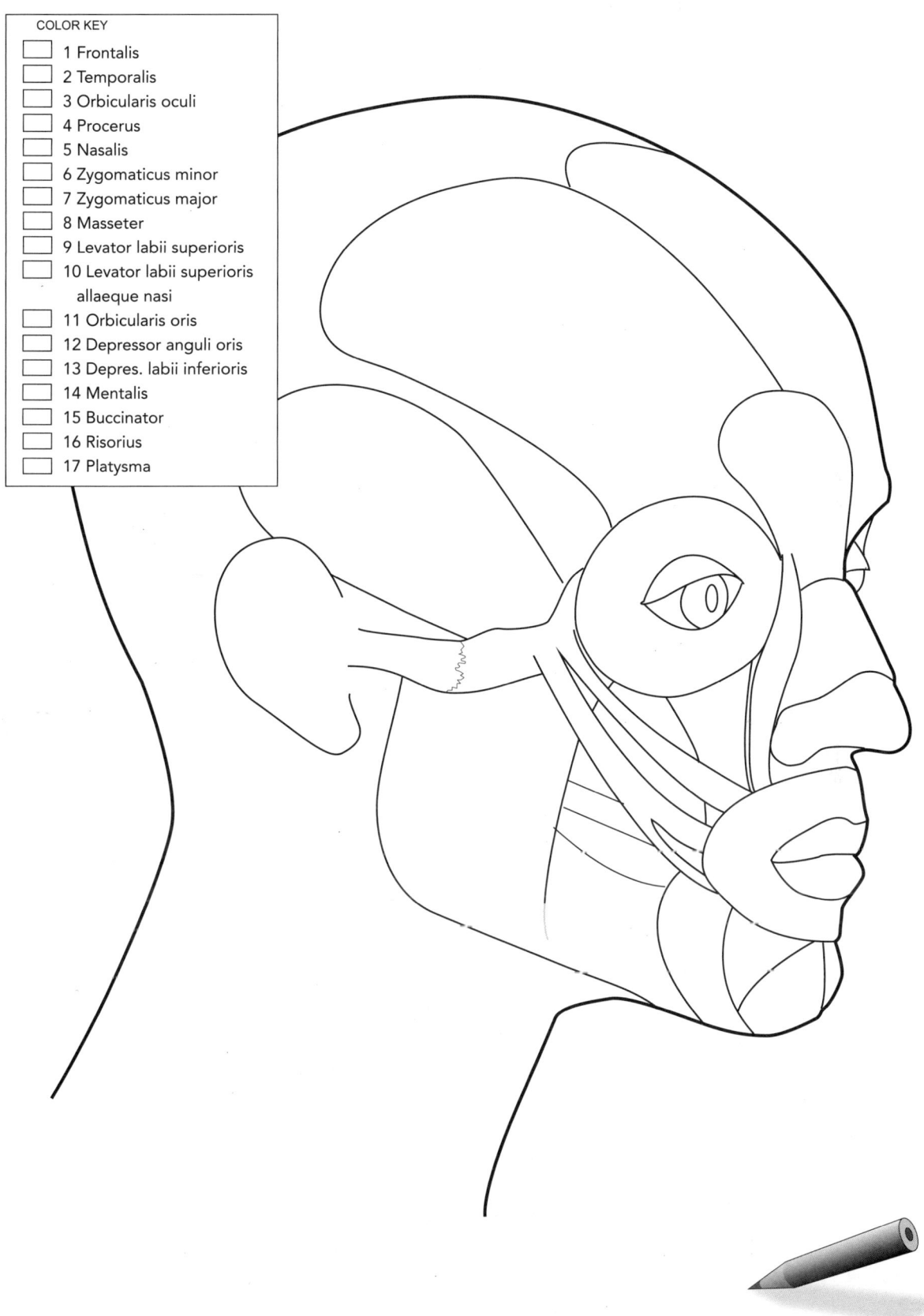

COLOR KEY
- [ ] 1 Frontalis
- [ ] 2 Temporalis
- [ ] 3 Orbicularis oculi
- [ ] 4 Procerus
- [ ] 5 Nasalis
- [ ] 6 Zygomaticus minor
- [ ] 7 Zygomaticus major
- [ ] 8 Masseter
- [ ] 9 Levator labii superioris
- [ ] 10 Levator labii superioris
     allaeque nasi
- [ ] 11 Orbicularis oris
- [ ] 12 Depressor anguli oris
- [ ] 13 Depres. labii inferioris
- [ ] 14 Mentalis
- [ ] 15 Buccinator
- [ ] 16 Risorius
- [ ] 17 Platysma

Draw your own: Mouth muscles

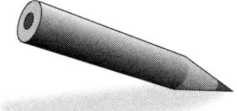

PHARYNX

The pharynx is a long hollow tube made of muscle, connective tissue, and mucous lining. It runs behind the nasal cavities, oral cavity, and larynx. The portion behind the larynx is called the laryngopharynx; the portion behind the oral cavity is the oropharynx; and the portion behind the nasal cavities is the nasopharynx or hypopharynx. The pharynx is about 12 cm long and about 4 cm wide at the top end. It narrows, until at its bottom end it is only about 2.5 cm in width. The laryngopharynx leads into the esophagus, posterior to the trachea. The esophagus is the part of the digestive system that leads into the stomach. The Eustachian tube joins the nasopharynx and the middle ear.

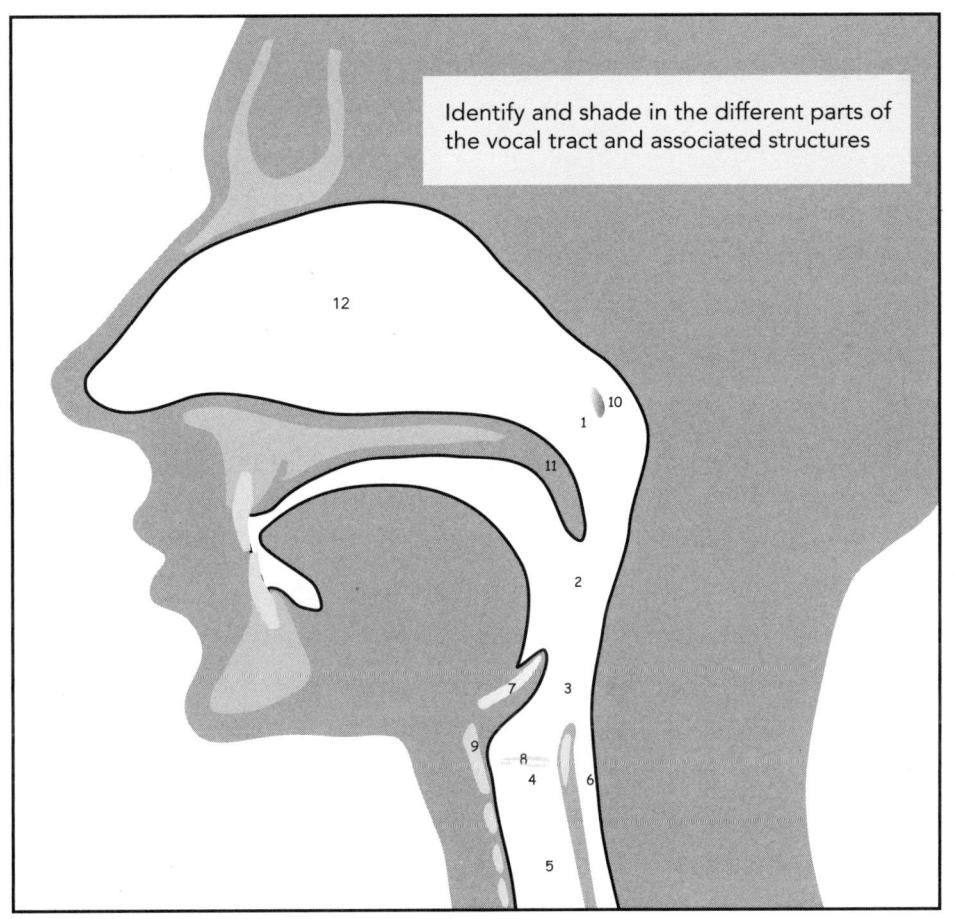

Identify and shade in the different parts of the vocal tract and associated structures

COLOR KEY

	1 Nasopharynx		5 Trachea		9 Thyroid cartilage
	2 Oropharynx		6 Esophagus		10 Eustachian tube orifice
	3 Laryngopharynx		7 Epiglottis		11 Velum (soft palate)
	4 Larynx		8 Vocal folds		12 Nasal cavity

Muscles of the pharynx

Pharyngeal constrictors: fan-shaped muscles that overlap one another. The inferior constrictor is the largest and strongest of the pharyngeal constrictors. It originates from the sides of the thyroid cartilage and then wraps around the lower to midregions of the pharynx. The middle constrictor extends from the hyoid bone and forms the middle portion of the pharynx. The superior constrictor originates from many locations in and around the soft palate and forms the topmost section of the pharynx. The pharynx constricts during swallowing and forces the bolus of food downward into the esophagus.

The three pharyngeal constrictors

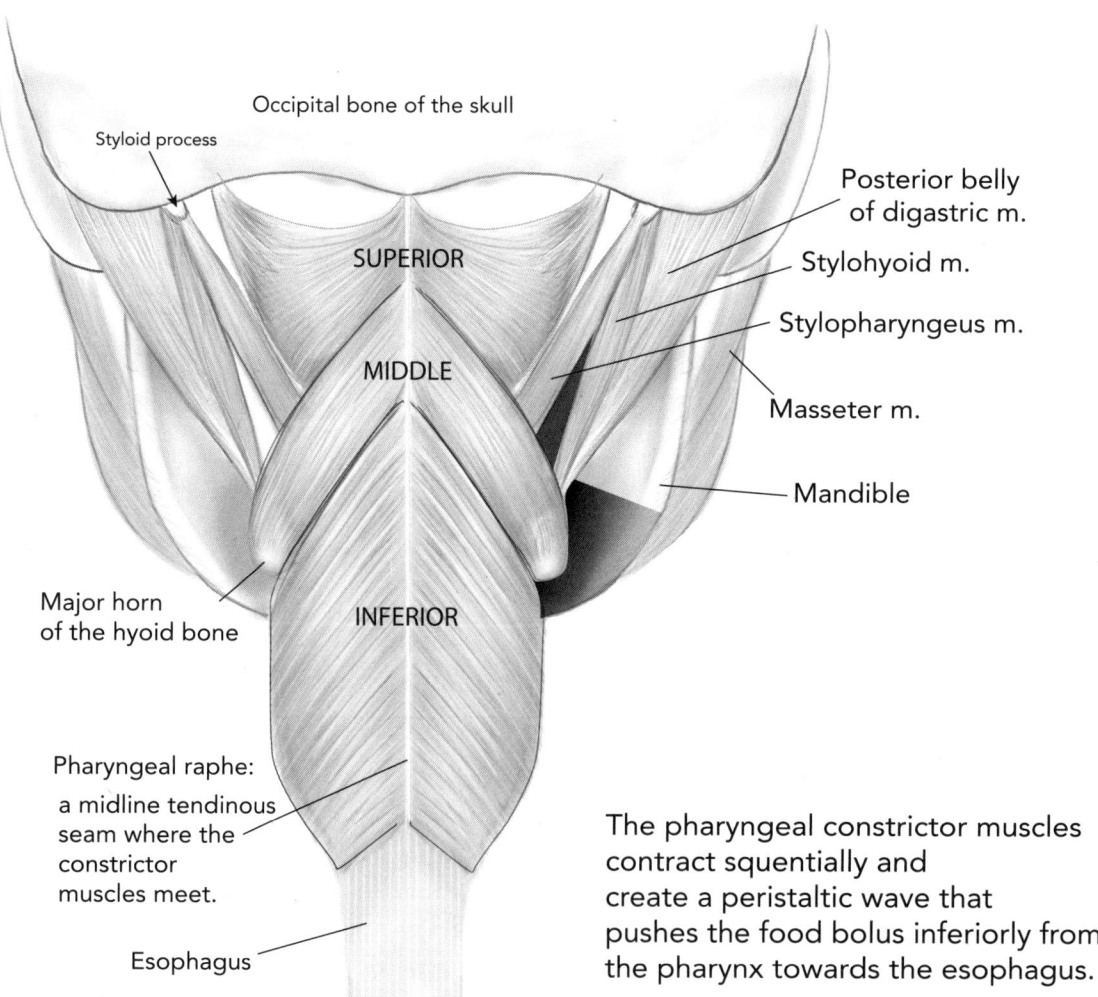

Occipital bone of the skull

Styloid process

SUPERIOR

Posterior belly of digastric m.

Stylohyoid m.

Stylopharyngeus m.

MIDDLE

Masseter m.

Mandible

Major horn of the hyoid bone

INFERIOR

Pharyngeal raphe: a midline tendinous seam where the constrictor muscles meet.

Esophagus

The pharyngeal constrictor muscles contract squentially and create a peristaltic wave that pushes the food bolus inferiorly from the pharynx towards the esophagus.

Cricopharyngeus: located at the lower margin of the inferior constrictor. This muscle arises from the cricoid cartilage and forms a ring around the top opening of the esophagus. The ring of muscle is called the pharyngoesophageal (PE) segment.

The PE segment remains contracted during rest and relaxes during swallowing to allow food to pass into the esophagus.

Stylopharyngeus: long thin muscle arising from the styloid process of the temporal bone. It runs inferiorly along the side of the pharynx between the superior and middle pharyngeal constrictors. Some of its fibers intermingle with the constrictors and others insert into the thyroid cartilage. The stylopharyngeus helps to elevate and open the pharynx

Pharyngeal constrictors and associated structures

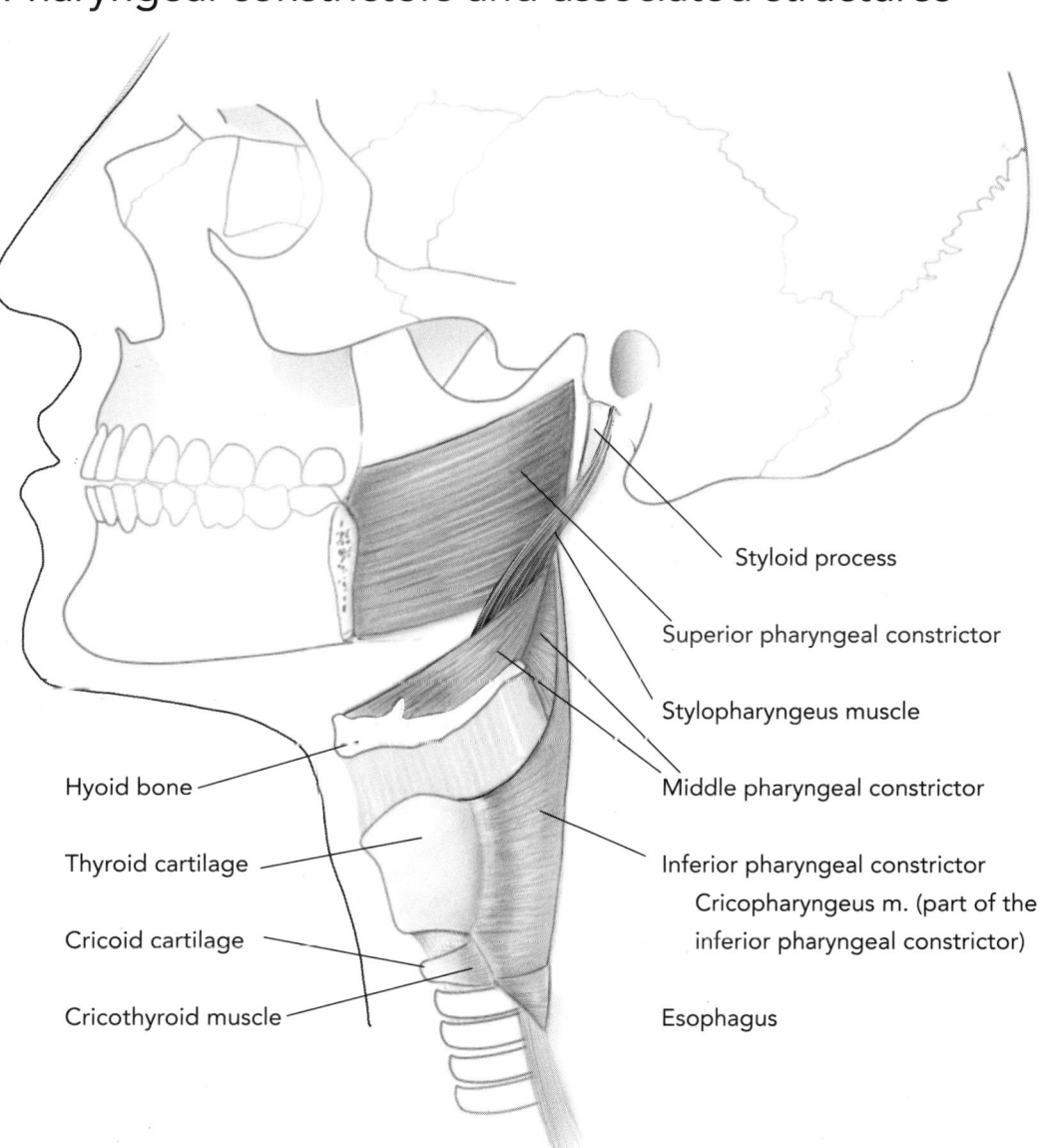

Styloid process

Superior pharyngeal constrictor

Stylopharyngeus muscle

Middle pharyngeal constrictor

Inferior pharyngeal constrictor
Cricopharyngeus m. (part of the
inferior pharyngeal constrictor)

Esophagus

Hyoid bone

Thyroid cartilage

Cricoid cartilage

Cricothyroid muscle

Salpingopharyngeus: arises from the cartilaginous portion of the Eustachian tube in the lateral walls of the nasopharynx. Its fibers run inferiorly and blend with the fibers of the palatopharyngeus muscle. The salpingopharyngeus helps to elevate and open the pharynx during swallowing.

Palatopharyngeus: arises from the palatal aponeurosis (the tendon that attaches the soft and hard palates) and the hard palate. It inserts into the superior border of the thyroid cartilage and the side of the pharynx. Contraction pulls the larynx and the pharynx superiorly, anteriorly, and medially. This muscle helps to elevate and open the pharynx during swallowing. It forms the posterior faucial pillar.

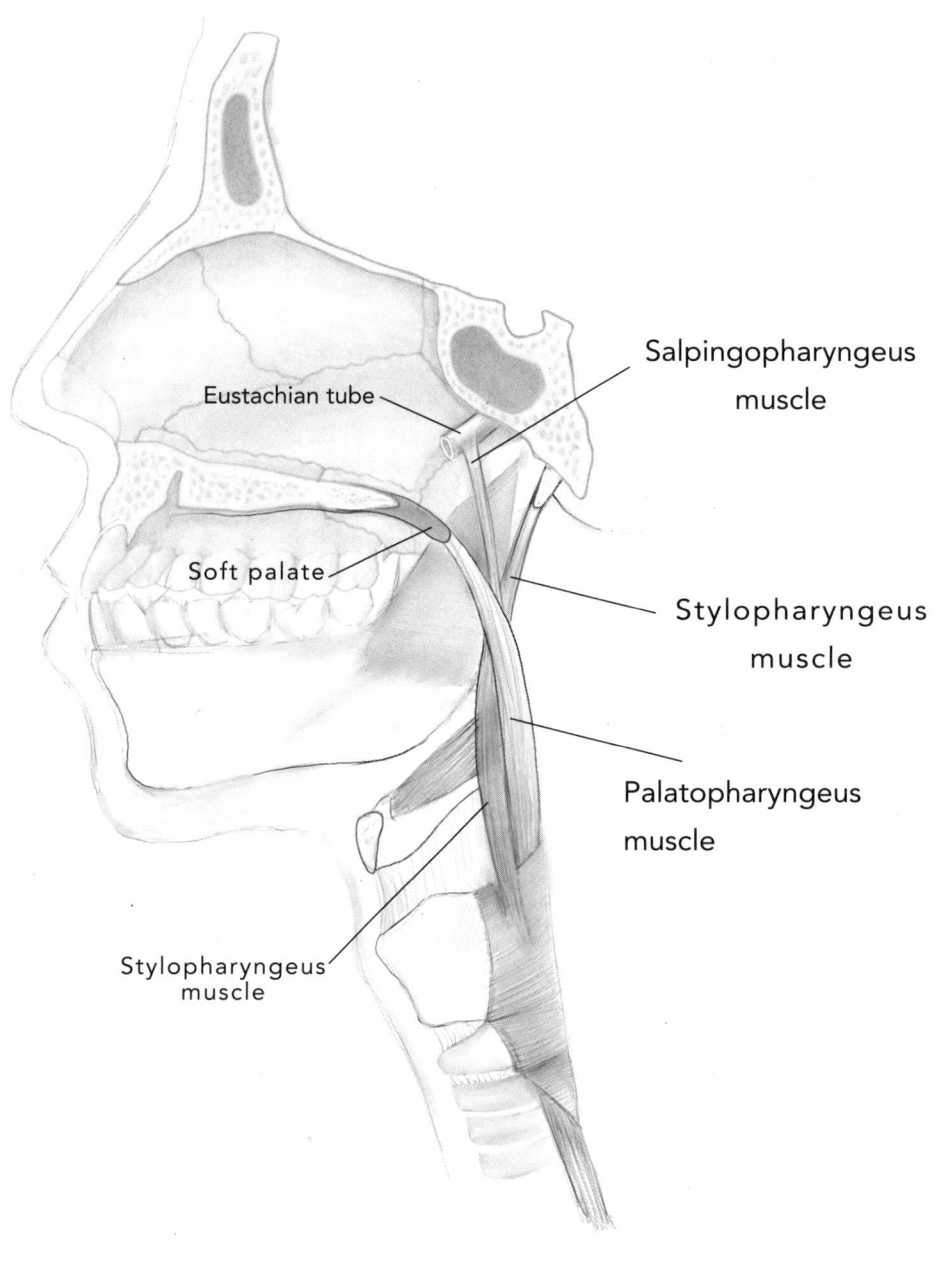

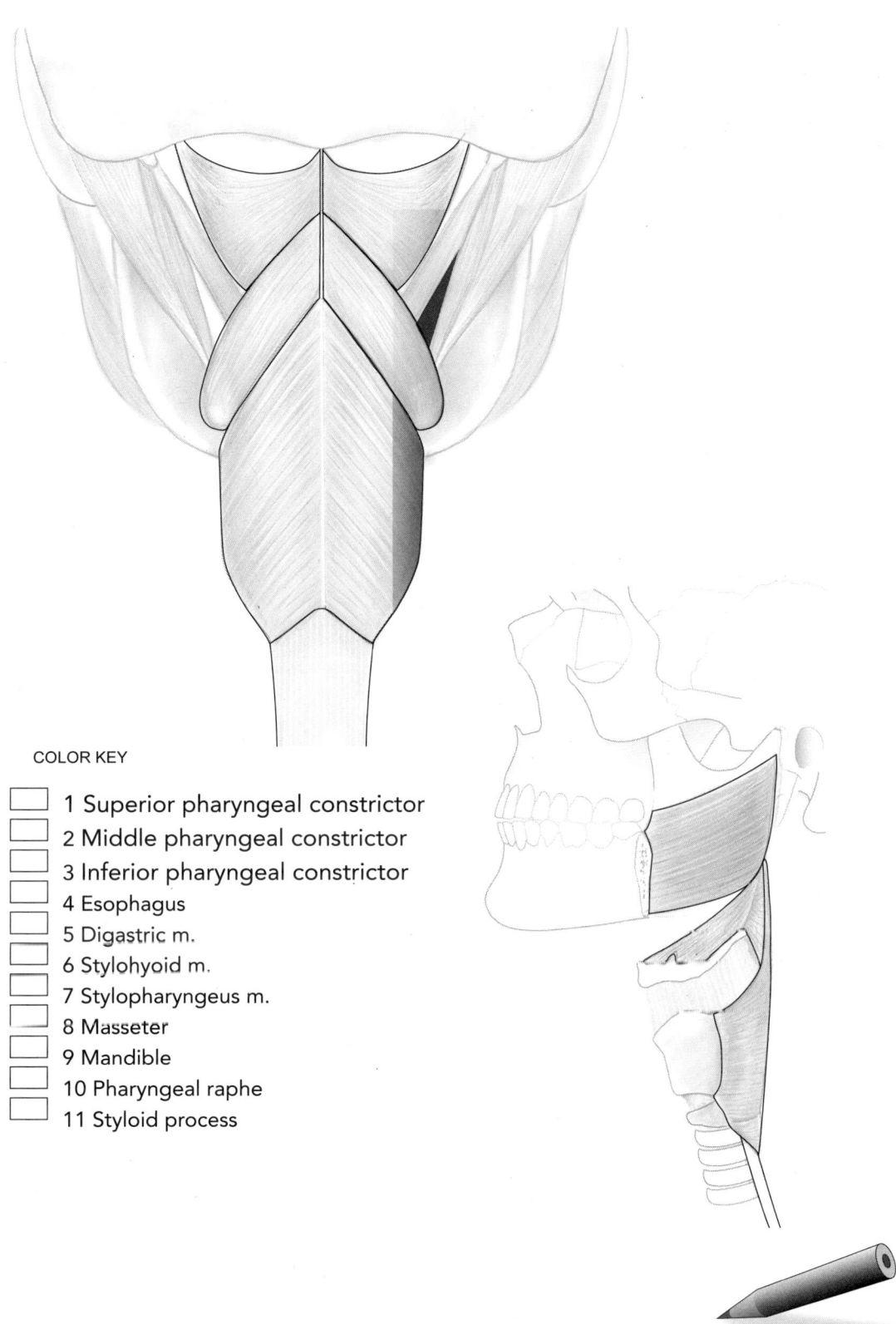

COLOR KEY

- 1 Superior pharyngeal constrictor
- 2 Middle pharyngeal constrictor
- 3 Inferior pharyngeal constrictor
- 4 Esophagus
- 5 Digastric m.
- 6 Stylohyoid m.
- 7 Stylopharyngeus m.
- 8 Masseter
- 9 Mandible
- 10 Pharyngeal raphe
- 11 Styloid process

Structures of the oral cavity

Lips

The lips are composed of muscle, mucous membrane, glandular tissues, and fat, and are covered by a layer of epithelium. The inner surface of the upper lip connects to the midline of the alveolar region by a small flap of tissue called the superior labial frenulum.

The lower lip is connected to the midline of the mandible by the inferior labial frenulum. The muscles of the lips give them an enormous amount of mobility, allowing them to open and close very rapidly, and to position themselves in many ways. This flexibility and speed of motion are very important in the articulation of such sounds as /p/, /b/, /m/, and /w/.

The lips are also crucial in mastication, acting to keep food and liquid within the mouth. Individuals with low muscle tone or with lip paralysis have difficulty in controlling the flow of saliva out of the mouth, as well as difficulty forming labial sounds.

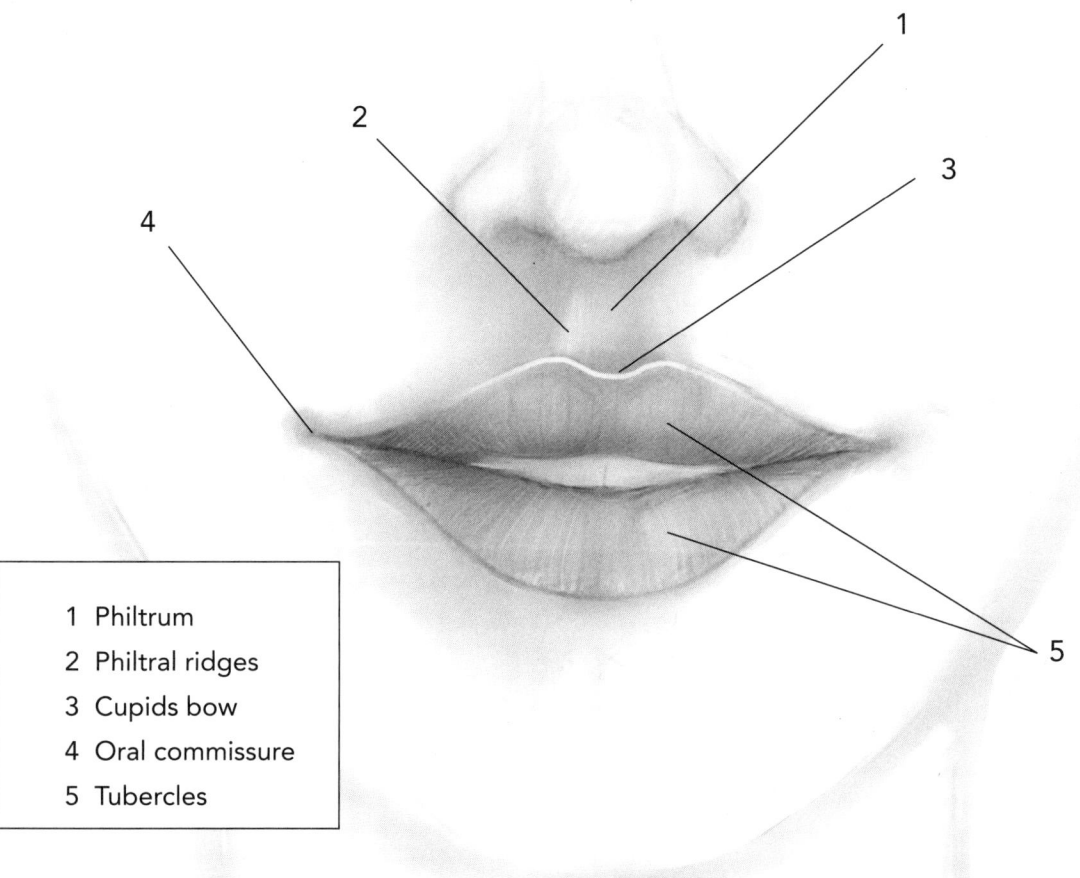

1 Philtrum
2 Philtral ridges
3 Cupids bow
4 Oral commissure
5 Tubercles

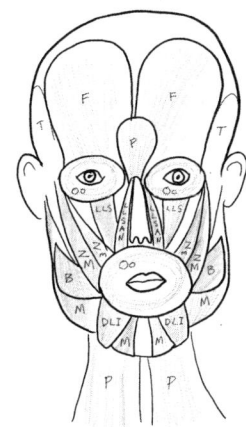

Draw your own: Face muscles

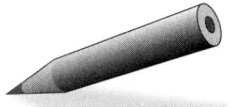

ORAL CAVITY

The oral cavity is a space bounded by the lips anteriorly, the cheeks laterally, and the palate superiorly. The tongue makes up the movable floor, and the back of the oral cavity opens into the oropharynx.

☐ 1 Upper labium
☐ 2 Gingivae (gums)
☐ 3 Superior labial frenulum
☐ 4 Hard palate
☐ 5 Soft palate
☐ 6 Uvula
☐ 7 Fauces (opening of pharynx)
☐ 8 Palatine tonsil
☐ 9 Palatoglossal arch
☐ 10 Palatopharyngeal arch
☐ 11 Inferior labial frenulum

☐ 12 Superior vestibule
☐ 13 Inferior vestibule
☐ 14 Palatine raphe
☐ 15 Lingual frenulum
☐ 16 Salivary ducts
☐ 17 Sublingual orifice s. duct
☐ 18 Submandibular orifice s.duct
☐ 19 Lower labium
☐ 20 Central incisors
☐ 21 Lateral incisors
☐ 22 Cuspids (canines)

☐ 23 1st bicuspids
☐ 24 2nd bicuspids
☐ 25 1st molars
☐ 26 2nd molars
☐ 27 3rd molars
   (wisdom teeth)

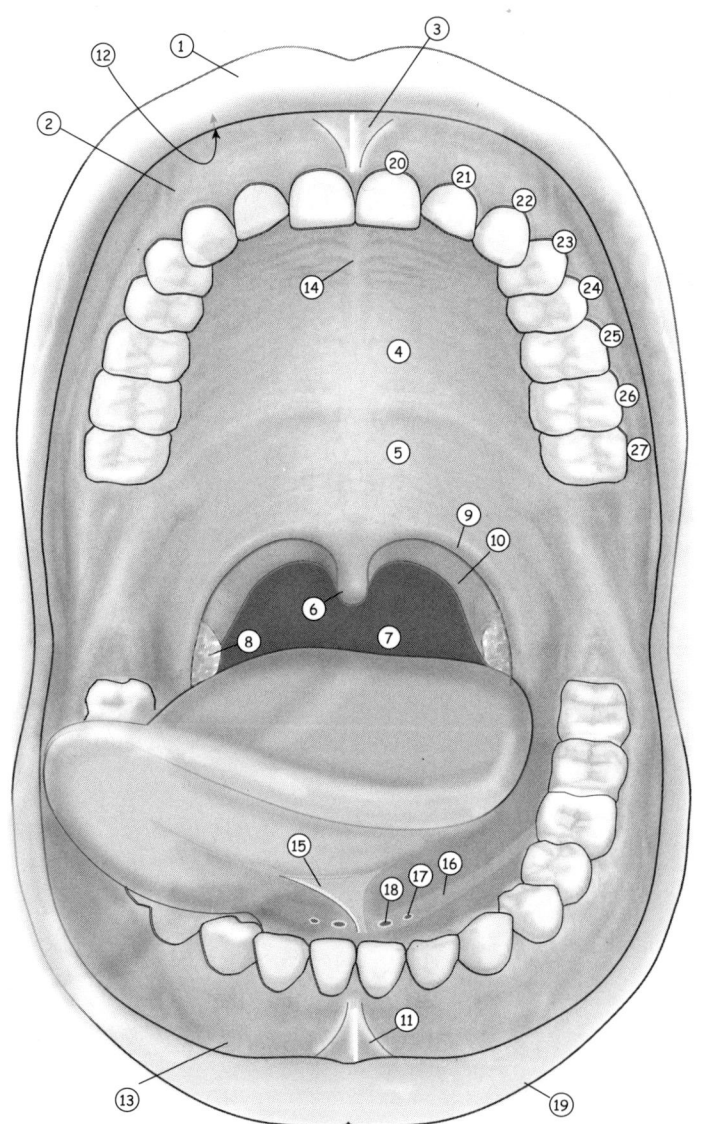

Shade in the illustration and label the structures

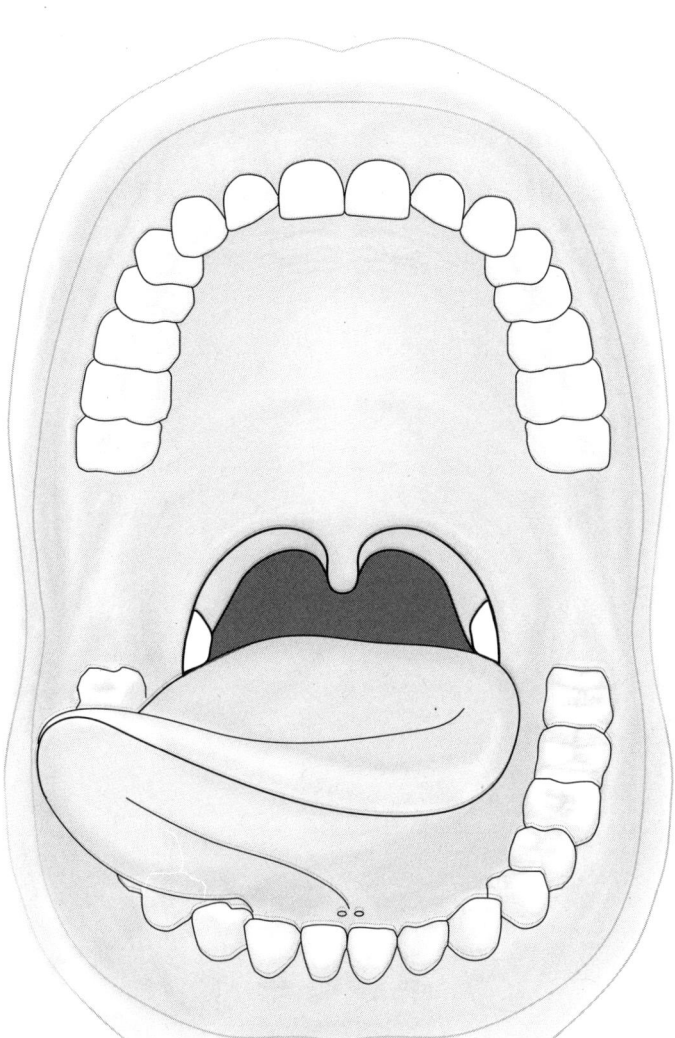

Teeth

Children have 20 teeth, 10 in the upper jaw (maxilla) and 10 in the lower jaw (mandible). Adults have 32 teeth, with 16 each in the upper and lower jaws. Humans have four types of teeth: incisors, canines, premolars, and molars. Teeth are essential for biting, cutting, and chewing food, and they also play an important role in speech production. They serve as an immovable articulator against which the tongue can form connections, and they also help to channel the flow of air and sound waves for some types of phonemes.

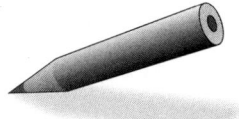

Draw your own: Skull

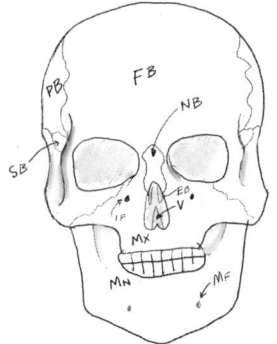

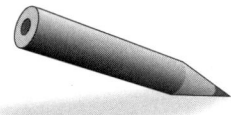

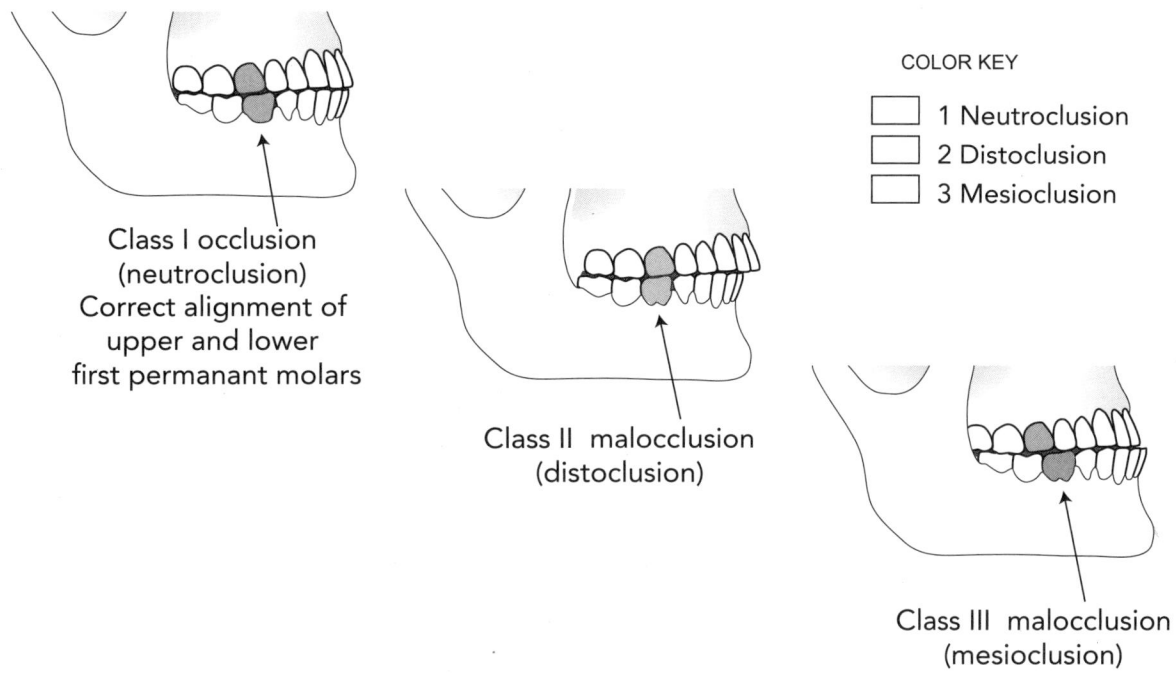

COLOR KEY

☐ 1 Neutroclusion
☐ 2 Distoclusion
☐ 3 Mesioclusion

Class I occlusion
(neutroclusion)
Correct alignment of
upper and lower
first permanant molars

Class II malocclusion
(distoclusion)

Class III malocclusion
(mesioclusion)

Dental Occlusion

The upper and lower teeth need to be in appropriate relationship to each other. If they are not, this can affect both eating and speech production. Occlusion refers to the relationship between the upper and lower dental arches and the positioning of individual teeth. Problems in upper and lower dental arch position and tooth relationships are called malocclusions.

Class I occlusion (neutroclusion): Class I occlusion refers to the normal occlusal relationship. In this position the first permanent molar of the upper jaw is positioned one half-tooth behind the first permanent molar of the lower jaw. The upper arch overlaps the lower one in front. The upper incisors hide the lower incisors so that only a little of the lower teeth show. Individual teeth may be misaligned or rotated, but the occlusion is normal.

Class II occlusion (distoclusion): the first molar of the lower jaw is posterior to the normal position. This results in the mandible being pulled back or retracted, a condition called overjet

Class III occlusion (mesioclusion): the first molar of the lower jaw is anterior to the normal position. The mandible protrudes too far forward, a condition called prognathic jaw.

Hard palate

The hard palate is a complex bony structure lined with epithelium. The hard palate makes up the roof of the oral cavity and the floor of the nasal cavity. It serves as a barrier between these two cavities, preventing food, air, and sound waves from escaping the oral cavity.

The anterior three-quarters of the hard palate are formed by the palatine processes of the maxilla. The processes join together at the midline and articulate at the intermaxillary suture. The posterior one-quarter of the hard palate is formed by the palatine bones of the skull. The meeting of the palatine bones and palatine processes forms a suture called the transverse palatine suture.

The raised ridge running from side to side toward the anterior of the hard palate, a few centimeters behind the upper teeth, is called the alveolar ridge, and is formed by the alveolar process of the maxilla. The alveolar ridge is the point of contact or approximation of the tongue for many of the speech sounds of English, including /t/, /d/, /s/, /z/, /l/, and /n/. The hard palate posterior to the alveolar ridge also serves as an immovable point of contact for the tongue in the articulation of many sounds, such as /ʃ/, /ʒ/, and /r/. Because the hard palate is instrumental in the production of many sounds, structural problems such as cleft palate can result in severe speech production difficulties

Velum

Posterior to the hard palate is the velum, also called the soft palate . The velum consists of several muscles and a large flat tendon, the palatal aponeurosis. The palatal aponeurosis attaches the velum to the posterior portion of the hard palate. Nerves, blood vessels, and glands are also located within the velum, which is covered by a mucous membrane.

The velum at rest hangs down into the pharynx. This creates a passageway between the velum and the posterior pharyngeal wall. The passageway is called the velopharyngeal passage or port. The velopharyngeal passage can be opened or closed by movement of the velum. When the velum is raised it forms a barrier between the oral and nasal cavities so that air, sound waves, and food are prevented from entering the nasal cavities. When the velopharyngeal passage is open, air is free to enter and exit the respiratory system through the nasal cavities. Sound waves are also free to travel into the nasal cavities. So is food, which can be a problem in cases of cleft palate or paralyzed velum. The velum is the point of articulation for the /k, g, and ŋ/ phonemes.

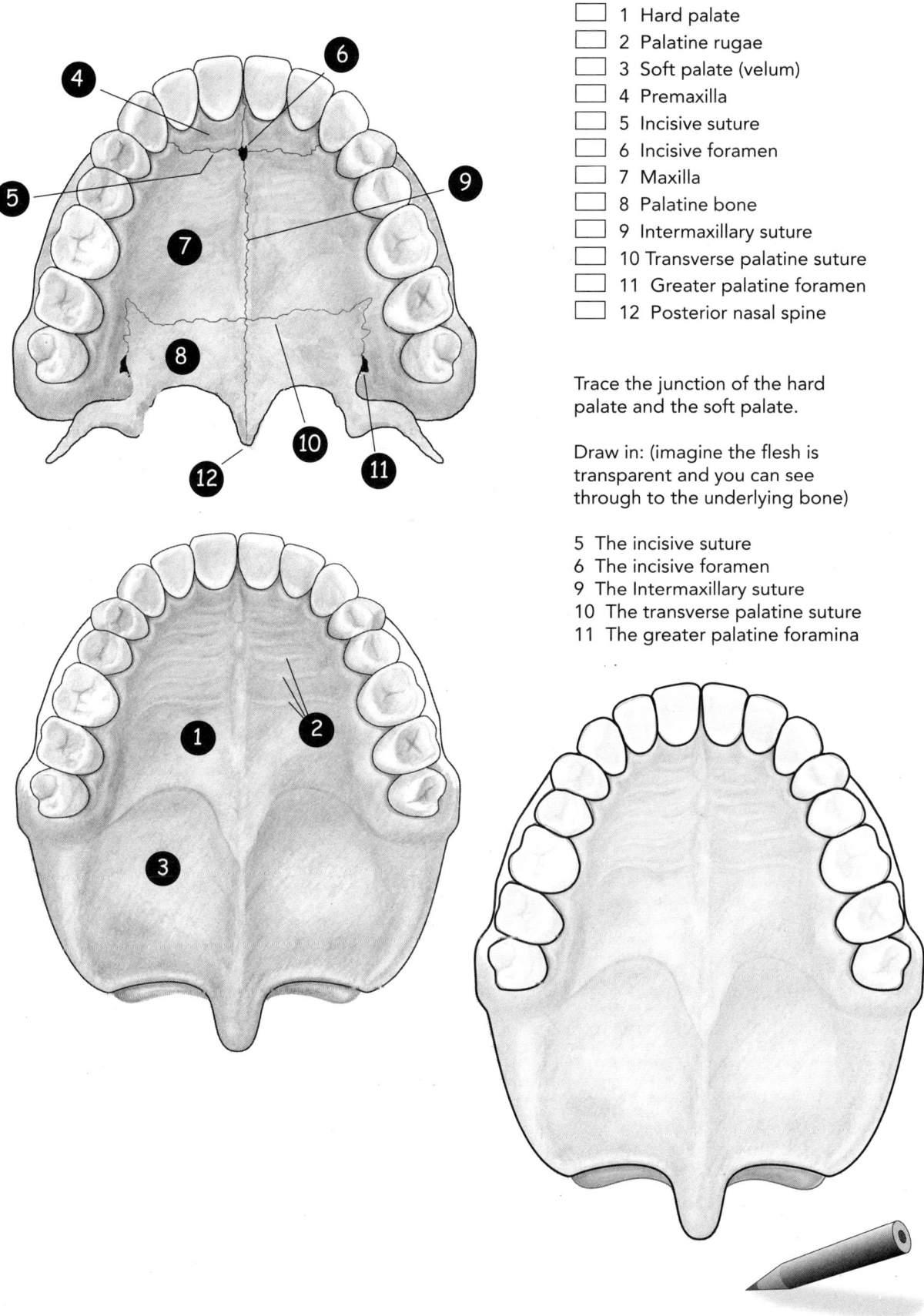

COLOR KEY

☐ 1 Hard palate
☐ 2 Palatine rugae
☐ 3 Soft palate (velum)
☐ 4 Premaxilla
☐ 5 Incisive suture
☐ 6 Incisive foramen
☐ 7 Maxilla
☐ 8 Palatine bone
☐ 9 Intermaxillary suture
☐ 10 Transverse palatine suture
☐ 11 Greater palatine foramen
☐ 12 Posterior nasal spine

Trace the junction of the hard palate and the soft palate.

Draw in: (imagine the flesh is transparent and you can see through to the underlying bone)

5 The incisive suture
6 The incisive foramen
9 The Intermaxillary suture
10 The transverse palatine suture
11 The greater palatine foramina

Muscles of the velum

Five muscles make up the velum; some elevate the velum and others depress it.

Levator veli palatini: arises from the temporal bone and Eustachian tube, and inserts into the palatal aponeurosis. This muscle makes up the bulk of the velum. Its fibers are arranged in a sling which helps to elevate the velum and close the velopharyngeal port.

Musculus uvuli: located on the nasal surface of the velum. It arises from the posterior nasal spine of the palatine bones as well as from the palatal aponeurosis and inserts into the uvula. This muscle bunches up the velum and helps to raise it.

Tensor veli palatini: originates from the base of the medial pterygoid plate of the sphenoid bone. Its fibers run downward and terminate in a tendon. The tendon winds around the hamulus of the medial pterygoid plate and then changes direction from downward to medial. The left and right sides of the tendon merge and expand to become the palatal aponeurosis. Contraction of the tensor veli palatini opens the Eustachian tube, which is normally closed. Opening of the Eustachian tube occurs during swallowing and allows air pressures within and outside the middle ear to equalize.

Palatoglossus: is a muscle of both the velum and the tongue. It arises from the palatal aponeurosis and inserts into the tongue posteriorly on each side. It elevates the dorsum of the tongue and depresses the soft palate. The muscle forms the anterior faucial pillar that is visible when looking in the oral cavity toward the throat. The anterior and posterior faucial pillars mark the posterior boundary of the oral cavity.

Palatopharyngeus: is a muscle of both the velum and the pharynx. It runs from the velum down the length of pharynx and mingles with fibers of the stylopharyngeus muscle. These fibers form the posterior faucial pillars. The palatopharyngeus narrows the pharyngeal cavity and thus helps to guide food into the lower pharynx during swallowing.

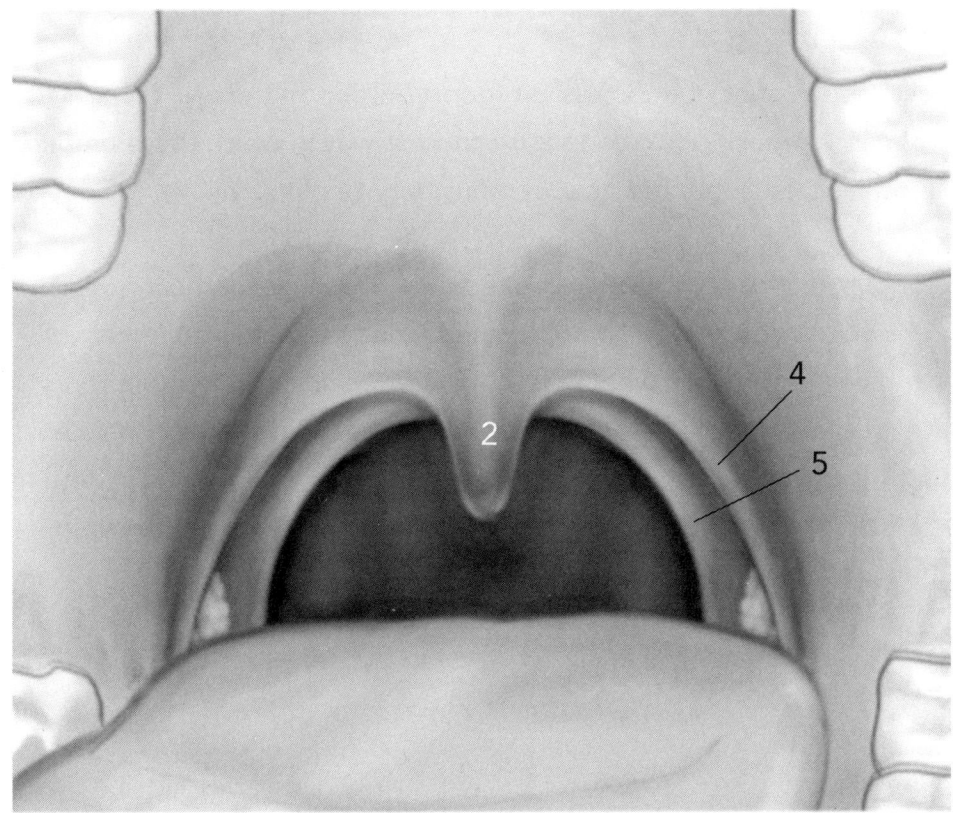

1 Levator veli palatini

2 Musculus uvuli

3 Tensor veli palatini

4 Palatoglossus

5 Palatopharyngeus

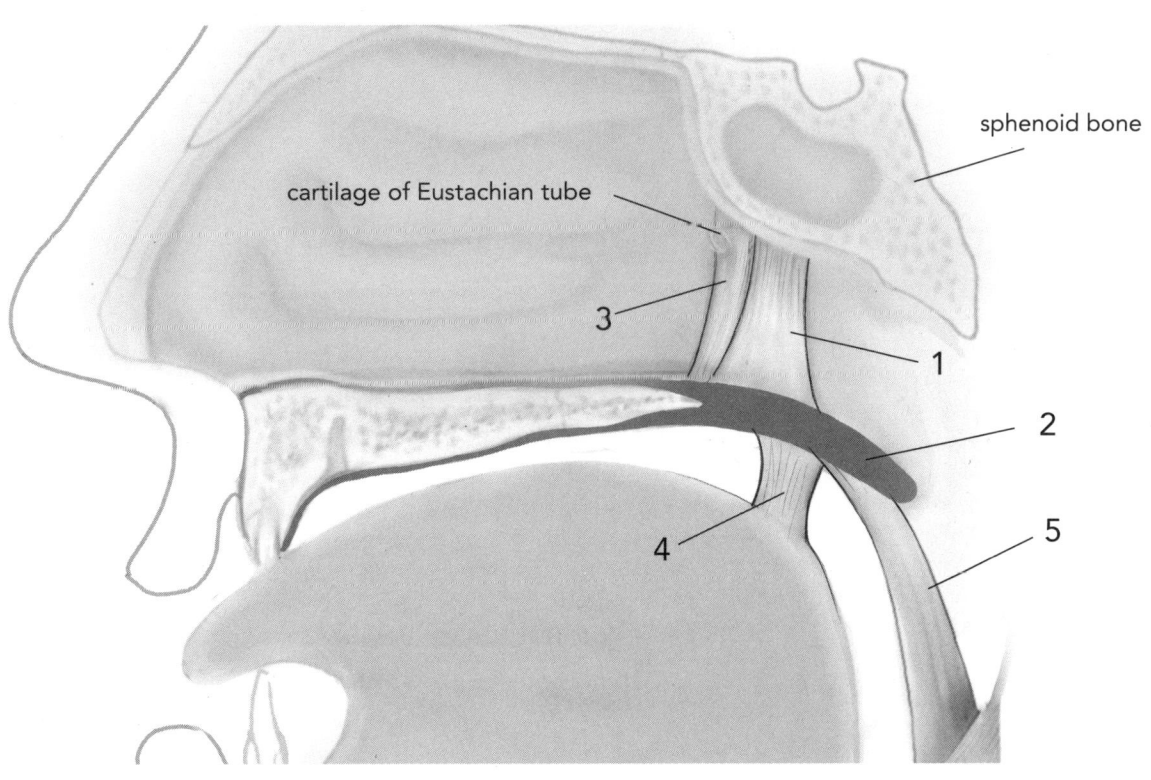

Tongue

The tongue is a large, muscular structure that occupies a good portion of the oral cavity. Because of the number of muscles making up the tongue and the way in which these muscles are intertwined with each other, the tongue has an enormous degree of flexibility and speed in its movements.

Different regions of the tongue can function semi-independently. The anterior most portion of the tongue is the tip, or apex. Just posterior to the tip is the blade. The blade is the part of the tongue that lies below the alveolar ridge when it is at rest. The part of the tongue lying just below the hard palate is called the front, and the part situated beneath the soft palate is called the back. The broad superior surface of the tongue is referred to as the dorsum, and the body refers to the major mass of the tongue. The root of the tongue attaches to the hyoid bone and extends along the pharynx.

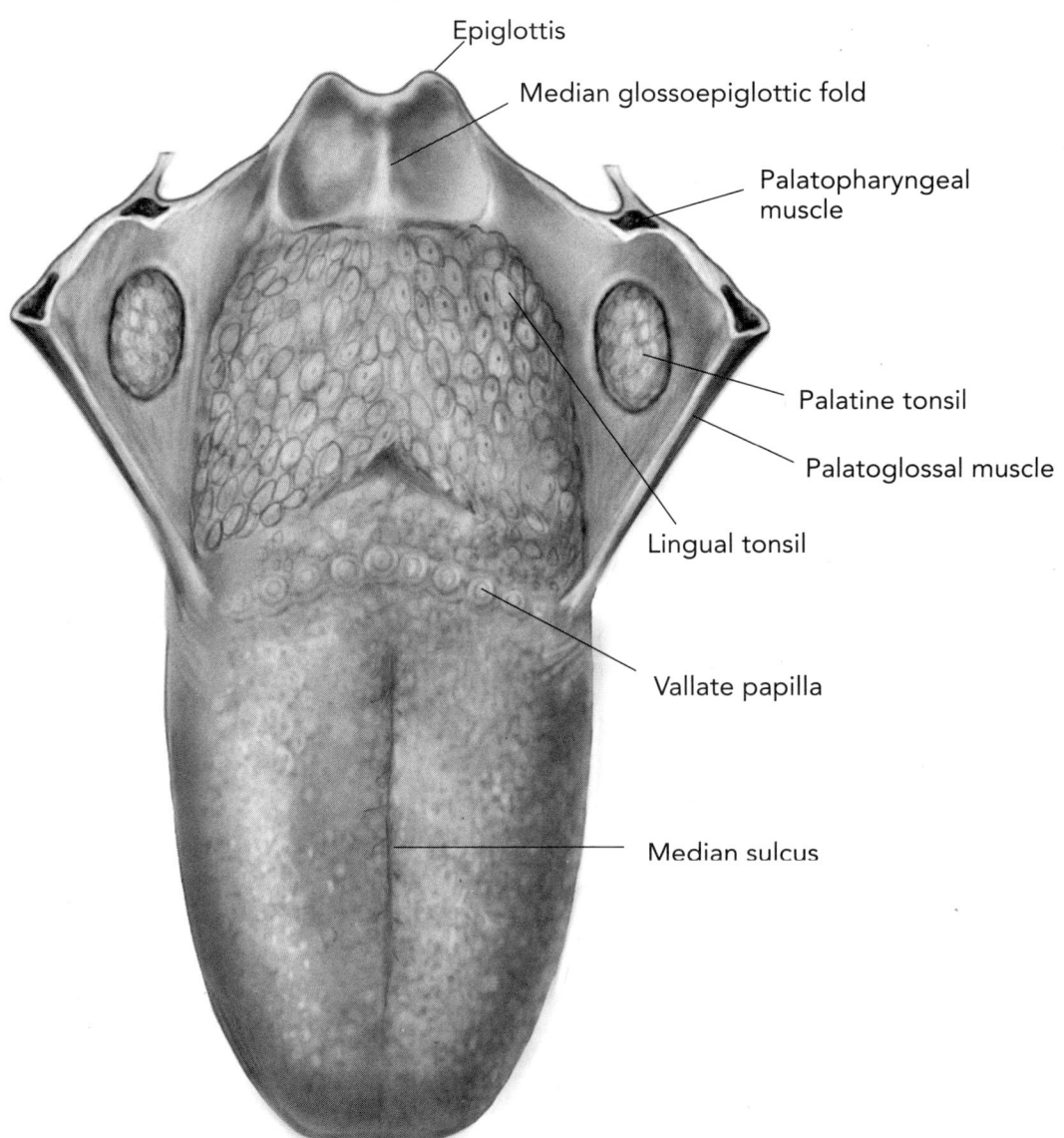

Epiglottis

Median glossoepiglottic fold

Palatopharyngeal muscle

Palatine tonsil

Palatoglossal muscle

Lingual tonsil

Vallate papilla

Median sulcus

The portion of the tongue lying in the pharynx is sometimes called the base, and the portion of the tongue surface within the oral cavity is referred to as the oral tongue. The oral surface makes up about two-thirds of the total surface of the tongue. The other third of the tongue surface lies within the pharynx and is also referred to as the pharyngeal surface.

The tongue is divided into left and right sides by the median sulcus, which provides the origination for some of the muscles. The lingual frenulum (or frenum) is a band of connective tissue joining the inferior tongue and the mandible.

Lingual papillae cover the dorsal side of the tongue.

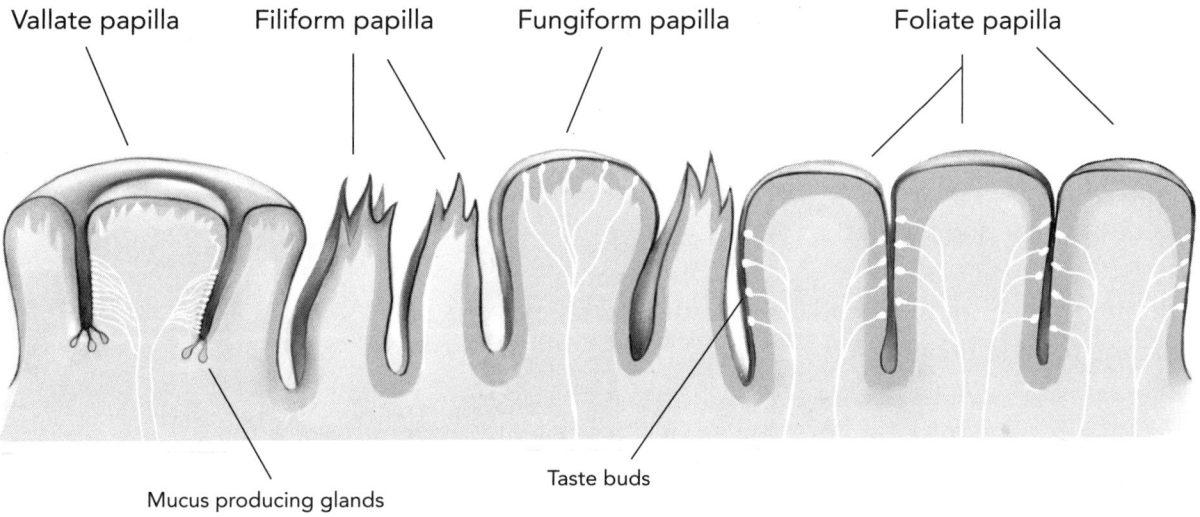

Vallate papilla   Filiform papilla   Fungiform papilla   Foliate papilla

Mucus producing glands

Taste buds

Draw your own: Papillae

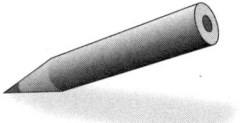

Muscles of the tongue

The tongue is suspended by muscles from the roof of the mouth and the base of the skull. It also attaches to the inner surface of the mandible, the hyoid bone, and the pharynx. The muscles of the tongue are classified according to whether they are intrinsic (both attachments within the tongue itself) or extrinsic (one attachment in the tongue and one in a structure external to the tongue). The intrinsic muscles are involved in adjusting the fine movements of shape and position. The intrinsic muscles are named for the direction that they run within the tongue. The extrinsic muscles move the tongue around to different positions within the oral cavity. The extrinsic muscles move the tongue as a unit and get the tongue into position for articulation. The extrinsic muscles are named for their attachments.

Extrinsic muscles of the tongue

Genioglossus: runs from the inner surface of the mandible to the tip and dorsum of the tongue and to the hyoid bone. It is the largest muscle and forms the main body of the tongue. Contraction of the anterior fibers retracts the tongue; contraction of the posterior fibers pulls the tongue forward.

Hyoglossus: runs from the hyoid bone to the lateral margins of the tongue and pulls the sides of the tongue downward.

Palatoglossus: runs from the front and sides of the palatal aponeurosis to the lateral margins of the tongue posteriorly. It elevates the back of the tongue.

Styloglossus: runs from the styloid process of the temporal bone to the lateral margins of the tongue. It elevates and retracts the tongue.

Intrinsic muscles of the tongue

Superior longitudinal: runs from the hyoid bone and median sulcus of the tongue to the lateral margins and apex of the tongue. This muscle elevates the tongue tip.

Inferior longitudinal: runs from the root of tongue and hyoid bone to the apex of the tongue. It pulls down the tip of the tongue; and retracts the tongue.

Transverse: runs from the median sulcus to the lateral margins of the tongue in the submucous tissue. Contraction pulls the edges of the tongue toward midline to narrow the tongue.

Vertical: runs from the mucous membrane of the tongue dorsum to the lateral and inferior surfaces of the tongue. Contraction pulls the tongue downward.

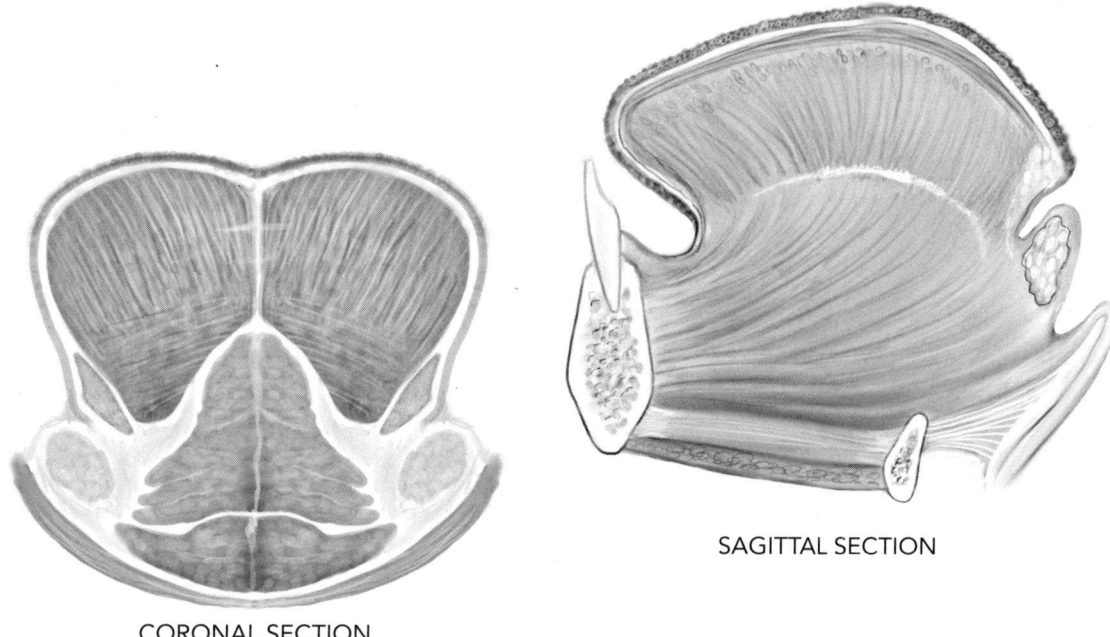

SAGITTAL SECTION

CORONAL SECTION

The above coronal section of the tongue
illustrates how the muscle fibers are intertwined.
Below is a more schematic representation.

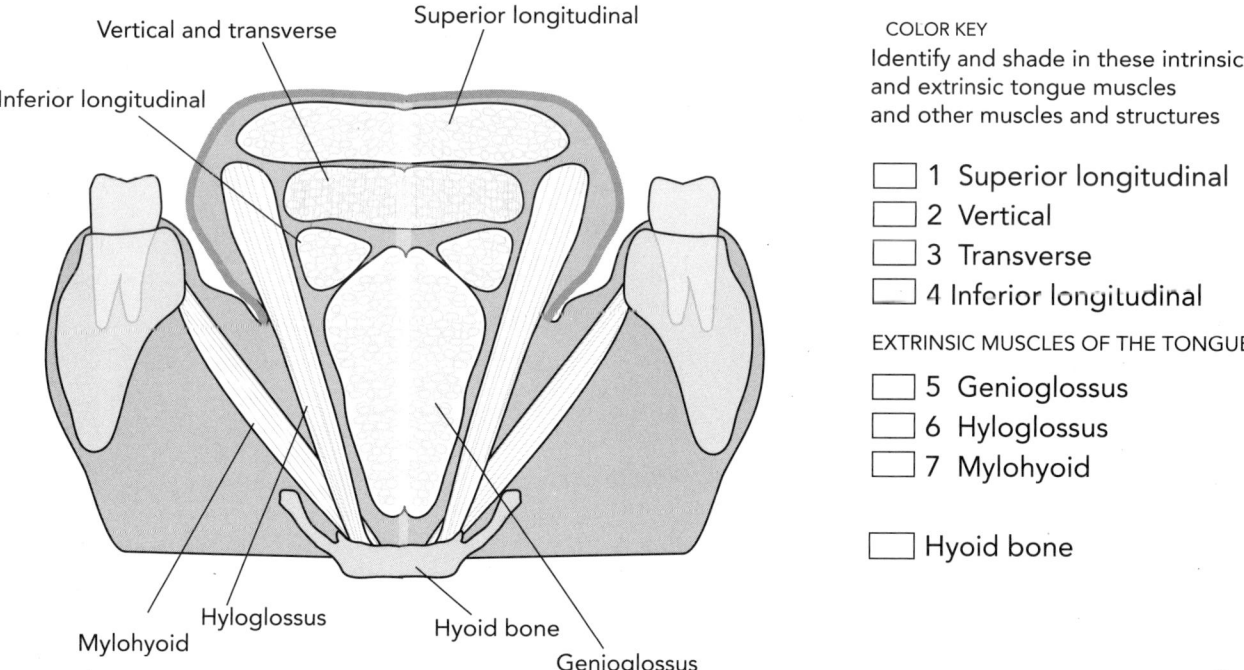

Vertical and transverse

Superior longitudinal

Inferior longitudinal

Mylohyoid

Hyloglossus

Hyoid bone

Genioglossus

Anterior coronal section through the tongue and mandible

COLOR KEY
Identify and shade in these intrinsic
and extrinsic tongue muscles
and other muscles and structures

☐ 1 Superior longitudinal
☐ 2 Vertical
☐ 3 Transverse
☐ 4 Inferior longitudinal

EXTRINSIC MUSCLES OF THE TONGUE

☐ 5 Genioglossus
☐ 6 Hyloglossus
☐ 7 Mylohyoid

☐ Hyoid bone

Extrinsic muscles of the tongue and other structures

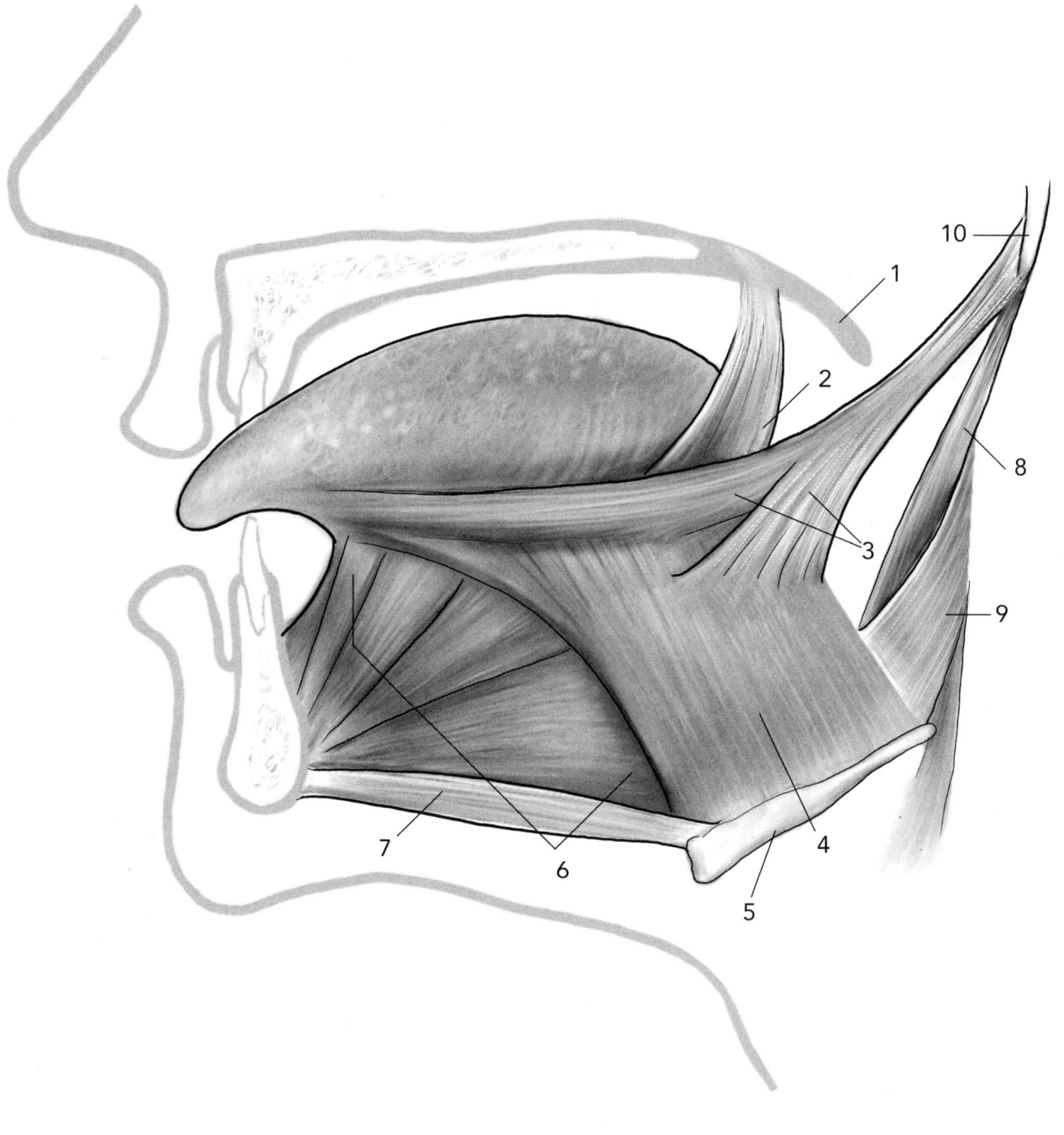

Extrinsic muscles of the tongue and other structures

COLOR KEY

- [ ] 1 Soft palate
- [ ] 2 Palatoglossus
- [ ] 3 Styloglossus
- [ ] 4 Hyoglossus
- [ ] 5 Hyoid bone
- [ ] 6 Genioglossus
- [ ] 7 Geniohyoid
- [ ] 8 Stylohyoid
- [ ] 9 Superior pharyngeal constrictor
- [ ] 10 Styloid process

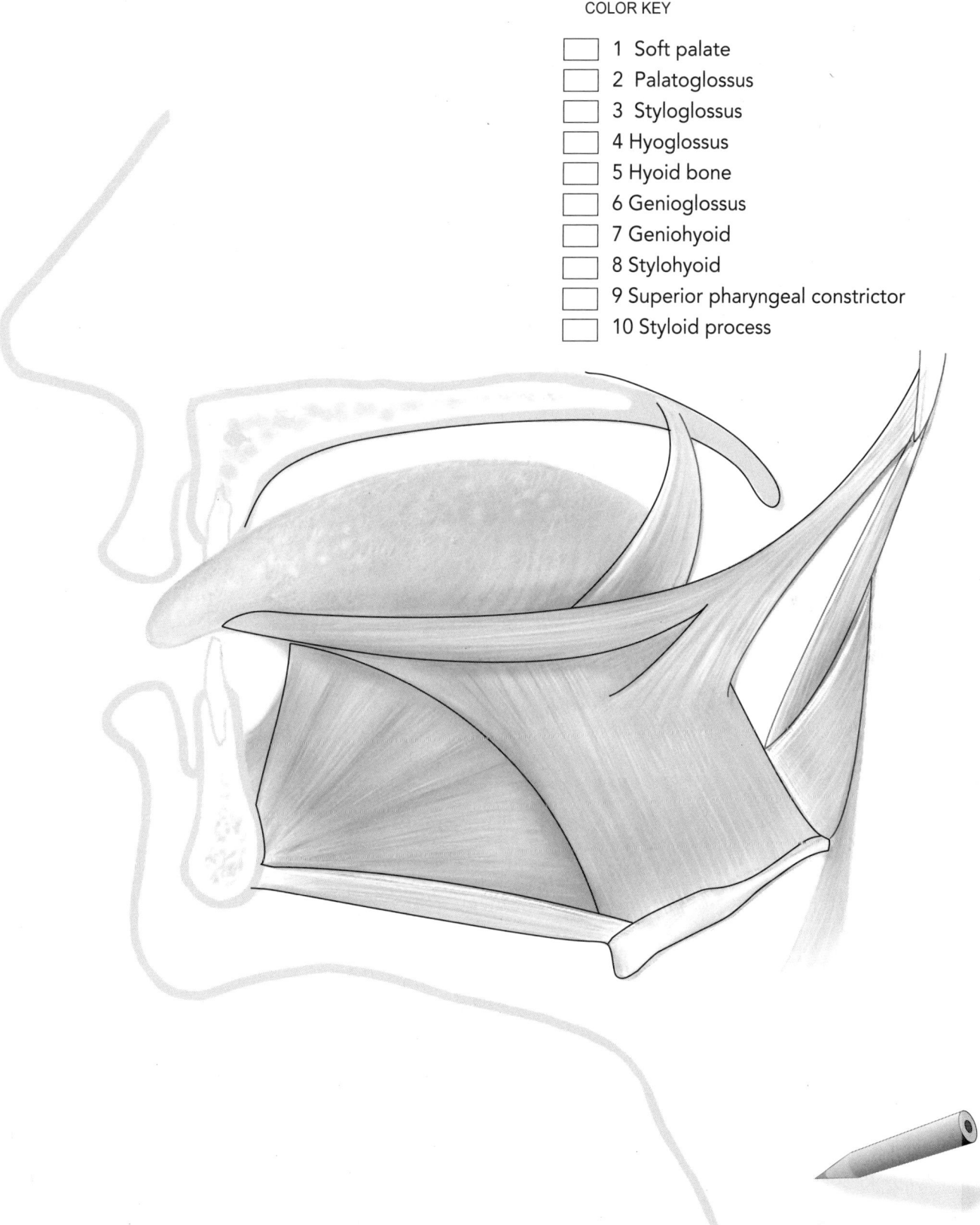

Nasal cavities

The structure of the nasal cavities is surprisingly complex. It is formed by the fusion of many of the bones of the skull. The nose is divided into two cavities by the nasal septum. The inferior, middle, and superior nasal conchae form each side of the nose. The posterior portions of the nasal cavities open into the nasopharynx. The nasal cavities are lined with mucous membrane that has cilia embedded in it. This helps to warm, moisturize, and filter inhaled air. The nasal cavity is important in the resonating of the nasal sounds in English (/m/, /n/, and /ŋ/).

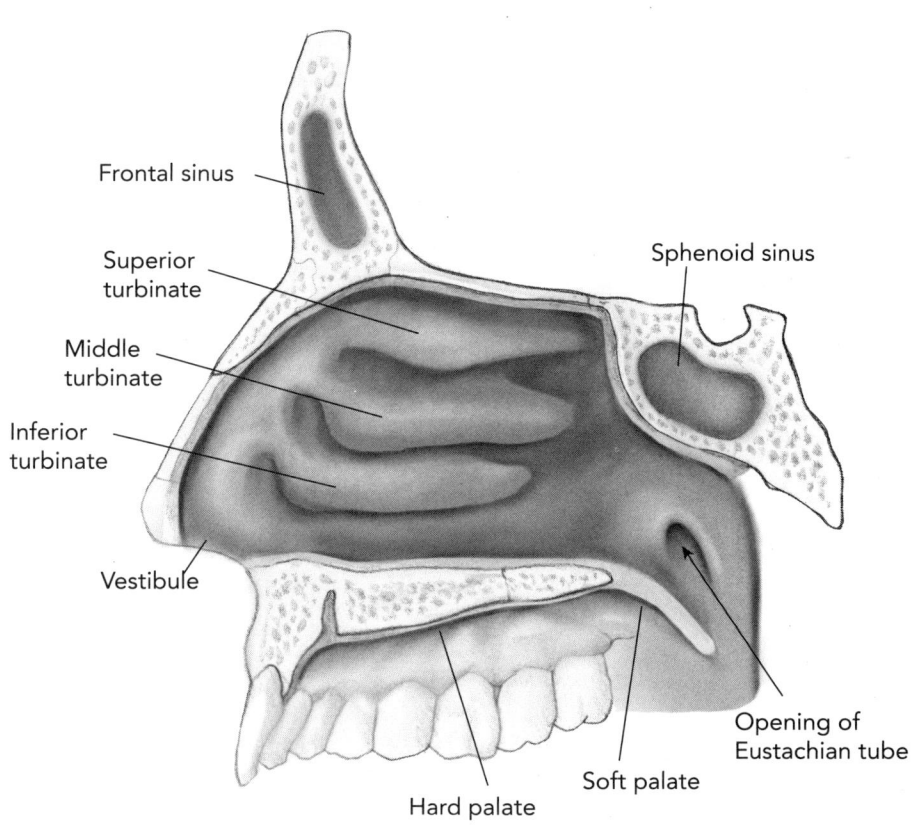

Frontal sinus

Sphenoid sinus

Superior turbinate

Middle turbinate

Inferior turbinate

Vestibule

Opening of Eustachian tube

Soft palate

Hard palate

Draw your own: Muscles of the tongue

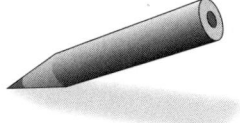

Sinuses, turbinates, bones

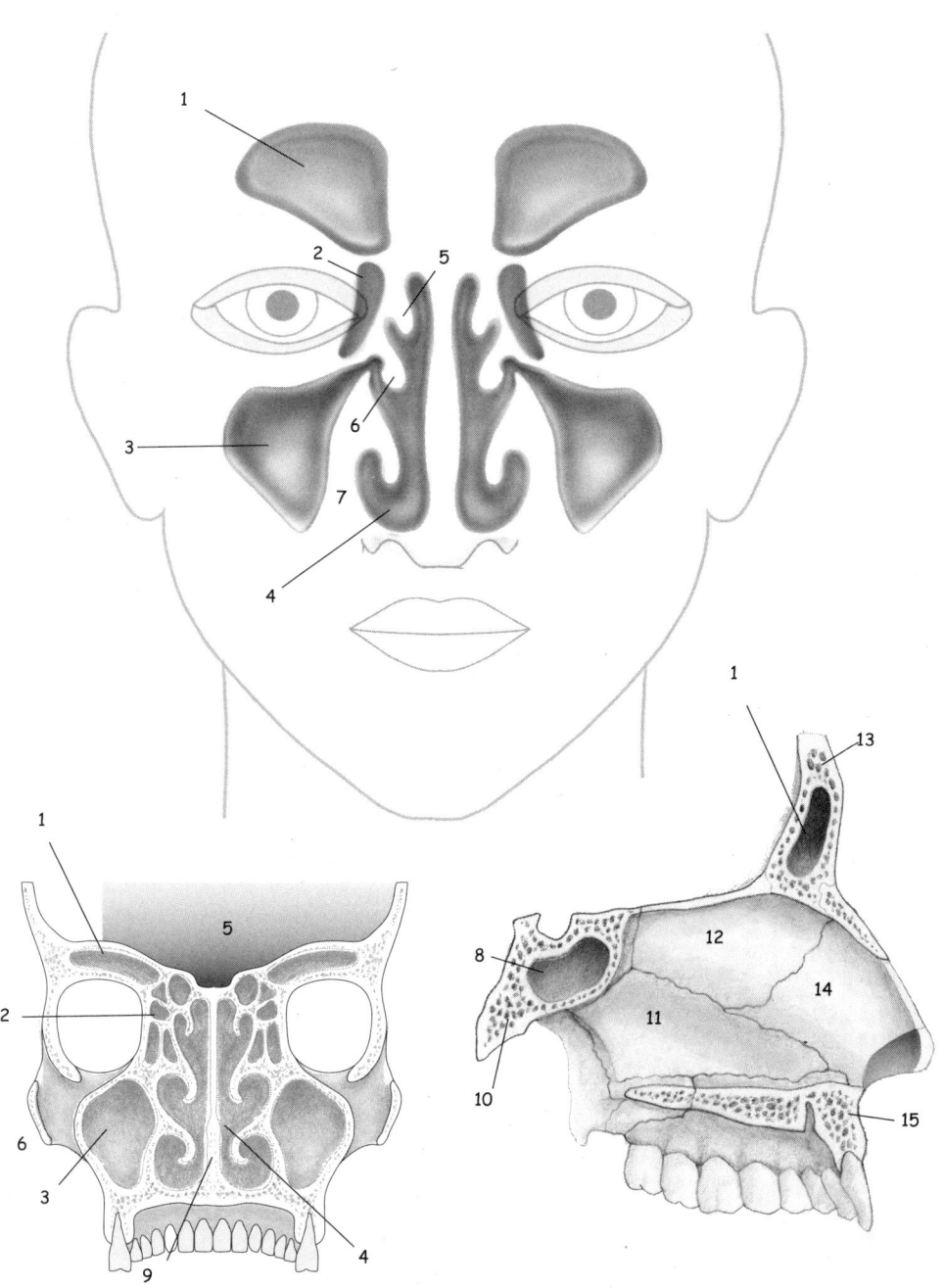

Sinuses, turbinates, bones

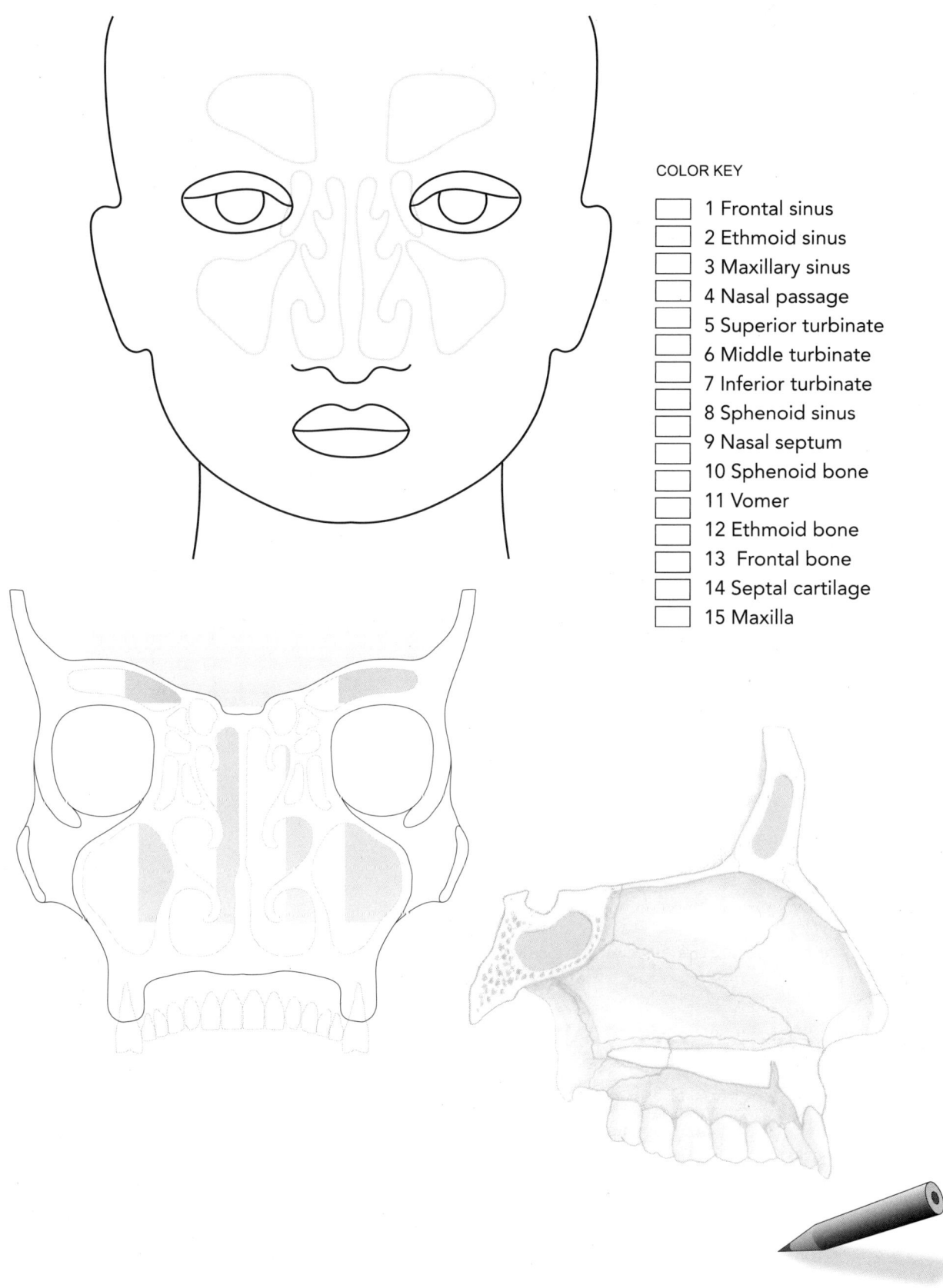

COLOR KEY

- [ ] 1 Frontal sinus
- [ ] 2 Ethmoid sinus
- [ ] 3 Maxillary sinus
- [ ] 4 Nasal passage
- [ ] 5 Superior turbinate
- [ ] 6 Middle turbinate
- [ ] 7 Inferior turbinate
- [ ] 8 Sphenoid sinus
- [ ] 9 Nasal septum
- [ ] 10 Sphenoid bone
- [ ] 11 Vomer
- [ ] 12 Ethmoid bone
- [ ] 13 Frontal bone
- [ ] 14 Septal cartilage
- [ ] 15 Maxilla

TEST YOURSELF: THE ARTICULATORY SYSTEM

MULTIPLE CHOICE: CRANIAL AND FACIAL BONES

1 ____ The foramen magnum is in which bone of the skull?
   a. Temporal
   b. Parietal
   c. Occipital
   d. Frontal

2 ____ Which of these features is present in the sphenoid bone?
   a. Crista galli
   b. Perpendicular plate
   c. Pterygoid processes
   d. Zygomatic processes

3 ____ Besides the maxilla, the hard palate is also composed of the
   a. Ethmoid bone
   b. Palatine bones
   c. Zygomatic bones
   d. Nasal bone

4 ____ Which two bones (or portions of bones) make up the posterior nasal septum?
   a. Perpendicular plate of the ethmoid; vomer
   b. Nasal; vomer
   c. Maxilla, sphenoid
   d. Inferior nasal concha; perpendicular plate of the ethmoid

5 ____ There are ___ cranial bones and ___ facial bones in the adult skull
   a. 6; 10
   b. 8; 14
   c. 12; 12
   d. 4; 8

6 ____ In which cranial bone is the inner ear located?
   a. Frontal
   b. Parietal
   c. Temporal
   d. Occipital

7 ____ Which bone forms the prominence of the cheek?
   a. Maxilla
   b. Nasal
   c. Palatine
   d. Zygomatic

8 _____ Which of the following statements (if any) is NOT true of the palatine bones?

    a. Situated at the posterior edge of the nasal cavity

    b. Form the anterior ¾ of the hard palate

    c. Consist of horizontal and perpendicular plates

    d. All the above are true

9 _____ The mastoid process is found in which bone?

    a. Occipital

    b. Parietal

    c. Temporal

    d. Frontal

10 _____ The coronoid and condylar processes are found on which bone?

    a. Maxilla

    b. Mandible

    c. Zygomatic

    d. Ethmoid

11 _____ Which statement best characterizes the nasal conchae?

    a. Thin, quadrilateral-shaped bone located midsagittally in the nasal cavity

    b. Paired small squarish bones situated at the upper and lateral part of the face

    c. Smallest and most fragile bones of the face

    d. Long, narrow, and curled like a seashell

12 _____ The maxilla

    a. Is composed of two irregularly shaped bones fused at the intermaxillary suture

    b. Contains the zygomatic, frontal, palatine, and alveolar processes

    c. Is fused with the palatine bones at the transverse palatine suture

    d. All the above

13 _____ People have different shaped noses because

    a. The nasal conchae vary among individuals

    b. The vomer is missing in some individuals

    c. The nasal bones vary in size and shape

    d. All the above

14 _____ The temporomandibular joint is formed between the

    a. Condylar process and temporal bone

    b. Coronoid process and temporal bone

    c. Condylar process and coronoid process

    d. None of the above

TRUE/FALSE: CRANIAL AND FACIAL BONES

1 _____   The vocal tract is a hollow muscular tube consisting of the larynx, pharynx, and oral cavity.

2 _____   The cranium is formed by 8 bones that are held together by synovial joints.

3 _____   The lower front of the skull is made up of 14 bones.

4 _____   The frontal bone forms the front portion of the skull above the eyes and includes the frontal sinuses.

5 _____   The frontal, sphenoid, ethmoid, and occipital bones are the only unpaired bones of the skull.

6 _____   All the bones of the skull except the mandible are joined by sutures and are therefore immovable.

7 _____   The two parietal bones form the sides and roof of the cranium.

8 _____   The mastoid process of the temporal bone protects the inner ear.

9 _____   The temporal bone contains the foramen magnum.

10 _____   The bone located at the back and lower part of the cranium is the occipital.

11 _____   The ethmoid bone consists of the perpendicular plate, the crista galli, the labyrinths, and the cribriform plate.

12 _____   The medial pterygoid plate of the sphenoid bone ends in the hamulus.

13 _____   Each ramus of the mandible ends in an anterior projection called the condyle, and a posterior projection called the coronoid process.

14 _____   The mandible is attached to the skull by a joint between the condylar process and the temporal bone.

15 _____   The mandible contains an alveolar process which holds the bottom teeth in place.

16 _____   The upper jaw is composed of two irregularly shaped bones that are fused at the intermaxillary suture.

17 _____   The two horizontal plates of the palatine bones form the anterior 1/4th of the hard palate.

18 _____   The palatine bones are fused with the maxilla at the transverse palatine suture.

19 _____   The vomer forms the posterior part of the nasal septum.

20 _____The nasal bones help to direct airflow, as well as humidify, warm, and filter air inhaled.

21 _____   The nasal turbinates vary in size and shape between individuals.

22 _____The zygomatic bones form the prominences of the cheek.

MATCHING   CRANIAL AND FACIAL BONES

Parietal	1 Forms the front portion of the skull above the eyes
Maxilla	2 Smallest bone of the face
Nasal	3 Long, narrow, and curled
Temporal	4 Form the prominences of the cheek
Mandible	5 Forms the back and lower part of the cranium
Ethmoid	6 Form the sides and roof of the cranium
Vomer	7 Forms the upper jaw
Lacrimal	8 Forms the roof of the nasal cavity
Frontal	9 Composed of the body and two rami
Sphenoid	10 Forms the posterior part of the nasal septum
Palatine	11 Consists of horizontal and perpendicular plates
Zygomatic	12 Form the bridge of the nose
Occipital	13 Contains the petrous portion
Turbinates	14 Contains the pterygoid processes

FILL IN THE BLANK   CRANIAL AND FACIAL BONES

1.   The _____ bone forms the prominences of the cheek.

2.   The largest immovable facial bone is the _____ .

3.   The _____   _____ bone is shaped like a butterfly.

4.   The _____   _____ bones make up the sides and roof of the cranium.

5.   The _____ makes up the posterior portion of the bony nasal septum.

6.   The _____ is the upper part of the cribriform plate.

7.   The _____ bone forms the posterior ¼ of the hard palate.

8.   The _____ bone separates the nasal cavity from the brain.

9.   The _____ separate each nasal cavity into four grooves.

10. The _____ protects the inner ear.

MULTIPLE CHOICE   FACIAL MUSCLES

1 _____   The muscle that moves the scalp and lifts the eyebrows is the
    a. Risorius
    b. Frontalis
    c. Platysma
    d. Temporalis

2 _____   The circular muscle surrounding the mouth is the
    a. Mentalis
    b. Levator anguli oris
    c. Orbicularis oris
    d. Auricularis anterior

3 _____   The lateral pterygoid muscle
    a. Is attached to the coronoid process and elevates the chin
    b. Is attached to the coronoid process and depresses the chin
    c. Is attached to the condylar process and elevates the chin
    d. Is attached to the condylar process and depresses the chin

4 _____   The muscle that closes the eyelids is the
    a. Orbicularis oculi
    b. Procerus
    c. Frontalis
    d. Auricularis posterior

5 _____   The risorius
    a. Elevates the upper lip
    b. Pulls the lower lip downward
    c. Stretches the mouth laterally
    d. Wrinkles the upper lip

6 _____   The levator labii superioris alaeque nasi
    a. Wrinkles the root of the nose
    b. Flares the nostrils
    c. Narrows the nose
    d. All the above

7 _____   Most of the muscles of the face
    a. Attach to the facial bones
    b. Are not very strong
    c. Are subcutaneous
    d. None of the above

8 _____ The muscle that produces a grinding motion of the jaw is the
  a. Medial pterygoid
  b. Lateral pterygoid
  c. Temporalis
  d. Masseter

9 _____ The muscles of the ear
  a. Also play a role in mastication
  b. Allow some individuals to hear better than others
  c. Allow some animals to adjust the direction of the pinna
  d. All the above

10 _____ The depressor anguli oris
  a. Is the most active of the facial muscles
  b. Protrudes the lower lip
  c. Produces a smile when activated
  d. Pulls the corner of the mouth downward

TRUE/FALSE   FACIAL MUSCLES

1 _____ Many facial muscles originate from the skull.

2 _____ The frontalis muscle produces winking and blinking.

3 _____ The orbicularis oculi is a circular muscle surrounding the upper and lower lips.

4 _____ The orbicularis oris contains the fibers of many other facial muscles.

5 _____ The anguli oris muscles pull the corner of the mouth upward or downward.

6 _____ The buccinator extends from the zygomatic arch to the corners of the mouth.

7 _____ The lower lip is protruded by contraction of the mentalis muscle.

8 _____ The masseter runs from the zygomatic arch and inserts into the condylar process of the mandible.

9 _____ The risorius stretches the mouth laterally.

10 _____ Fibers from the platysma blend with fibers around the angle of the mouth and the upper and lower lip.

11 _____ The auricularis muscles are subdivided into superficial and deep portions.

12 _____ Contraction of the lateral pterygoid can be unilateral or bilateral.

13 _____ The temporalis muscle raises the eyebrows.

FILL IN THE BLANK   FACIAL MUSCLES

1.   The _____ surrounds the outer ear and draws it forward and upward.

2.   The posterior fibers of the _____ muscle retract the mandible.

3.   The _____ elevates the upper lip.

4.   The _____ pulls the lower lip downward.

5.   The _____ allows us to smile.

6.   The main muscle of the lip is the _____.

7.   The _____ runs from the temporal bone and inserts into the

coronoid process and ramus of the mandible.

8.   Side-to-side movements of the jaw are produced by the _____.

9.   The _____ draws the outer ear backward.

10.   The muscle that protrudes the lower lip is the _____.

11.   The _____ allows the cheeks to draw inwards.

12.   The upper lip is elevated by the _____.

13.   Contraction of the _____ can be bilateral or unilateral.

14.   The _____ elevates the mandible.

Name the structures

1_____

2_____

3_____

4_____

5_____

Place the appropriate number next to each muscle

_____Levator anguli oris

_____Levator
labii superioris

_____Buccinator

_____Masseter

_____ Depressor
anguli oris

_____ Levator labii
superioris alaeque nasi

_____ Zygomaticus minor

_____ Orbicularis oris

_____ Zygomaticus major

_____ Mentalis

_____ Temporalis

_____ Depressor
labii inferioris

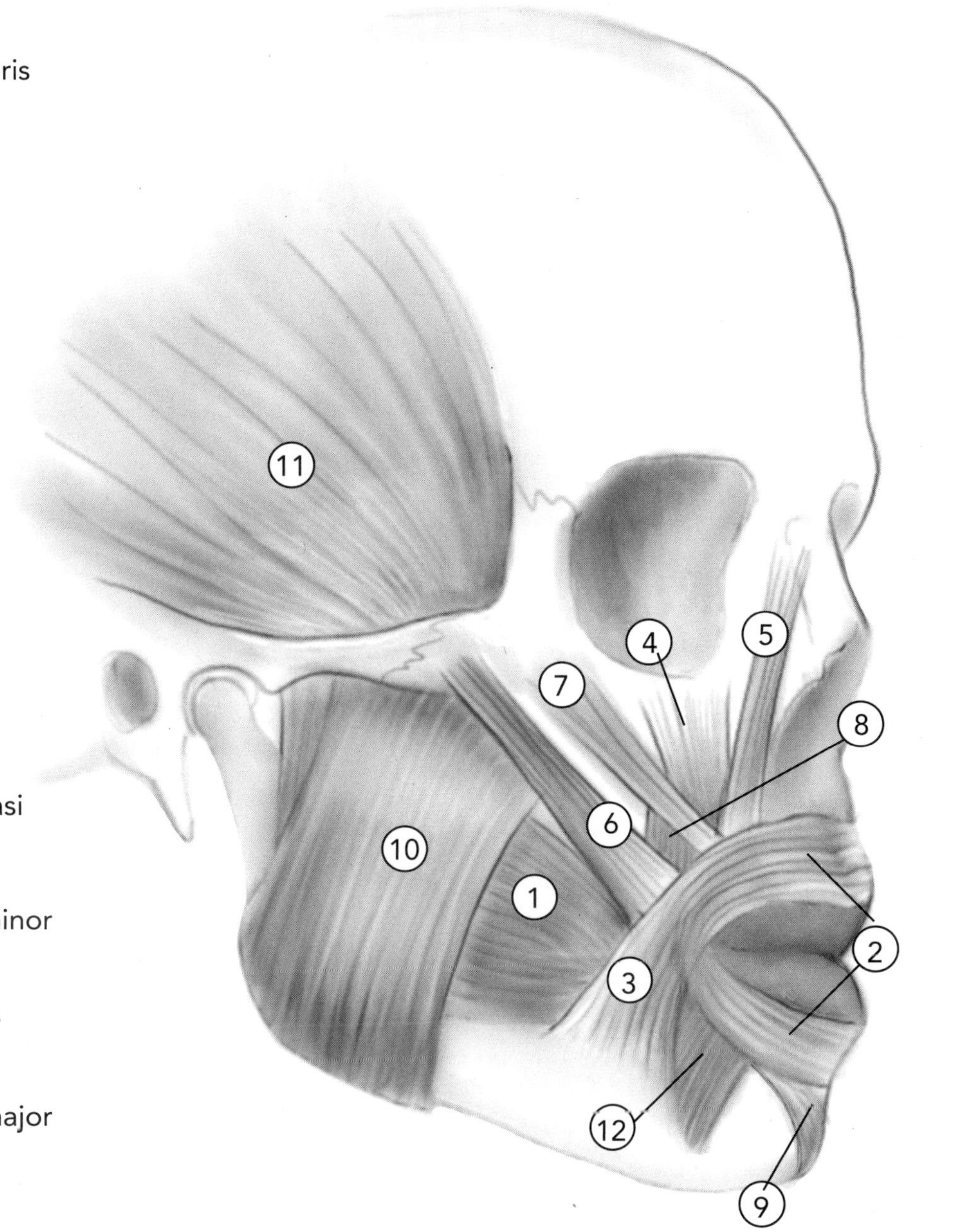

MULTIPLE CHOICE   PHARYNX

1 _____   The pharynx
    a. Is narrower at its top end and wider at its bottom end
    b. Is descriptively divided into naso-, oro-, and laryngopharyngeal portions
    c. Is continuous with the trachea
    d. All of the above

2 _____   Which muscle originates from the sides of the thyroid cartilage and wraps around the lower to midregions of the pharynx?
    a. Stylopharyngeus
    b. Cricopharyngeus
    c. Inferior pharyngeal constrictor
    d. Palatopharyngeus

3 _____   The cricopharyngeus muscle
    a. Arises from the cricoid cartilage
    b. Forms a ring around the superior opening of the esophagus
    c. Relaxes during swallowing
    d. All the above

4 _____   Which of the following statements (if any) is NOT true of the stylopharyngeus muscle?
    a. Originates from the styloid process of the temporal bone
    b. Some fibers insert into the thyroid cartilage
    c. Helps to elevate and open the pharynx during swallowing
    d. All the above statements are true

TRUE/FALSE   PHARYNX

1 _____   The laryngopharynx leads into the trachea.

2 _____   The Eustachian tube joins the nasopharynx and the middle ear.

3 _____   The superior constrictor is the largest and strongest of the pharyngeal constrictors.

4 _____   The middle constrictor originates from the hyoid bone.

5 _____   The cricopharyngeus is located at the lower margin of the inferior constrictor.

6 _____   The stylopharyngeus arises from the cartilaginous portion of the Eustachian tube.

7 _____   The salpingopharyngeus forms the posterior faucial pillars.

8 _____   The palatopharyngeus arises from the palatal aponeurosis and the hard palate.

FILL IN THE BLANK   PHARYNX

1.   The muscle that forms the posterior faucial pillar is the _____.

2.   The largest and strongest of the constrictors is the _____.

3.   The topmost portion of the pharynx is formed by the _____ muscle.

4.   The _____ muscle remains contracted during rest and relaxes during swallowing.

5.   The muscle that runs inferiorly along the side of the pharynx between the superior and

middle pharyngeal constrictors is the _____.

6.   Fibers of the _____ muscle blend with the fibers of the

palatopharyngeus muscle.

7.   Contraction of the _____ muscle pulls the larynx and the pharynx

superiorly, anteriorly, and medially.

MATCHING: PHARYNX

	Cricopharyngeus	1 Arises from the cartilaginous portion of the Eustachian tube
	Palatopharyngeus	2 Arises from the styloid process of the temporal bone
	Salpingopharyngeus	3 Located at the lower margin of the inferior constrictor
	Inferior pharyngeal constrictor	4 Arises from the hyoid bone
	Stylopharyngeus	5 Arises from the sides of the thyroid cartilage
	Superior pharyngeal constrictor	6 Arises from the palatal aponeurosis
	Middle pharyngeal constrictor	7 Has multiple origins in and around the soft palate

MULTIPLE CHOICE   TEETH, TONGUE, PALATE

1 _____   The flap of tissue connecting the inner surface of the upper lip to the midline of the
alveolar region in the upper jaw is called the
a. Superior alveolar flap
b. Superior labial frenulum
c. Superior dental occlusion
d. None of the above

2 _____   Which of the following statements (if any) is NOT true of human teeth?
a. Types of teeth include incisors, canines, premolars, and molars
b. Teeth are important in both mastication and speech
c. Both children and adults have 32 teeth
d. All the above are true

3 _____   In a normal occlusal relationship
a. The first permanent molar of the upper jaw is positioned one half-tooth behind
the first permanent molar of the lower jaw
b. The first permanent molar of the upper jaw is positioned one half-tooth in front
of the first permanent molar of the lower jaw
c. The first permanent molars of the upper and lower jaw are aligned exactly with each other
d. None of the above

4 _____   When the first molar of the lower jaw is posterior to the normal position this is called
a. Neutroclusion
b. Distoclusion
c. Mesioclusion
d. Alliocclusion

5 _____   When the first molar of the lower jaw is anterior to the normal position this is called
a. Neutroclusion
b. Distoclusion
c. Mesioclusion
d. Alliocclusion

6 _____   The palatine processes of the maxilla articulate at the
a. Transverse palatine suture
b. Intermaxillary suture
c. Alveolar ridge
d. Palatal aponeurosis

7 _____   The posterior one-quarter of the hard palate is formed by the
a. Palatine processes of the maxilla
b. Alveolar processes of the maxilla
c. Palatine bones of the skull
d. Temporal processes of the zygomatic bone

8 _____   The velopharyngeal passageway
      a. Can be opened or closed by movement of the velum
      b. Can form a barrier between the oral and nasal cavities
      c. Can allow air and sound waves to enter the nasal cavities
      d. All the above

9 _____   The muscle which has a sling like arrangement of fibers and is instrumental in elevating the velum is the
      a. Tensor veli palatini
      b. Musculus uvuli
      c. Levator veli palatini
      d. None of the above

10 _____   Which of the following statements (if any) is not true of the musculus uvuli?
      a. Right and left sides merge to become the palatal aponeurosis
      b. Located on the nasal surface of the velum
      c. Bunches up the velum and helps to raise it
      d. All the above are true

11 _____   Contraction of the tensor veli palatini
      a. Elevates the velum
      b. Depresses the velum
      c. Opens the Eustachian tube
      d. None of the above

12 _____   The muscle that functions to elevate the dorsum of the tongue and to depress the soft palate is the
      a. Palatopharyngeus
      b. Palatoglossus
      c. Levator veli palatini
      d. Tensor veli palatini

13 _____   The anterior most portion of the tongue is the
      a. Blade
      b. Dorsum
      c. Front
      d. Apex

14 _____   The dorsum of the tongue refers to the
      a. Superior surface of the tongue
      b. Major mass of the tongue
      c. Base of the tongue
      d. Back of the tongue

15 _____   The oral surface makes up about _____ of the total surface of the tongue
     a. One third
     b. Two thirds
     c. One quarter
     d. One half

16 _____   The muscle that pulls the edges of the tongue toward midline is the
     a. Vertical
     b. Superior longitudinal
     c. Hyoglossus
     d. None of the above

17 _____   The inferior longitudinal muscle
     a. Pulls the tongue forward
     b. Narrows the tongue
     c. Elevates the tongue tip
     d. Depresses the tongue tip

18 _____   The muscle that elevates and retracts the tongue is the
     a. Palatoglossus
     b. Styloglossus
     c. Genioglossus
     d. Hyoglossus

19 _____   The tongue is divided into right and left sides by the
     a. Median sulcus
     b. Lingual frenulum
     c. Lateral sulcus
     d. Labial frenulum

20 _____The nasal cavities
     a. Are formed by the fusion of many bones of the skull
     b. Are divided into left and right by the nasal septum
     c. Contain the turbinates which form each side of the nose
     d. All the above

TRUE/FALSE   TEETH, TONGUE, PALATE

1 _____   The floor of the oral cavity is formed by the tongue.

2 _____   The inner surface of the upper lip connects to the midline of the alveolar

region by a small flap of tissue called the lingual frenulum.

3 _____   Human teeth include incisors, canines, premolars, and molars.

4 _____   In a normal occlusal relationship, the first permanent molar of the upper jaw is positioned

one half-tooth behind the first permanent molar of the lower jaw.

5 _____   In mesioclusion the first molar of the lower jaw is posterior to the normal position.

6 _____   The posterior one-quarter of the hard palate is formed by the palatine bones of the skull.

7 _____   The palatine bones and palatine processes meet at the intermaxillary suture.

8 _____   When the velopharyngeal passageway is open air is forced to exit through the oral cavity.

9 _____   The tensor veli palatini muscle elevates the velum to close the velopharyngeal passageway.

10 _____   The palatoglossus is a muscle of both the velum and the tongue.

11 _____   The levator veli palatini muscle inserts into the palatal aponeurosis.

12 _____   The palatopharyngeus muscle narrows the pharyngeal cavity.

13 _____   The pharyngeal surface of the tongue makes up two thirds of the tongue body.

14 _____   The tongue is divided into anterior and posterior portions by the median sulcus.

15 _____   The intrinsic muscles of the tongue are involved in adjusting the fine movements of shape and position.

16 _____   The inferior longitudinal muscle pulls the tip of the tongue upward.

17 _____   The genioglossus muscle pulls the tip of the tongue downward.

18 _____   The hyoglossus muscle runs from the hyoid bone to the lateral margins of the tongue.

19 _____   The vertical muscle pulls the tongue downward.

20 _____The styloglossus muscle narrows the tongue.

FILL-IN THE BLANK   TEETH, TONGUE, PALATE

1   _____ is when the first molar of the lower jaw is anterior to the normal position.

2   _____ is when the first molar of the lower jaw is posterior to the normal position.

3   The palatine processes of the maxilla articulate at the _____.

4   The posterior one-quarter of the hard palate is formed by the _____.

5   The muscle that bunches up the velum and helps to raise it is the _____.

6   The _____ is the muscle that opens the Eustachian tube.

7   The _____ elevates the velum.

8   The _____ and _____ form the

        anterior and posterior faucial pillars.

9   The muscle that elevates the dorsum of the tongue and depresses the soft palate

        is the _____.

10   The _____ is the part of the tongue that lies below the

        alveolar ridge when it is at rest.

11   The superior surface of the tongue is referred to as the _____.

12   The root of the tongue attaches to the _____.

13   The _____ divides the tongue into right and left sides.

14   The muscle that pulls down the tip of the tongue is the _____.

15   The _____ muscle elevates the back of the tongue.

16   The _____ muscle runs from the median septum to lateral

        margins in the submucous tissue of the tongue.

17   Contraction of the _____ muscle pulls the tongue downward.

18   The _____ muscle elevates and retracts the tongue.

19   The _____ muscle pulls the sides of the tongue downward.

20   Contraction of the _____ muscle can either

        retract or pull the tongue forward depending on which fibers are activated .

MATCHING: TEETH, TONGUE, PALATE

Transverse muscles	1 Pulls tongue downward
Neutroclusion	2 Large flat tendon connecting the hard and soft palates
Intermaxillary suture	3 Opens the Eustachian tube
Genioglossus muscle	4 Narrows the tongue
Tensor veli palatini muscle	5 Bunches up the velum and helps to raise it
Superior longitudinal muscle	6 First permanent molar of the upper jaw is positioned one half-tooth behind the first permanent molar of the lower jaw
Palatoglossus muscle	7 Palatine processes of the maxilla join at the midline
Distoclusion	8 Main body of the tongue
Palatal aponeurosis	9 Forms the anterior faucial pillars
Vertical muscle	10 Pulls the sides of the tongue downward
Transverse palatine suture	11 First molar of the lower jaw is posterior to the normal position
Levator veli palatini muscle	12 Elevates tongue tip
Mesioclusion	13 First molar of the lower jaw is anterior to normal position
Inferior longitudinal muscle	14 Meeting of the palatine bones and palatine processes
Musculus uvuli	15 Elevates the velum to close the velopharyngeal port
Hyoglossus muscle	16 Forms the posterior faucial pillars
Palatopharyngeus muscle	17 Pulls down tongue tip
Styloglossus muscle	18 Elevates and retracts the tongue

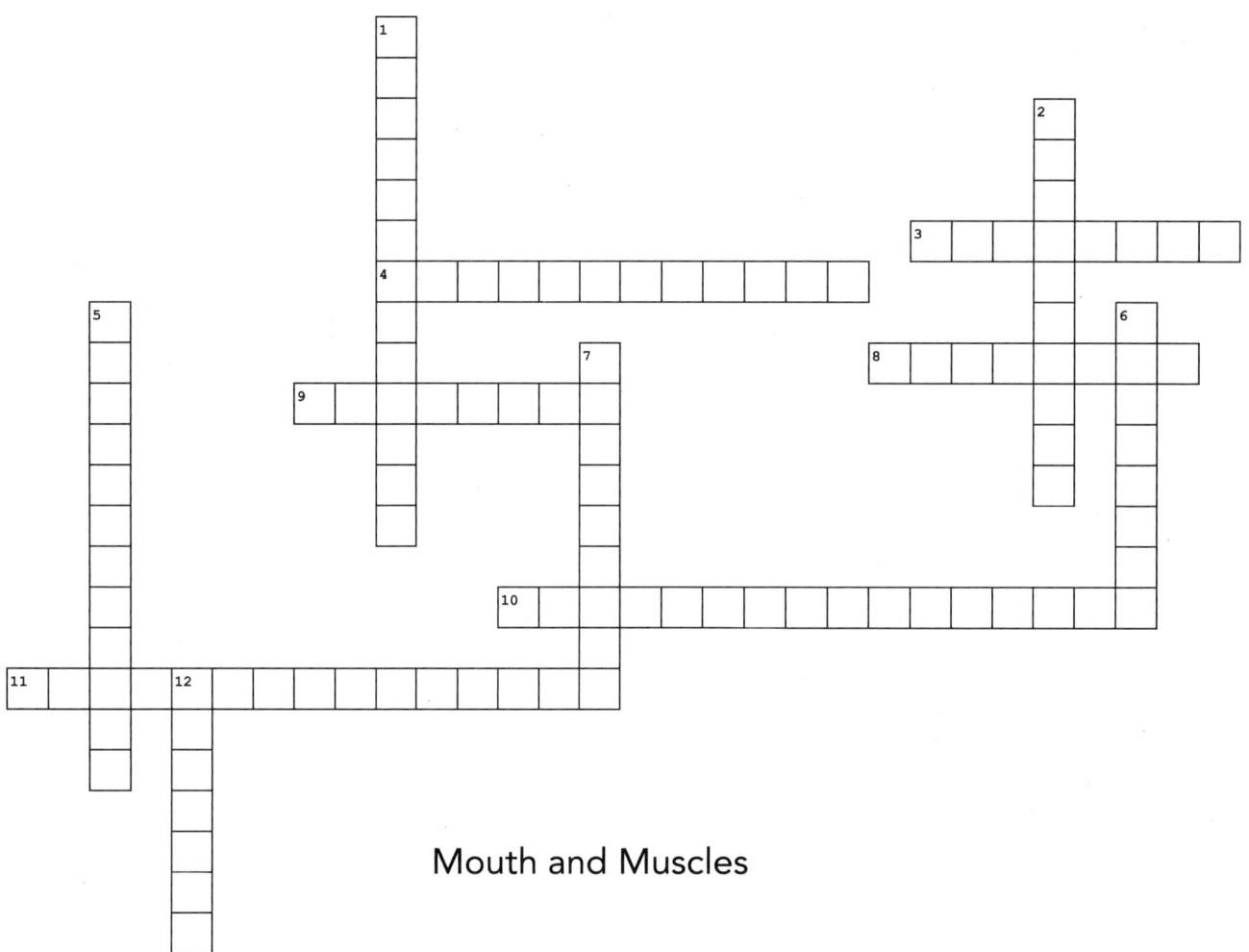

Mouth and Muscles

Across

3. Nose wrinkler
4. You need these pharyngeal muscles to swallow your food
8. Sounds like an intelligent muscle
9. Elevates and protrudes the mandible
10. Muscle forms the posterior faucial pillar
11. Forms a ring of muscle around the top opening of the esophagus

Down

1. Normal relationship between upper and lower jaws
2. Food will escape from your molars without this muscle
5. Synonym for Class III occlusion
6. Can't smile without this muscle
7. Muscle that elevates the eyebrows and forehead
12. This condition occurs when the mandible is retracted

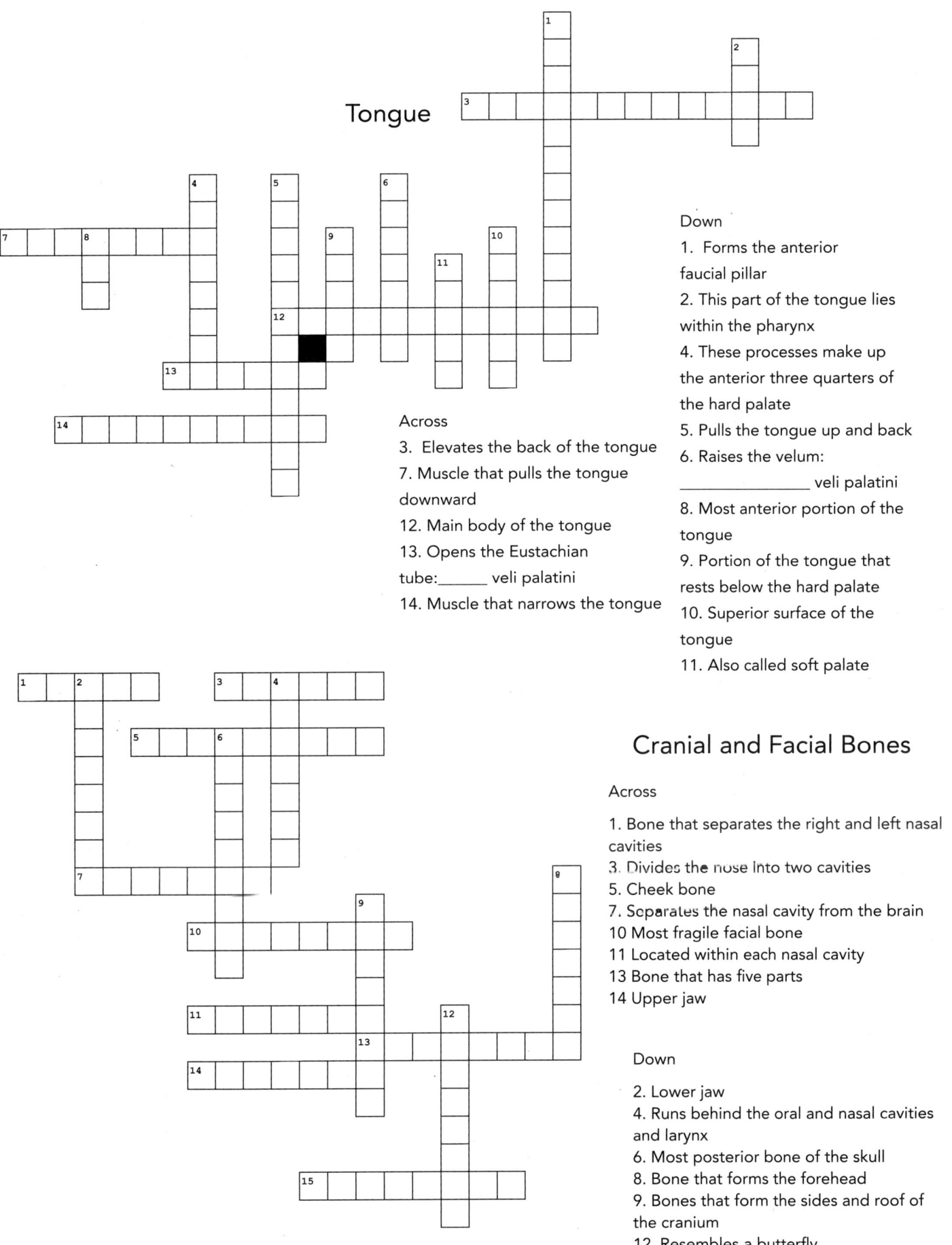

Tongue

Down

1. Forms the anterior faucial pillar
2. This part of the tongue lies within the pharynx
4. These processes make up the anterior three quarters of the hard palate
5. Pulls the tongue up and back
6. Raises the velum: _____ veli palatini
8. Most anterior portion of the tongue
9. Portion of the tongue that rests below the hard palate
10. Superior surface of the tongue
11. Also called soft palate

Across

3. Elevates the back of the tongue
7. Muscle that pulls the tongue downward
12. Main body of the tongue
13. Opens the Eustachian tube:_____ veli palatini
14. Muscle that narrows the tongue

Cranial and Facial Bones

Across

1. Bone that separates the right and left nasal cavities
3. Divides the nose into two cavities
5. Cheek bone
7. Separates the nasal cavity from the brain
10 Most fragile facial bone
11 Located within each nasal cavity
13 Bone that has five parts
14 Upper jaw

Down

2. Lower jaw
4. Runs behind the oral and nasal cavities and larynx
6. Most posterior bone of the skull
8. Bone that forms the forehead
9. Bones that form the sides and roof of the cranium
12. Resembles a butterfly

Section Five

The Auditory System

The auditory system consists of the outer,
middle, and inner ears.
It converts acoustic pressure waves to mechanical energy
in the middle ear, and mechanical to
electrical energy in the inner ear.
The electrical energy is sent to the brain
in the form of nerve impulses and
is interpreted as sound.

OUTER EAR

Two parts make up the outer ear, the pinna (auricle) and the external auditory meatus (ear canal).

Pinna

The pinna is the external "flap" on the side of the head. It is made of flexible elastic cartilage and attaches to the side of the cranium by ligaments. The main function of the pinna is to help channel sound waves into the ear canal. The pinna also helps to localize sounds, and protects the entrance to the external auditory meatus.

Parts of the pinna include:

Helix: fold of tissue that forms the outer margin of the pinna.

Antihelix: fold of tissue anterior to the helix.

Scapha: groove between the helix and the antihelix.

Tragus: slight protrusion of cartilage anterior to the auditory meatus.

Triangular fossa: concave space between the antihelix and the ascending portion of the helix.

Antitragus: cartilaginous protrusion that is smaller and opposite to the tragus. It forms the inferior boundary of the concha.

Intertragal notch: space between the tragus and antitragus.

Concha: entrance to the external auditory meatus.

Lobule: non-cartilaginous inferior portion of the pinna.

External auditory meatus (ear canal)

The external auditory meatus leads from the pinna to the tympanic membrane. In adults, the meatus is an S-shaped tube about 2.5 to 3.5 cm long and about 6 mm in diameter. The lateral one-third to one-half of the canal is cartilaginous, and the medial one-half to two-thirds is bone. The entire canal is lined with a layer of epidermis. The cartilaginous part of the canal contains glands that secrete oil and a waxy substance called cerumen which lubricate the ear canal. The lateral part of the canal also contains cilia.

The cilia move in a wavelike fashion, which helps to propel the cerumen, together with small particles of dust or other substances, toward the outside. The external auditory meatus resonates and boosts the amplitude of high-frequency sounds entering the ear.

Outer ear

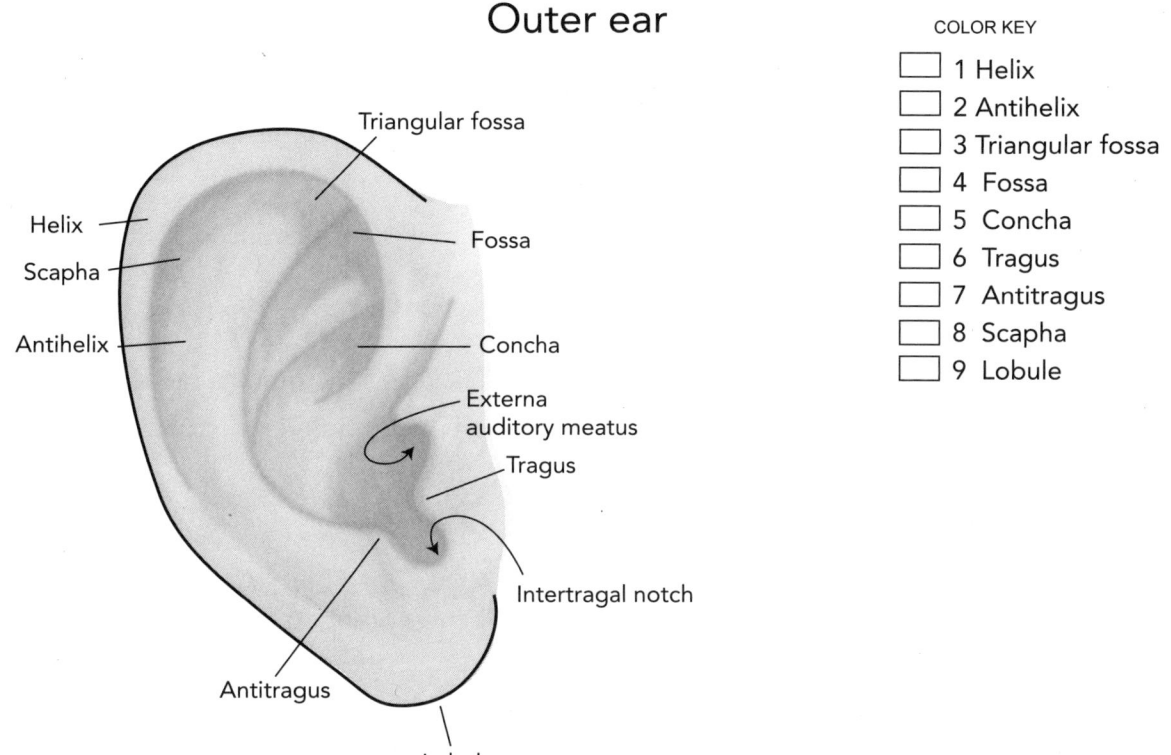

COLOR KEY

- [ ] 1 Helix
- [ ] 2 Antihelix
- [ ] 3 Triangular fossa
- [ ] 4 Fossa
- [ ] 5 Concha
- [ ] 6 Tragus
- [ ] 7 Antitragus
- [ ] 8 Scapha
- [ ] 9 Lobule

Draw your own: Outer ear

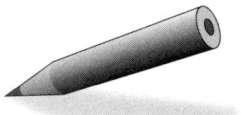

Tympanic membrane

The tympanic membrane (TM) is the interface between the outer ear and the middle ear. It is a semi-transparent, oval-shaped sheet of membrane that is concave on its external (lateral) surface. This gives the TM a conical shape, with the point of the cone facing the middle ear space. The membrane is composed of external, middle, and internal layers.

External (lateral) layer: connected to the epidermis of the external auditory meatus.

Internal (medial) layer: composed of mucous membrane and is continuous with the mucous membrane that lines the cavity of the middle ear.

Fibrous layer: located between the external and internal layers and contains radial and circular fibers. These fibers provide support to the tympanic membrane structure.

Umbo: tip of the cone.

Pars flaccida: the small, superior section of the tympanic membrane. It contains fewer fibers than the pars tensa.

Pars tensa: forms the remaining section of the tympanic membrane.

Cone of light: when light from an otoscope is directed on the tympanic membrane a cone-shaped reflection can be seen at around the 5 o' clock position on the right tympanic membrane and around the 7 o' clock position on the left tympanic membrane.

Function of the tympanic membrane

The primary function of the tympanic membrane is to vibrate when acoustic pressure waves impinge on it. Part of the malleus (one of the ossicles - see below) is embedded within the tympanic membrane. Therefore, the vibration of the tympanic membrane is transmitted to the malleus and to the other two bones in the middle ear, the incus and the stapes. The tympanic membrane is extremely sensitive to tiny variations in pressure. It responds to an extraordinary range of pressures across a wide range of frequencies. Thus, the tympanic membrane is involved in the process of transducing pressure waves to mechanical vibration.

Tympanic membrane

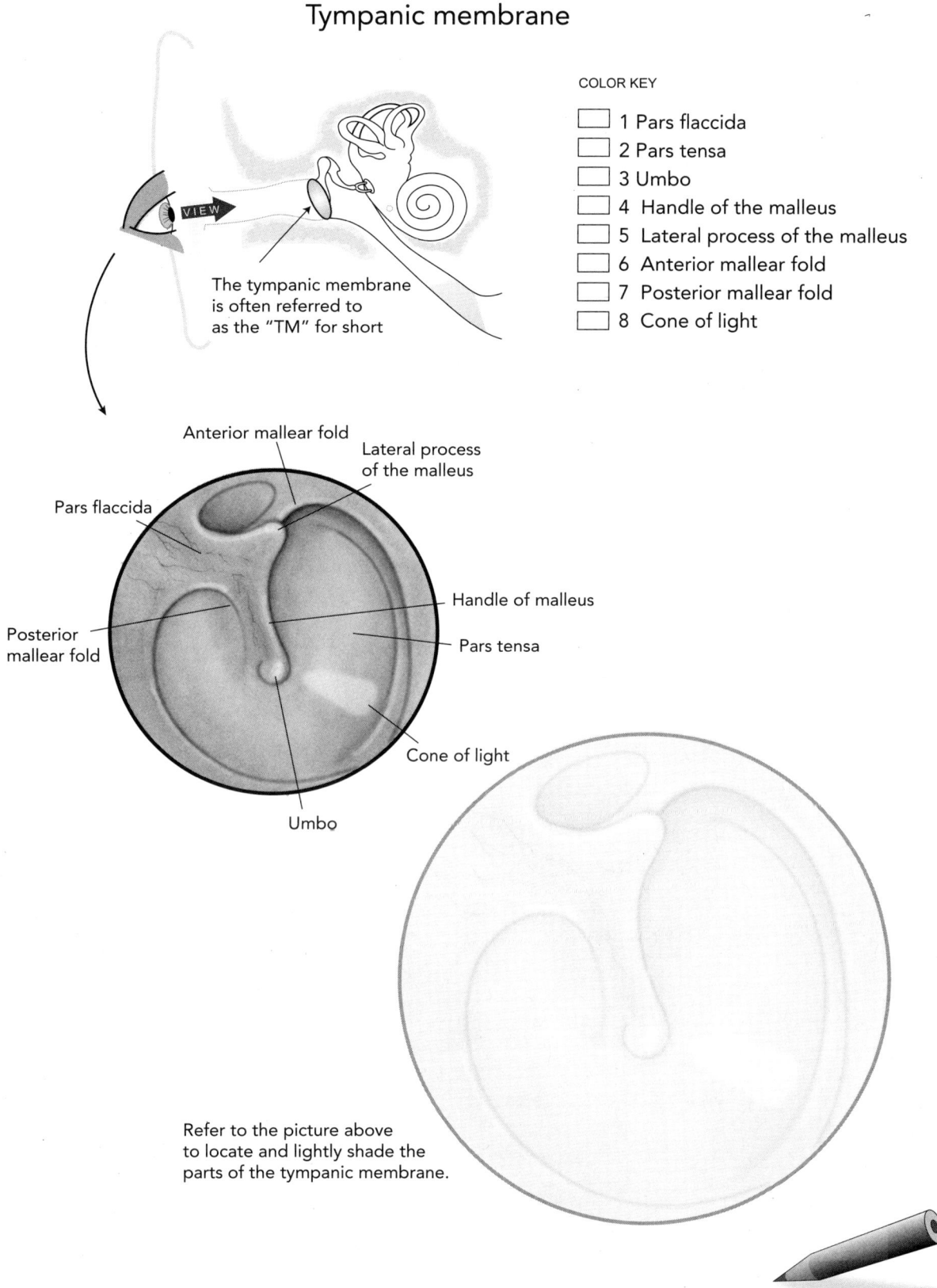

The tympanic membrane is often referred to as the "TM" for short

COLOR KEY

1 Pars flaccida
2 Pars tensa
3 Umbo
4 Handle of the malleus
5 Lateral process of the malleus
6 Anterior mallear fold
7 Posterior mallear fold
8 Cone of light

Anterior mallear fold

Lateral process of the malleus

Pars flaccida

Posterior mallear fold

Handle of malleus

Pars tensa

Cone of light

Umbo

Refer to the picture above to locate and lightly shade the parts of the tympanic membrane.

MIDDLE EAR

The middle ear lies directly behind the tympanic membrane. The middle ear is a tiny space, about 6 mm wide and about 4 mm deep with a volume of about 2 ml. The space is divided into two sections—the tympanic cavity (tympanum), and the epitympanic recess (attic). In the normal ear, the middle ear is an air-filled cavity. It is ventilated and drained by the Eustachian tube. It contains three small bones, the malleus, incus, and stapes, collectively referred to as the ossicles; ligaments that hold the ossicles in place; and two muscles.

Eustachian tube

The Eustachian tube runs from the nasopharynx to the middle ear. The tube is about 35 mm in length. The anterior two-thirds of the tube lies within a canal made of cartilage, and the posterior one-third lies within a bony canal. The pharyngeal opening of the tube is a slit approximately 8 mm high and 1 mm wide. This end of the tube is normally closed, except when one swallows or yawns, when it opens through the action of the tensor veli palatini muscle. The opening to the bony section is normally open. The inside of the tube is lined with epithelium.

Functions of the Eustachian tube

The Eustachian tube serves to keep the middle ear space ventilated and drained through two functions. First, it equalizes the air pressure between the otherwise closed middle ear and the external atmosphere because air from the atmosphere enters the middle ear when the tube opens. Second, it helps to clear mucus from the middle ear by draining the mucus to the pharynx, where it is swallowed.

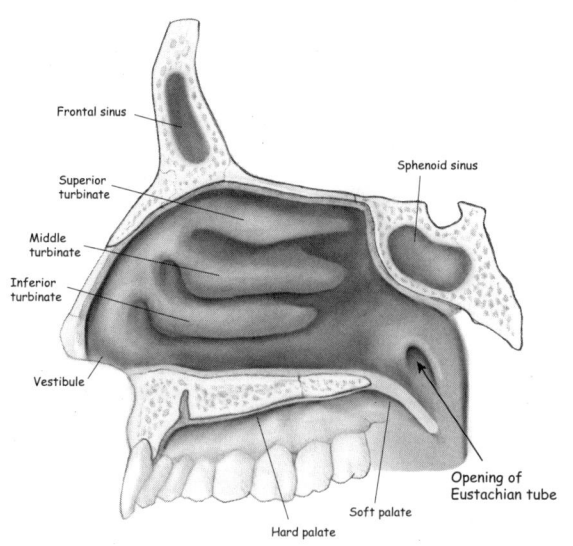

Middle ear structures

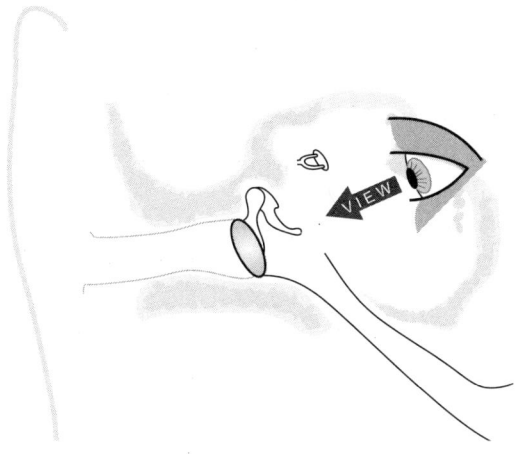

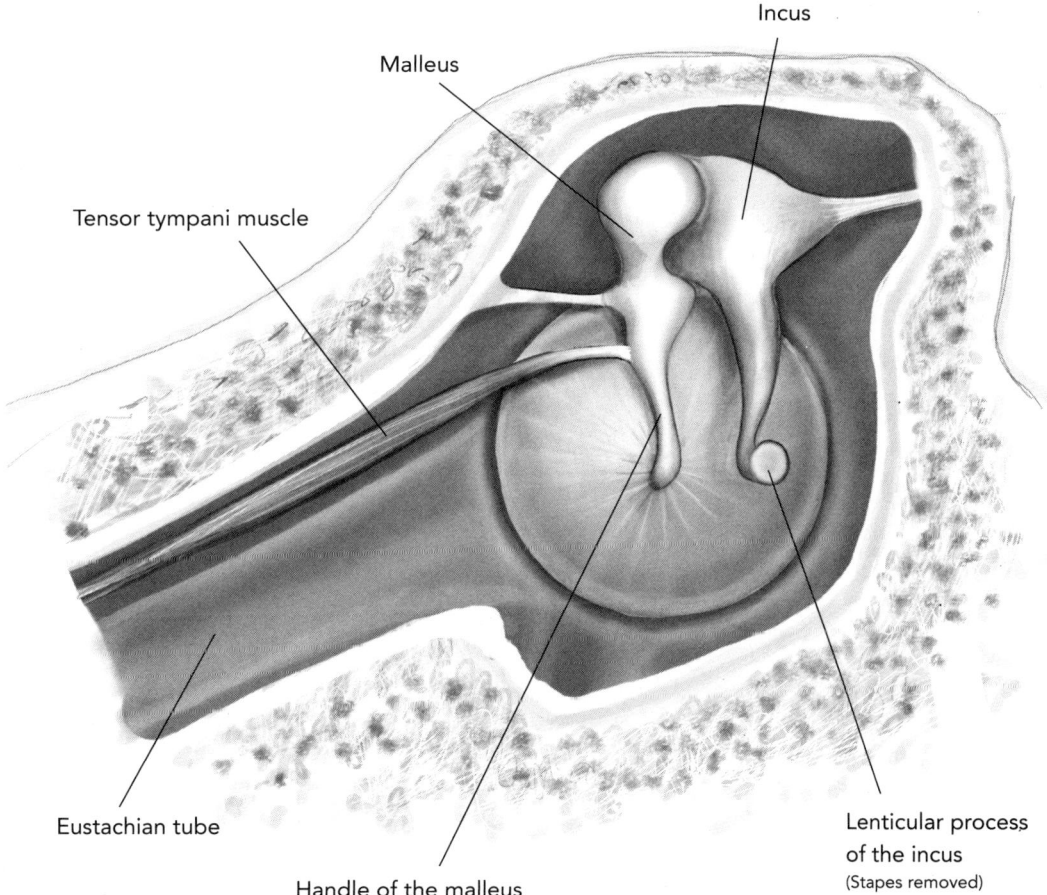

Incus

Malleus

Tensor tympani muscle

Eustachian tube

Handle of the malleus

Lenticular process
of the incus
(Stapes removed)

Ossicles

The ossicles are the three smallest bones in the human body – malleus, incus, and stapes. They are connected to each other, to the tympanic membrane on one side, and to a part of the inner ear called the oval window on the other (most medial) side.

Malleus: has two parts—the head and the manubrium. The manubrium is embedded in the tympanic membrane. The head extends into the epitympanic recess.

Incus: connected to the malleus. Consists of a body and several processes.

Stapes : attached to the incus and to the oval window. Has a footplate and a horseshoe-shaped body.

Windows from the middle ear to the inner ear

Oval window: opening covered by a membrane. The oval window leads from the middle ear to the vestibule of the inner ear.

Round window: membrane-covered opening between the middle and inner ears.

Muscles of the middle ear

Tensor tympani: runs parallel to the Eustachian tube. It originates at the tendon of the tensor veli palatini muscle. From there the fibers pass through a bony canal in the temporal bone of the cranium. The muscle then emerges into the tympanic cavity and connects with the manubrium of the malleus. Contraction pulls the malleus inward (medially).

Stapedius: runs from the posterior wall of the tympanic cavity to the head of the stapes. Contraction pulls the stapes posteriorly. The stapedius muscle is involved in a reflex known as the acoustic, or stapedial, reflex. This reflex occurs when the stapedius muscle contracts strongly in response to intense sound of 80 dB HL (hearing level) or more, stiffening the ossicular chain and the tympanic membrane. This has the effect of reducing the pressure applied to the oval window, which reduces the sound intensity by around 10-20 dB.

Ossicles

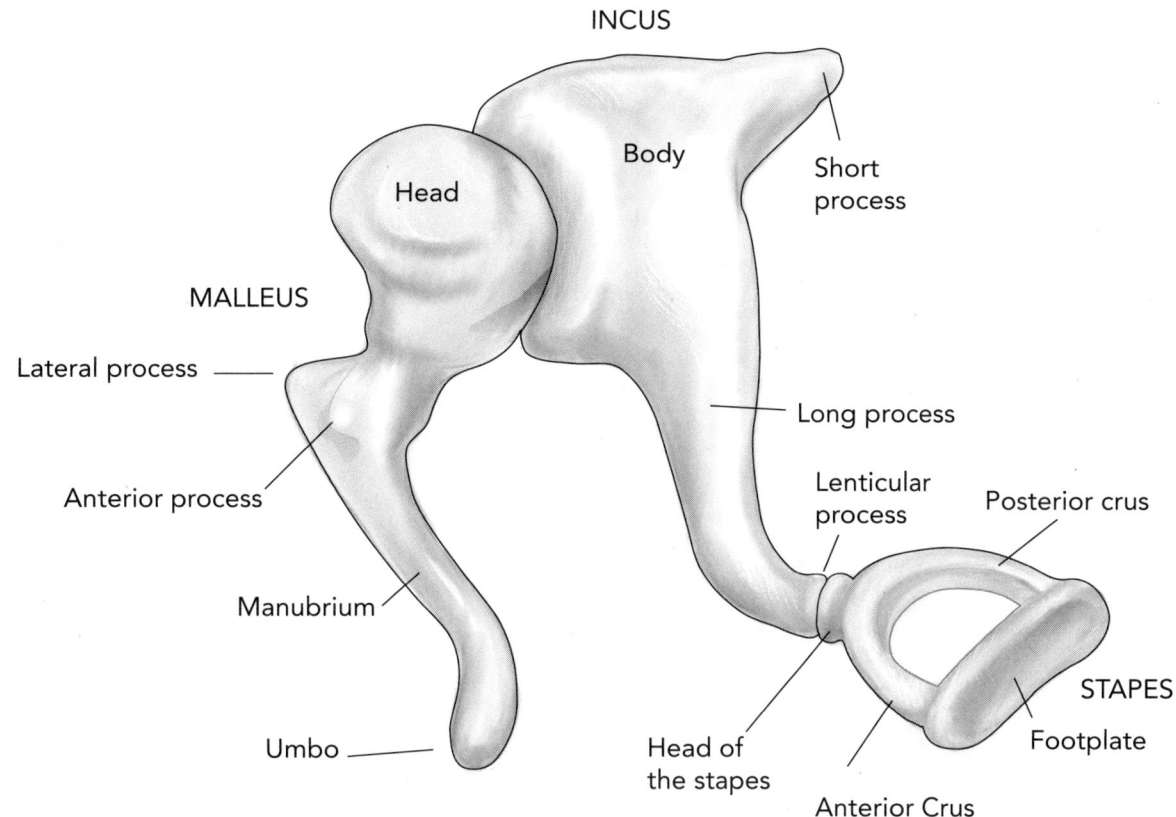

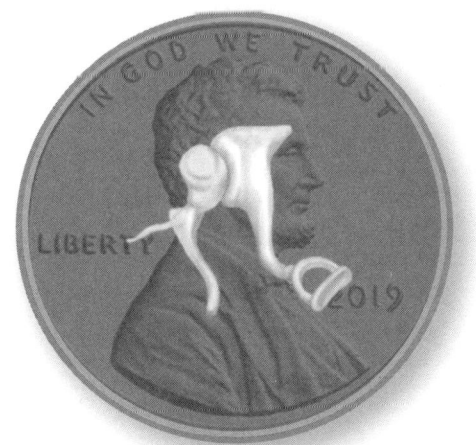

Size of ossicles compared to US one cent piece

Ossicles and their attachments

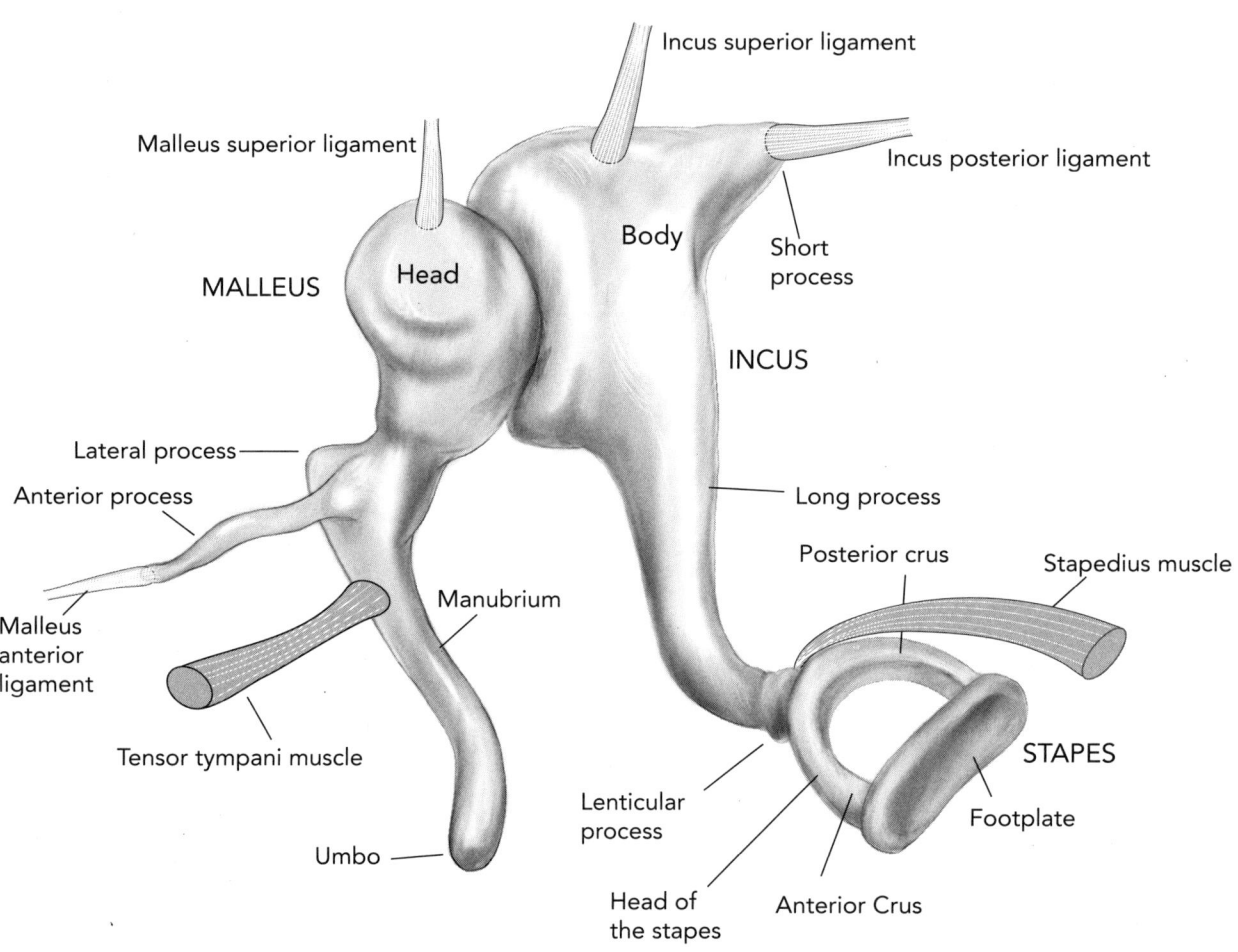

Ossicles and their attachments

COLOR KEY

- [ ] 1 Malleus
- [ ] 2 Incus
- [ ] 3 Stapes
- [ ] 4 Tensor tympani muscle
- [ ] 5 Stapedius muscle
- [ ] 6 Malleus superior ligament
- [ ] 7 Malleus anterior ligament
- [ ] 8 Incus posterior ligament
- [ ] 9 Incus superior ligament

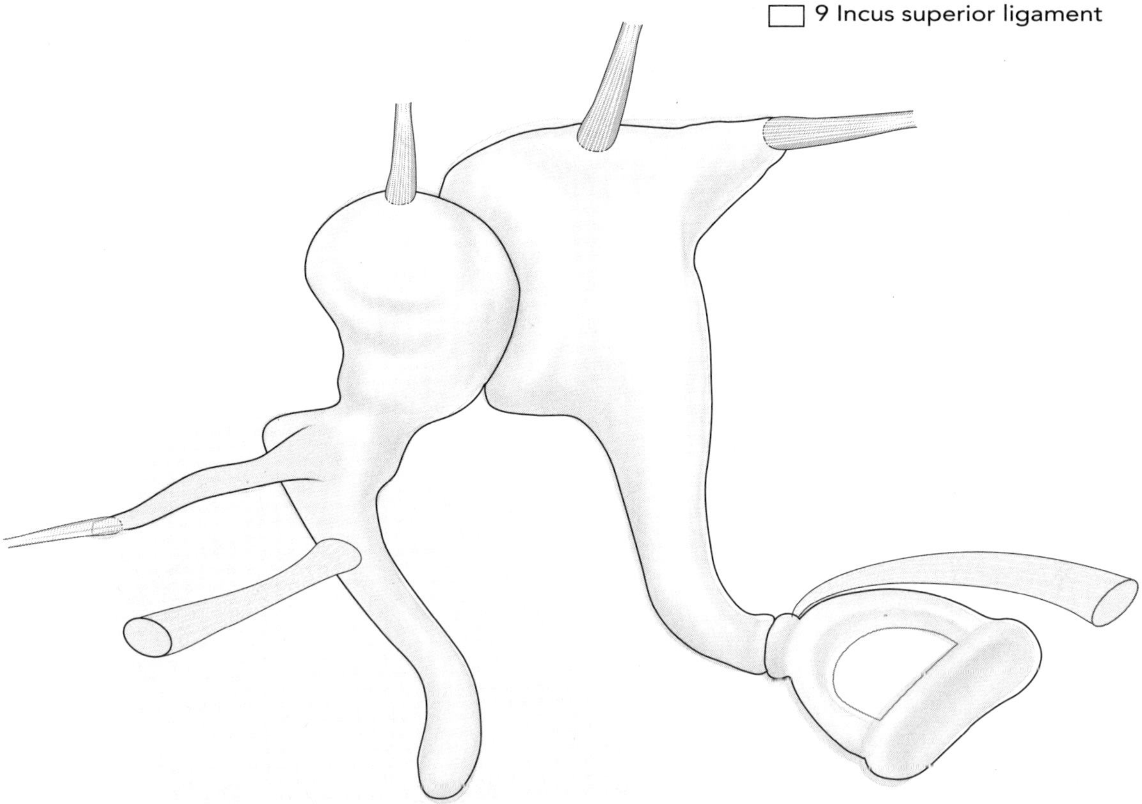

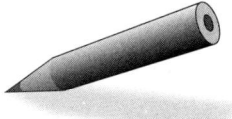

INNER EAR

The inner ear lies deep within the temporal bone and is composed of the cochlea, the semicircular canals, and a connecting vestibule between them. The cochlea is involved with hearing. The semicircular canals and vestibule are important for balance.

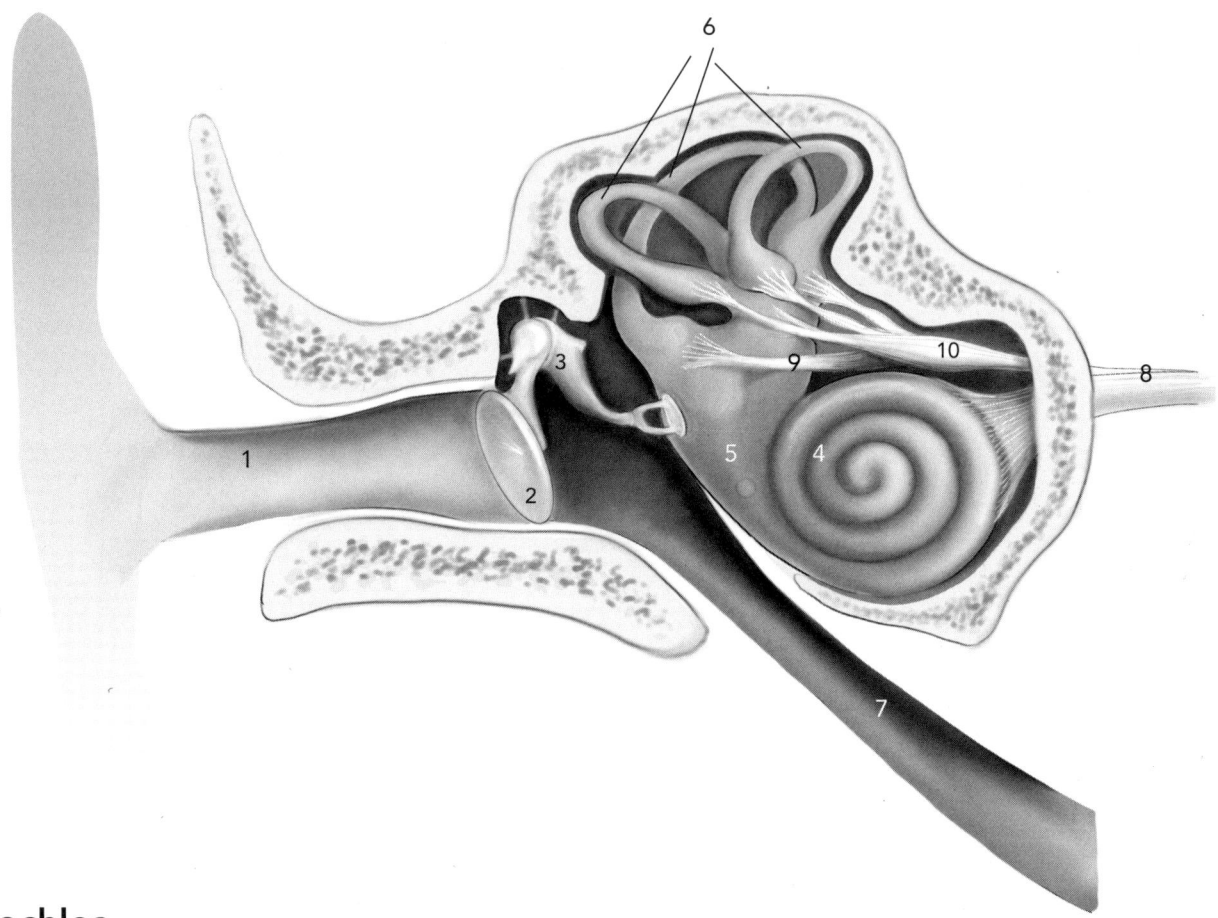

Cochlea

The cochlea is housed in the petrous portion of the temporal bone, just medial to the tympanic cavity. It is a snail-shaped, bony, spiral canal that makes two- and three-quarter turns around a bony core. Parts of the cochlea include:

Modiolus: bony core of the cochlea.

Osseous spiral lamina: bony shelf that projects from the modiolus like the turns of a screw. The cochlear turns decrease in size from the base to the apex.

Apex: point of the canal farthest from the middle ear.

Cochlear duct: membranous canal that lies inside the bony canal. It takes the same snail shape as the bony canal. The cochlear duct is attached to the osseous spiral lamina and to the outer wall of the bony canal.

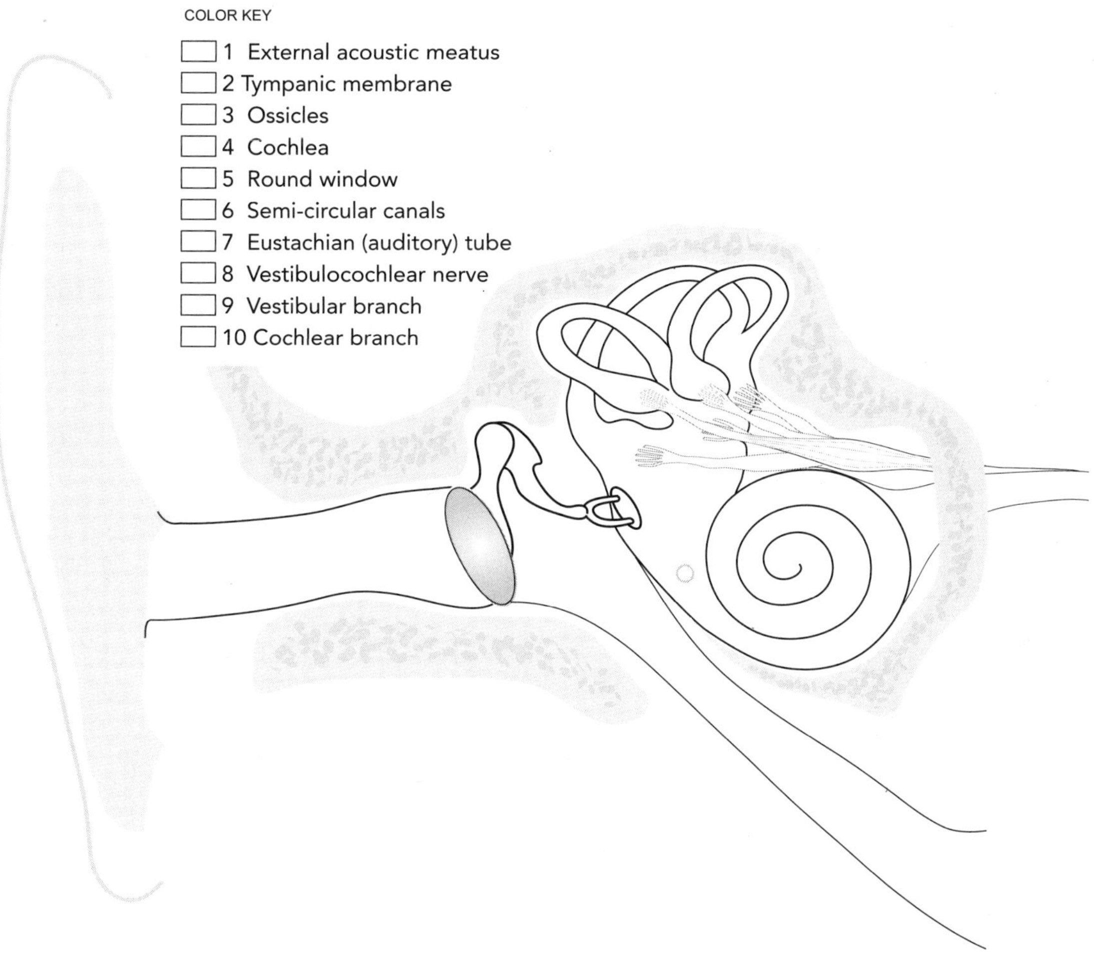

COLOR KEY

☐ 1 External acoustic meatus
☐ 2 Tympanic membrane
☐ 3 Ossicles
☐ 4 Cochlea
☐ 5 Round window
☐ 6 Semi-circular canals
☐ 7 Eustachian (auditory) tube
☐ 8 Vestibulocochlear nerve
☐ 9 Vestibular branch
☐ 10 Cochlear branch

Basilar membrane: forms the base of the cochlear duct. The basilar membrane is important in the cochlea's ability to perform a frequency and intensity analysis of all incoming sounds. The membrane is not equally wide along its entire length. It is narrowest at its base closest to the middle ear. It increases in width and stiffness at its apex, farthest from the middle ear. The membrane is more responsive to high frequencies at the base and lower frequencies at the apex.

Traveling wave: vibration of the basilar membrane produces a traveling wave, which always moves from the base to the apex. As the wave travels along the basilar membrane, it increases in amplitude to a peak that corresponds to the frequency of stimulation. At the peak the hair cells in the Organ of Corti (see below) are activated. The activation stimulates the auditory nerve to fire at that frequency.

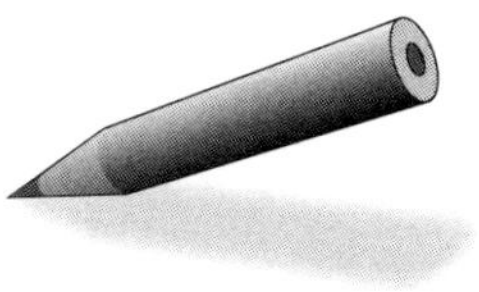

Vestibular duct: filled with perilymph. It is separated from the the cochlear duct by the vestibular membrane (also called Reissner's membrane).

Vestibular canal: space above the vestibular membrane. The vestibular canal terminates at the oval window.

Tympanic canal: space below the basilar membrane. The tympanic canal terminates at the round window.

Helicotrema: point of communication where the vestibular and tympanic canals meet each other at the end of the cochlear duct.

Perilymph: fluid that lies between the bony canal and the cochlear duct.

Endolymph: fluid within the cochlear duct.

Organ of Corti

The Organ of Corti contains the sensory cells for hearing. These cells are called inner and outer hair cells, named for the tiny hair-like projections that extend from their tops into the cochlear duct. The organ also contains pillar cells. The Organ of Corti is situated within the cochlear duct. It sits on the basilar membrane and runs along its entire length.

Outer hair cells: about 12,000 tube-shaped outer hair cells arranged in three to five rows along the basilar membrane. These cells amplify sounds entering the cochlea.

Inner hair cells: about 3500 flask-shaped inner hair cells arranged in a single row along the length of the basilar membrane. The inner hair cells transform the sound vibrations in the fluid-filled cochlea into electrical nerve impulses that are then relayed to the nervous system.

Tunnel of Corti: formed by two rows of pillar cells. These cells separate the inner and outer hair cells.

Tectorial membrane: gelatinous structure that forms the roof of the cochlear duct. The tips of the outer hair cells are embedded in the tectorial membrane.

Vestibular apparatus

The organ of balance within the inner ear is the vestibular apparatus. It consists of the semicircular ducts, utricle, and saccule.

Semicircular canals: 3 interconnecting semicircular canals within the inner ear: horizontal, superior, and posterior. Each canal is at a right angle to the others, and each senses a different plane of movement of the body. Each canal is lined with cilia and filled with endolymph. Every time the head moves, the endolymph moves the cilia, generating a signal that is transmitted to the brain. The horizontal canal detects horizontal head movements; the superior and posterior canals detect vertical head movements.

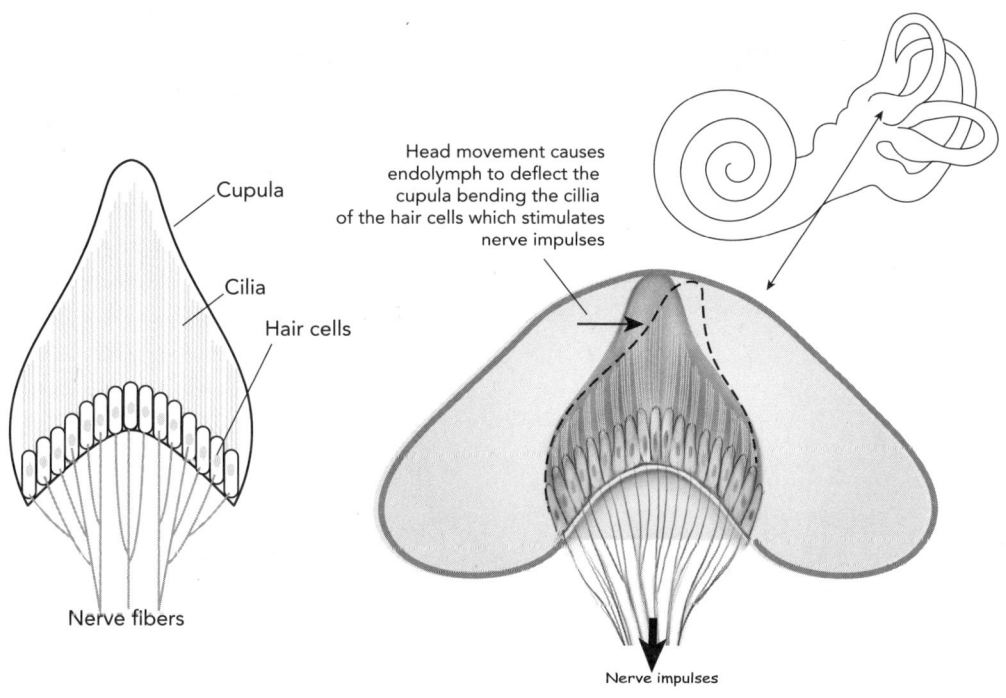

Ampulla: enlargement of each bony canal. The ampulla contains hair cells embedded in a gelatinous structure called the cupola.

Utricle: adjacent to the semi-circular canals and is lined with membrane. It senses acceleration in the horizontal plane.

Saccule: adjacent to the cochlea and senses acceleration in the vertical plane.

Inner ear

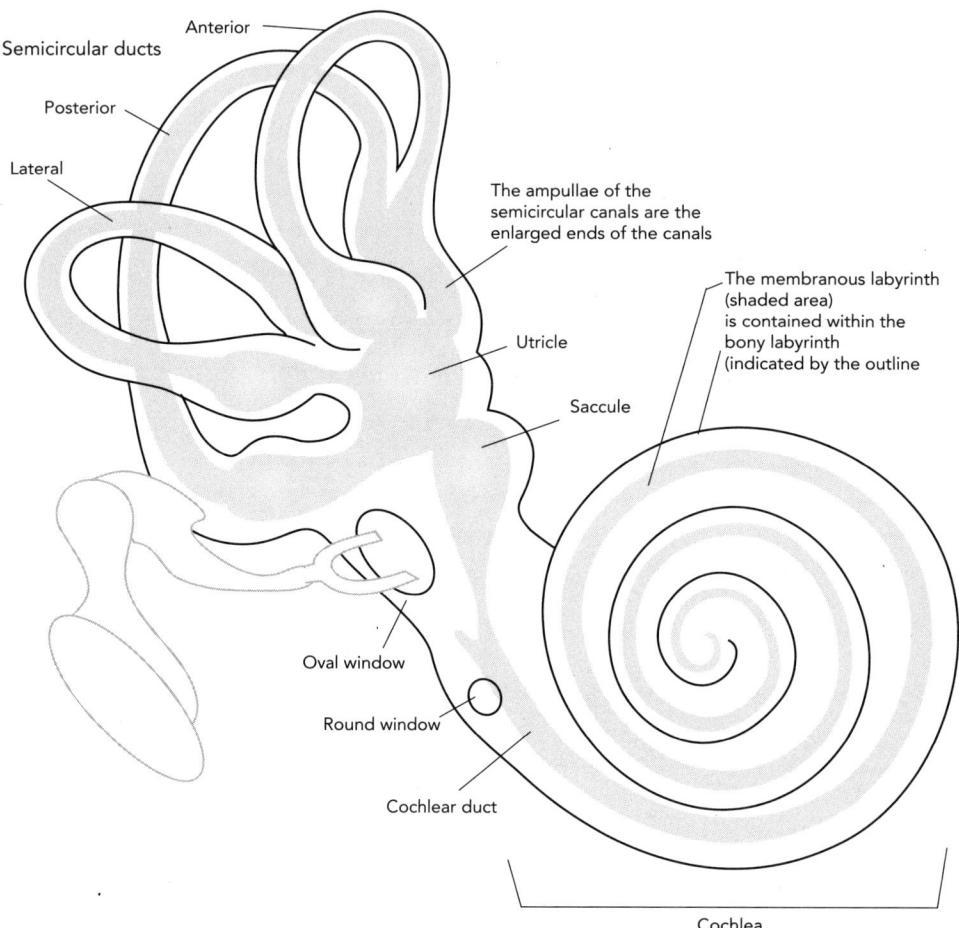

Semicircular ducts

Anterior

Posterior

Lateral

The ampullae of the semicircular canals are the enlarged ends of the canals

The membranous labyrinth (shaded area) is contained within the bony labyrinth (indicated by the outline

Utricle

Saccule

Oval window

Round window

Cochlear duct

Cochlea

Auditory nerve

The auditory nerve is composed of two branches. The cochlear branch transmits hearing information from the cochlea to the nervous system. The vestibular branch transmits information about balance to the nervous system.

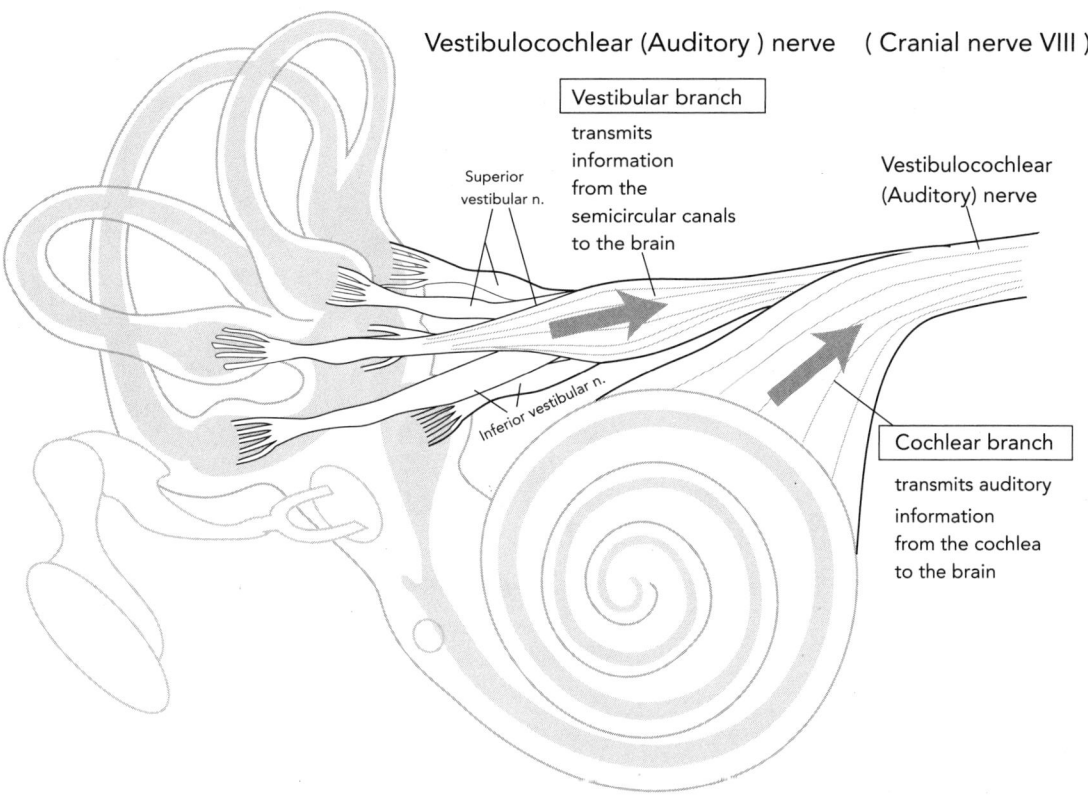

Vestibulocochlear (Auditory) nerve   (Cranial nerve VIII)

Vestibular branch

transmits information from the semicircular canals to the brain

Superior vestibular n.

Inferior vestibular n.

Vestibulocochlear (Auditory) nerve

Cochlear branch

transmits auditory information from the cochlea to the brain

Cochlear duct and organ of Corti

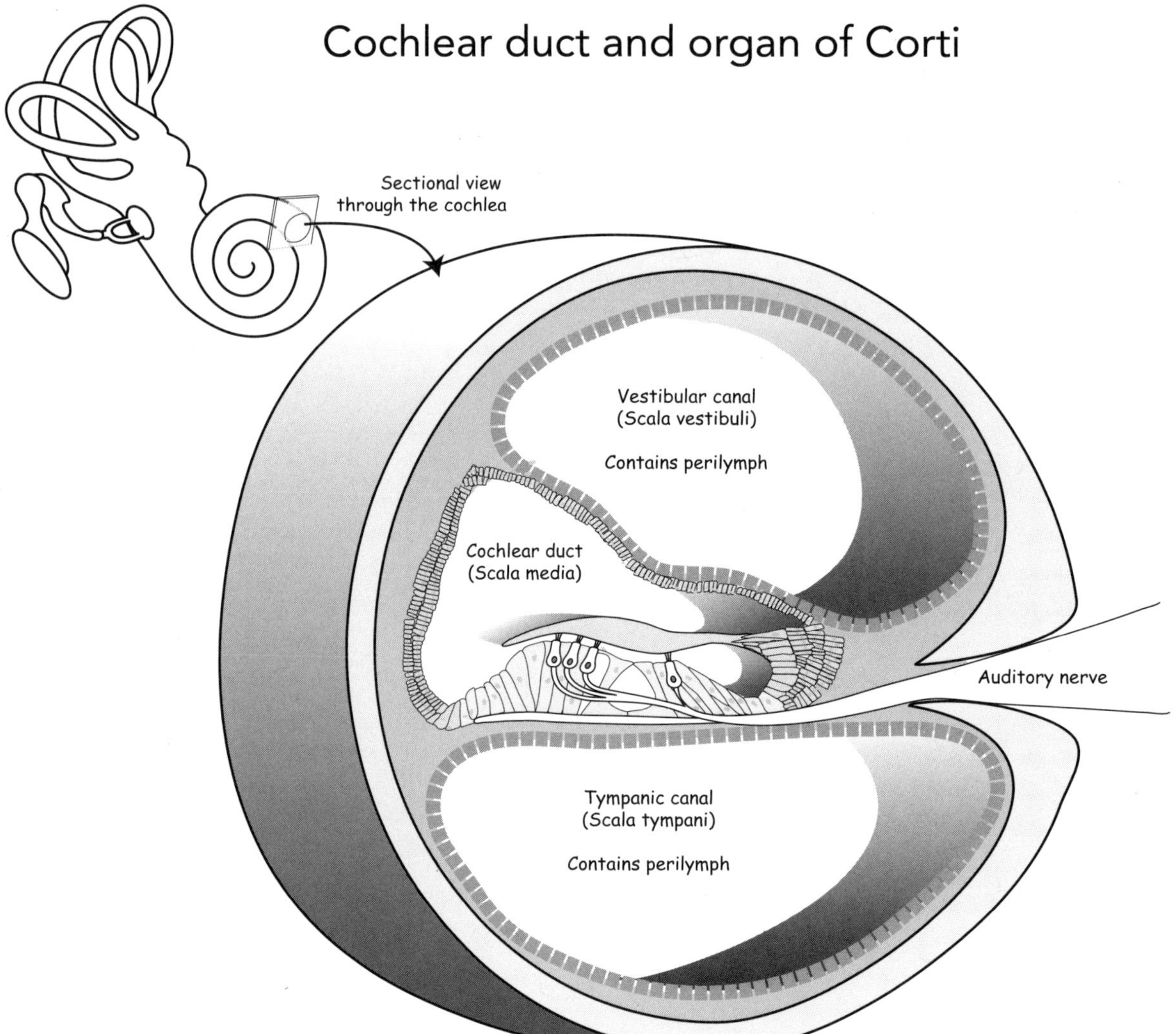

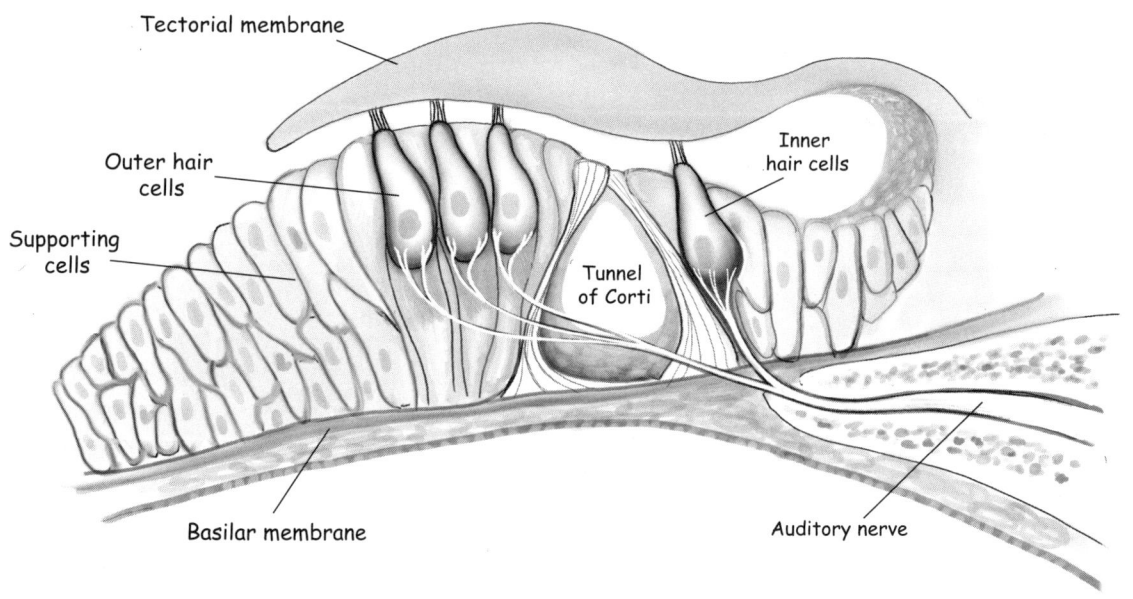

Sectional view through the cochlea

Vestibular canal
(Scala vestibuli)

Contains perilymph

Cochlear duct
(Scala media)

Auditory nerve

Tympanic canal
(Scala tympani)

Contains perilymph

Tectorial membrane

Outer hair cells

Inner hair cells

Supporting cells

Tunnel of Corti

Basilar membrane

Auditory nerve

COLOR KEY

☐ 1 Tectorial membrane
☐ 2 Inner hair cells
☐ 3 Outer hair cell
☐ 4 Basilar membrane
☐ 5 Tunnel of Corti
☐ 6 Cochlear nerve

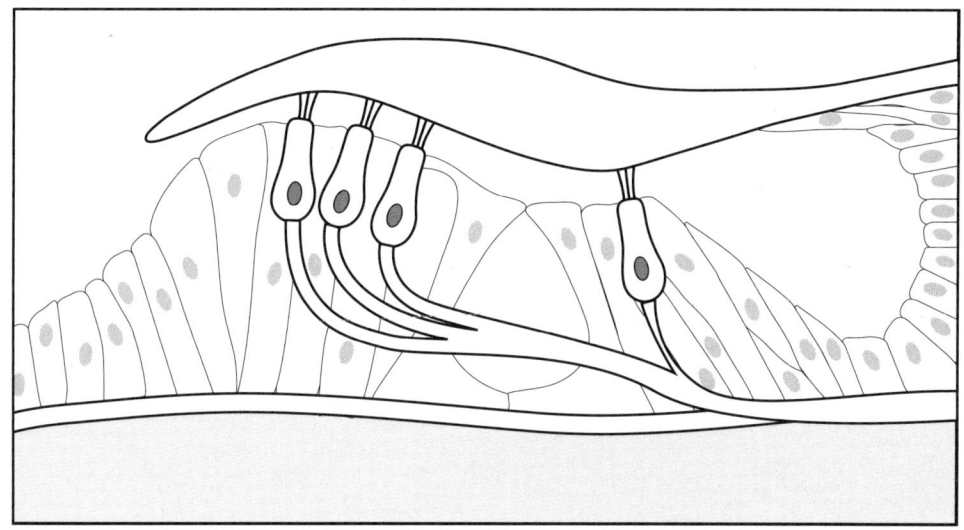

COLOR KEY

☐ 1 Bony labyrinth
☐ 2 Vestibular canal
   (Scala vestibuli)
☐ 3 Cochlear duct
☐ 4 Tympanic canal
   (Scala tympani)
☐ 5 Cochlear nerve

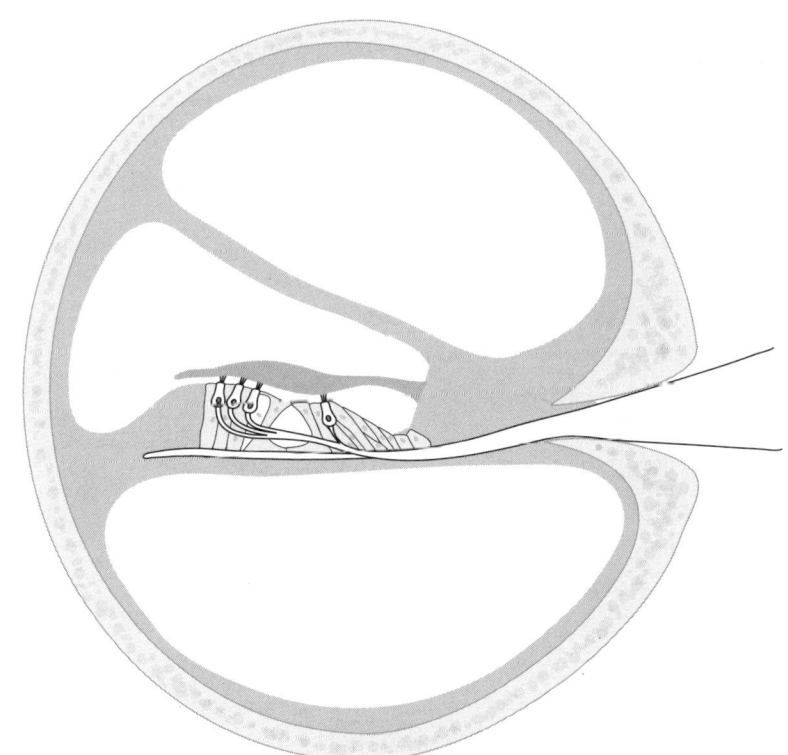

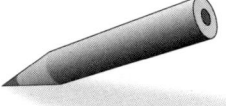

TEST YOURSELF: THE AUDITORY SYSTEM

MULTIPLE CHOICE   OUTER AND MIDDLE EAR

1 _____   The ear
   a. Acts as a transducer
   b. Converts acoustic pressure waves to mechanical energy
   c. Converts mechanical energy to electrical energy
   d. All the above

2 _____   Which of the following (if any) is NOT a function of the pinna?
   a. Convert mechanical to electrical energy
   b. Funnel sound waves into the ear
   c. Help to localize sound
   d. All the above are functions of the pinna

3 _____   Another word for the eardrum is
   a. Auricle
   b. Pinna
   c. External auditory meatus
   d. Tympanic membrane

4 _____   The helix is the
   a. Fold of tissue forming the outer margin of the pinna
   b. Entrance to the external auditory meatus
   c. Inferior portion of the pinna
   d. None of the above

5 _____   The concha is the
   a. Fold of tissue forming the outer margin of the pinna
   b. Entrance to the external auditory meatus
   c. Inferior portion of the pinna
   d. None of the above

6 _____   Which of the following structures (if any) is NOT part of the pinna?
   a. Scapha
   b. Tragus
   c. Triangular fossa
   d. All the above are part of the pinna

7 _____   The antitragus
   a. Forms the superior boundary of the concha
   b. Is the groove between the helix and the antihelix
   c. Forms the inferior boundary of the concha
   d. None of the above

8 _____   The external auditory meatus
      a. Is about 35 mm in length
      b. Opens through the action of the tensor veli palatini muscle
      c. Resonates and boosts the amplitude of high-frequency sounds
      d. Is extremely sensitive to tiny variations in pressure

9 _____   The ossicles of the middle ear are the
      a. Malleus, incus, stapes
      b. Malleus, incus, pinna
      c. Malleus, pinna, stapes
      d. Malleus, tympanus, stapes

10 _____   The tube that runs from the nasopharynx to the middle ear is the
      a. External auditory meatus
      b. Tympanic tube
      c. Eustachian tube
      d. None of the above

11 _____   What structure provides the boundary between the outer and middle ear?
      a. Oval window
      b. Cochlea
      c. Pinna
      d. Tympanic membrane

12 _____   What are the ossicles?
      a. Fluid-filled canals that extend into the cochlea
      b. Small bones that provide firmness to the pinna
      c. Fine hairs within the external auditory meatus
      d. None of the above

13 _____   The external auditory meatus is lined with fine hairs and glands that produce
      a. Cochlear fluid
      b. Cerumen
      c. Eustachian fluid
      d. All the above

14 _____   The acoustic reflex can reduce loud sound by how many decibels?
      a. 70-80
      b. 50-60
      c. 0-10
      d. 10-20

15 ____ The helix and antihelix are located within the
- a. Ossicles
- b. Pinna
- c. Eustachian tube
- d. Tympanic cavity

16 ____ The malleus is pulled inward by which muscle?
- a. Tensor veli palatini
- b. Tensor tympani
- c. Stapedius
- d. None of the above

TRUE/FALSE   OUTER AND MIDDLE EAR

1 ____ The outer ear is made up of the pinna and the tympanic membrane

2 ____ The main function of the pinna is to help channel soundwaves into the external auditory meatus

3 ____ The concha is the fold of tissue that forms the outer part of the pinna

4 ____ The helix is the entrance to the external auditory meatus

5 ____ The external auditory meatus is made up of both cartilage and bone

6 ____ Cilia within the external auditory meatus move in a wavelike fashion which propels cerumen

7 ____ The external auditory meatus boosts the amplitude of high-frequency sounds entering the ear

8 ____ The tympanic membrane is composed of two layers

9 ____ The fibrous layer of the tympanic membrane contains radial and circular fibers

10 ____ A part of the incus is embedded in the tympanic membrane

11 ____ The middle ear is divided into the tympanic cavity and the epitympanic recess

12 ____ The Eustachian tube runs from the nasopharynx to the inner ear

13 ____ The oval window leads from the middle ear to the inner ear

14 ____ The tensor tympani muscle is involved in the acoustic reflex

15 ____The intertragal notch is the space between the tragus and antitragus

16 ____The tragus is a slight protrusion of cartilage posterior to the auditory meatus

FILL IN THE BLANK   OUTER AND MIDDLE EAR

1.   The _____ is the entrance to the external auditory meatus.

2.   The fold of tissue that forms the outer margin of the pinna is the _____.

3.   The _____ is the inferior non-cartilaginous portion of the pinna.

4.   The external auditory meatus is about _____ long and about _____ in diameter.

5.   The meatus is lined with a layer of _____.

6.   The meatus is lubricated by _____.

7.   The conical tip of the tympanic membrane is called the _____.

8.   The Eustachian tube is opened by the _____ muscle.

9.   The _____ is attached to the oval window.

10.   The acoustic reflex is mediated by the _____ muscle.

11.   The _____ is a concave space between the antihelix and the

      ascending portion of the helix.

12.   The groove between the helix and the antihelix is the _____.

13.   The _____ is a small cartilaginous protrusion that forms the

      inferior boundary of the concha.

MATCH THE LETTERS AND NUMBERS

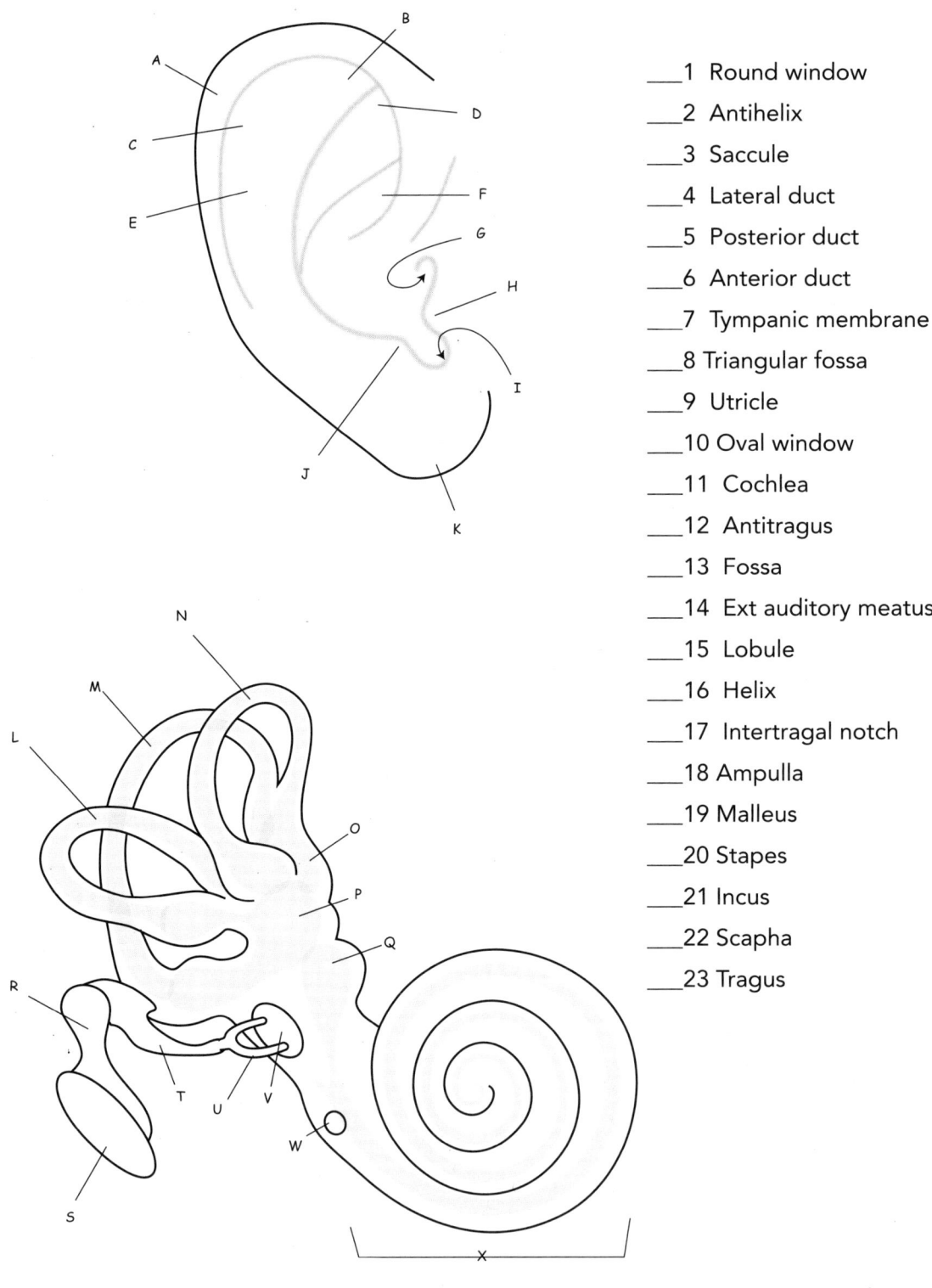

___1 Round window

___2 Antihelix

___3 Saccule

___4 Lateral duct

___5 Posterior duct

___6 Anterior duct

___7 Tympanic membrane

___8 Triangular fossa

___9 Utricle

___10 Oval window

___11 Cochlea

___12 Antitragus

___13 Fossa

___14 Ext auditory meatus

___15 Lobule

___16 Helix

___17 Intertragal notch

___18 Ampulla

___19 Malleus

___20 Stapes

___21 Incus

___22 Scapha

___23 Tragus

MATCHING: OUTER AND MIDDLE EAR

Umbo	1 Larger portion of the tympanic membrane
Antihelix	2 Fold of tissue forming the outer margin of the pinna
Lobule	3 Part of the malleus
Pars flaccida	4 Opening from the middle ear to the inner ear
Helix	5 Entrance to the external auditory meatus
Epitympanic recess	6 Waxy substance secreted within the external auditory meatus
Manubrium	7 Portion of the middle ear
Cerumen	8 Fold of tissue anterior to the helix
Pars tensa	9 Non-cartilaginous inferior portion of pinna
Oval window	10 Superior section of the tympanic membrane
Concha	11 Tip of the cone of the tympanic membrane
Scapha	12 Groove between the helix and the antihelix
Triangular fossa	13 Concave space between the antihelix and the ascending portion of the helix

MATCH THE LETTERS AND NUMBERS

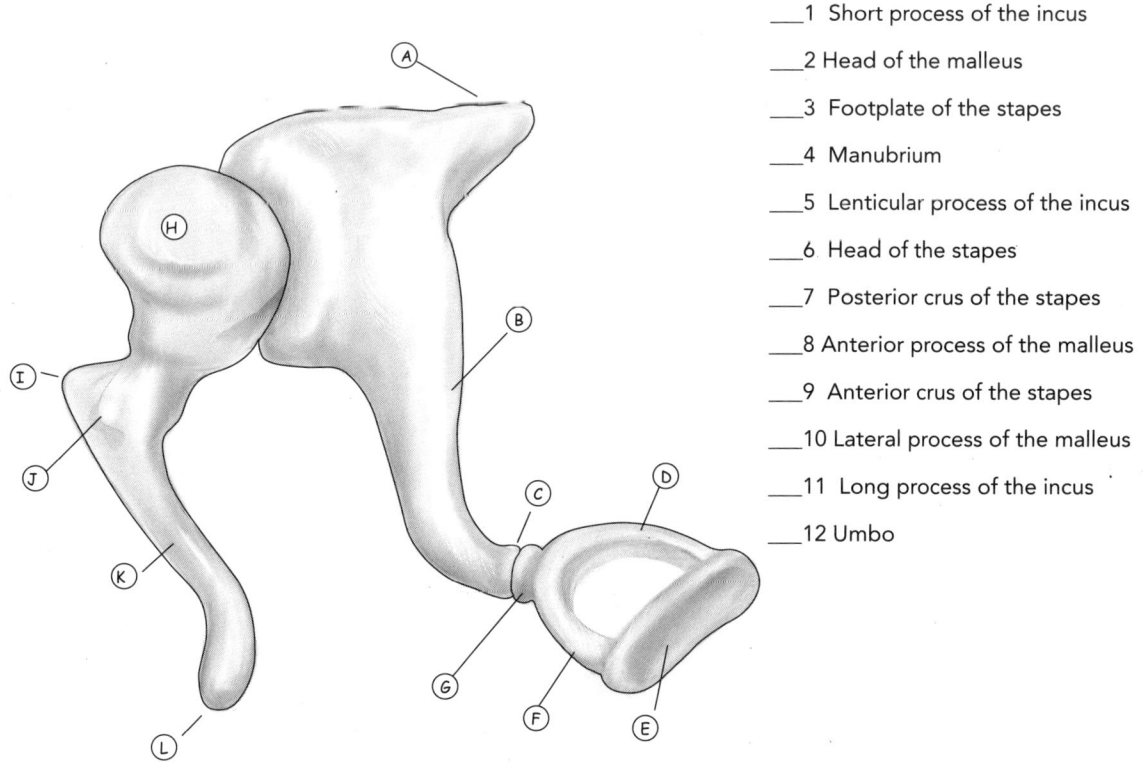

___1 Short process of the incus

___2 Head of the malleus

___3 Footplate of the stapes

___4 Manubrium

___5 Lenticular process of the incus

___6 Head of the stapes

___7 Posterior crus of the stapes

___8 Anterior process of the malleus

___9 Anterior crus of the stapes

___10 Lateral process of the malleus

___11 Long process of the incus

___12 Umbo

MULTIPLE CHOICE   INNER EAR

1 _____   The organs in the inner ear involved with balance are the
   a. Vestibule and semi-circular canals
   b. Vestibule and cochlea
   c. Semi-circular canals and cochlea
   d. Cochlea and organ of Corti

2 _____   Sound vibrations from the tympanic membrane are transmitted to the inner ear via the
   a. Oval window
   b. Semi-circular canals
   c. Eustachian tube
   d. External auditory meatus

3 _____   The structures in the inner ear involved with hearing are the
   a. Vestibule and semi-circular canals
   b. Vestibule and cochlea
   c. Semi-circular canals and cochlea
   d. Cochlea and organ of Corti

4 _____   The ___ is a spiral shaped chamber that looks like a snail
   a. Vestibule
   b. Cochlea
   c. Semi-circular canals
   d. All the above

5 _____   The inner ear
   a. Is an air-filled cavity
   b. Receives vibrations from the middle ear
   c. Transmits vibrations to the middle ear
   d. Connects the Eustachian tube to the pharynx

6 _____ Which is located between the bony canal and the membranous canal?
   a. Cartilage
   b. Endolymph
   c. Mesolymph
   d. Perilymph

7 _____   Which structure projects from the modiolus?
   a. Basilar membrane
   b. Semicircular canals
   c. Tectorial membrane
   d. Osseous spiral lamina

8 _____   The roof of the cochlear duct is formed by the
        a. Tectorial membrane
        b. Basilar membrane
        c. Vestibular membrane
        d. Tympanic membrane

9 _____   The vestibular canal terminates at the
        a. Round window
        b. Helicotrema
        c. Oval window
        d. Organ of Corti

10 _____   The hearing receptors in the inner ear are called the
        a. Organ of Corti
        b. Malleus
        c. Basilar membrane
        d. Semi-circular canals

11 _____   Which of the following structures is not found in the inner ear?
        a. Semi-circular canals
        b. Basilar membrane
        c. Organ of Corti
        d. Stapedius muscle

12 _____   Where is the tectorial membrane found?
        a. Middle ear
        b. Organ of Corti
        c. Basilar membrane
        d. Tympanic membrane

13 _____   The utricle and saccule are in the
        a. Eustachian tube
        b. Semi-circular canal
        c. Organ of Corti
        d. Vestibule

14 _____   Which membrane forms the base of the cochlear duct?
        a. Semi-circular
        b. Tectorial
        c. Basilar
        d. Tympanic

15 ____   The function of the organ of Corti is to
    a. Protect the tympanic membrane
    b. Send nerve impulses to the brain
    c. Direct sound waves to the tympanic membrane
    d. Balance air pressure on both sides of the tympanic membrane

16 ____   Each part of the basilar membrane is sensitive to different
    a. Intensities
    b. Qualities
    c. Frequencies
    d. All the above

17 ____   All of these are true of the ampulla EXCEPT
    a. Is an enlargement of each semi-circular canal
    b. Contains hair cells
    c. Contains the basilar membrane
    d. Contains the cupola

18 ____   The point of communication between the scala vestibuli and scala tympani is the
    a. Round window
    b. Oval window
    c. Helicotrema
    d. Cupola

19____ The outer hair cells
    a. Transform fluid vibrations into nerve impulses
    b. Amplify sounds entering the cochlea
    c. Form part of the tunnel of Corti
    d. None of the above

20____ Which of the following statements (if any) is NOT true of the inner hair cells?
    a. There are around 12,000 inner hair cells
    b. The cells are arranged in a single row along the length of the basilar membrane
    c. The cells transform fluid vibrations into nerve impulses
    d. All the above are true

MATCHING: INNER EAR

	Tectorial membrane	1 Senses acceleration in the horizontal plane
	Ampulla	2 Sensory cells for hearing
	Organ of Corti	3 Space above the vestibular membrane
	Osseous spiral lamina	4 Bony core of the cochlea
	Cochlear duct	5 Space below the basilar membrane
	Cupola	6 Bony shelf projecting from the modiolus
	Basilar membrane	7 Senses acceleration in the vertical plane
	Helicotrema	8 Membranous canal inside the bony canal
	Vestibular canal	9 Base of the cochlear duct
	Utricle	10 Point of communication between the vestibular and tympanic canals
	Modiolus	11 Roof of the cochlear duct
	Tympanic canal	12 Enlargement of each semicircular canal
	Saccule	13 Gelatinous structure with embedded hair cells
	Tunnel of Corti	14 Arranged in three to five rows along the basilar membrane
	Outer hair cells	15 Separate inner and outer hair cells

TRUE/FALSE   INNER EAR

1 ____   The cochlea is housed in the petrous portion of the temporal bone.

2 ____   The cochlea makes one and one half turns around the modiolus.

3 ____   The cochlear turns increase in size from the base to the apex.

4 ____   The apex is the point of the canal nearest to the middle ear.

5 ____   Perilymph lies between the bony canal and the membranous canal and endolymph lies within the

    membranous canal.

6 ____   Reissner's membrane separates the cochlear and vestibular ducts.

7 ____   The vestibular canal terminates at the round window and the tympanic canal terminates

    at the oval window.

8 ____   The organ of Corti consists of the sensory cells for hearing.

9 ____   The tips of the stereocilia of the outer hair cells are embedded in the tectorial membrane.

10 ____   The basilar membrane is narrowest at its base and wider at its apex.

11 ____   The basilar membrane is more responsive to low frequencies at the base.

12 ____   Vibration of the basilar membrane produces a wave which always moves from the apex to the base.

13 _____ The 3 semi-circular canals are the horizontal, superior, and posterior.

14 _____ The semi-circular canals detect head movements while the utricle and saccule detect acceleration.

15 _____ At the point of maximum displacement of the basilar membrane, the stereocilia of the hair cells are

activated, which stimulates the auditory nerve to fire at that frequency.

16_____ The Organ of Corti contains inner and outer hair cells and pillar cells.

17_____There are about 12,000 tube-shaped inner hair cells.

18_____The outer hair cells amplify sounds entering the cochlea.

FILL IN THE BLANK   INNER EAR

1   The cochlea is housed in the _____.

2   The _____ is the bony core of the cochlea.

3   The _____ lies within the bony canal.

4   _____ lies between the bony and membranous canals.

5   The base of the cochlear duct is the _____.

6   The _____ forms the roof of the cochlear duct.

7   The _____ separates the cochlear duct from the vestibular duct.

8   The point of communication between the vestibular and tympanic canals is the

       _____.

9   The organ of Corti sits on the _____.

10   Each semi-circular canal opens into an enlargement of the bony canal called the

       _____ which contains hair cells embedded in a

       gelatinous structure called the _____.

11   The utricle senses acceleration in the _____ plane.

12   The saccule senses acceleration in the _____ plane.

13   The _____ is formed by two rows of pillar cells.

14   The _____ hair cells transform the sound

       vibrations in the fluid-filled cochlea into electrical nerve impulses.

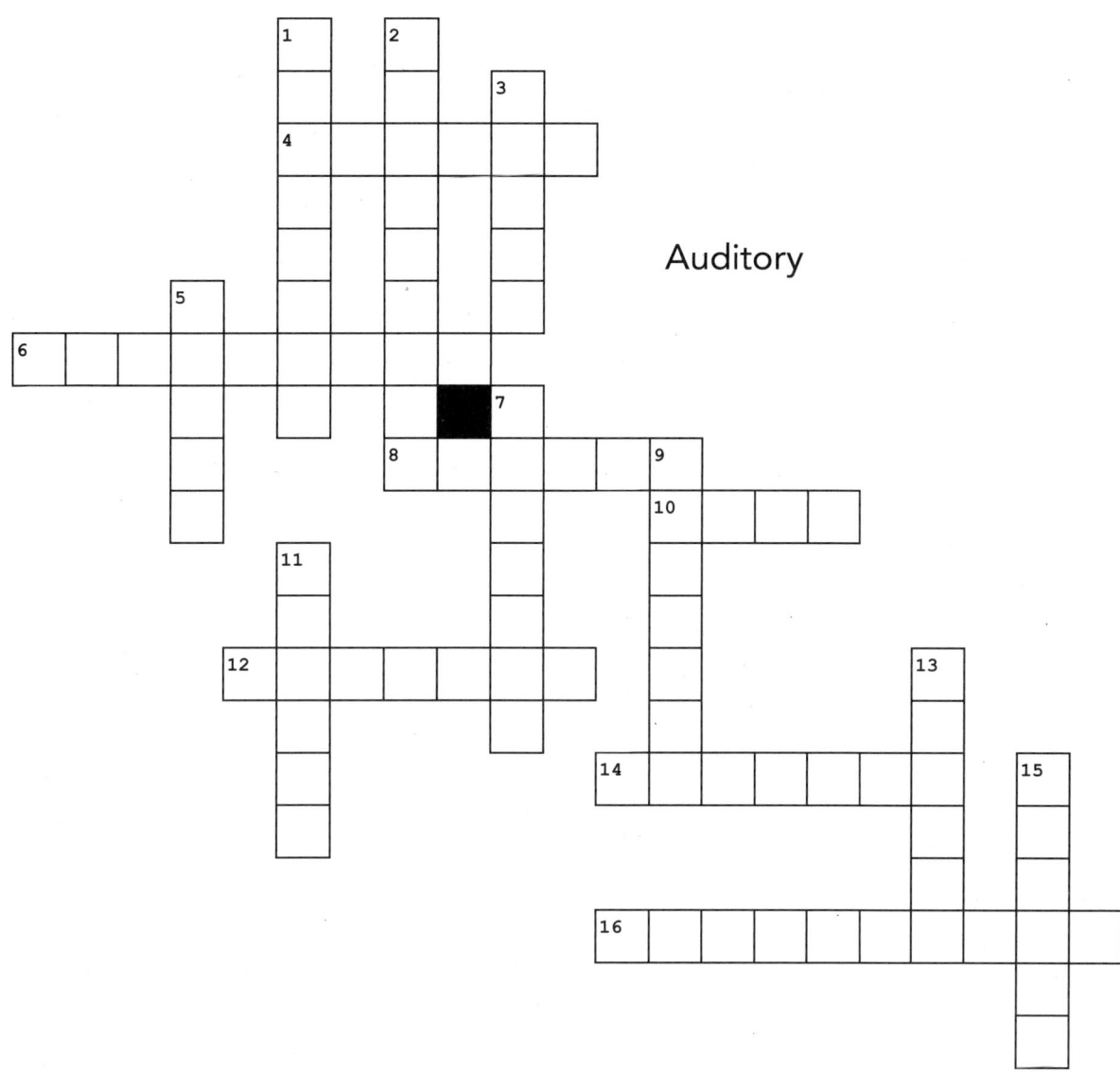

Auditory

Across
4. This bone attaches to the oval window
6. Opposite of helix
8. A groovy part of the pinna
10. Tip of the cone
12. Same as tympanic membrane
14. Secreted in the ear canal
16. Opposite of tragus

Down
1. Smallest bones in the body
2. This muscle is involved in the acoustic reflex
3. This fold of tissue forms the outer margin of the pinna
5. Flap on the outside of the head
7. The manubrium is part of this bone
9. Another word for pinna
11. Rhymes with vagus
13. Entrance to the ear canal
15. Common place for ear piercing

The Nervous System

The nervous system (NS) serves as the control system of the body and regulates all movements including those involved in speech production. The nervous system is divided into central and peripheral portions. The central nervous system consists of the brain and spinal cord. The peripheral nervous system consists of cranial and spinal nerves.

CENTRAL AND PERIPHERAL NERVOUS SYSTEMS

The NS is divided into the central nervous system (CNS) and peripheral nervous system (PNS). The CNS consists of the brain and spinal cord. The PNS is further divided into the somatic system and the autonomic system. The somatic division of the PNS consists of the cranial and spinal nerves that transmit and receive nerve impulses to and from all the muscles and glands of the body. The autonomic system supplies the internal organs, including the blood vessels, stomach, intestine, liver, kidneys, bladder, genitals, lungs, pupils, heart, and sweat, salivary, and digestive glands.

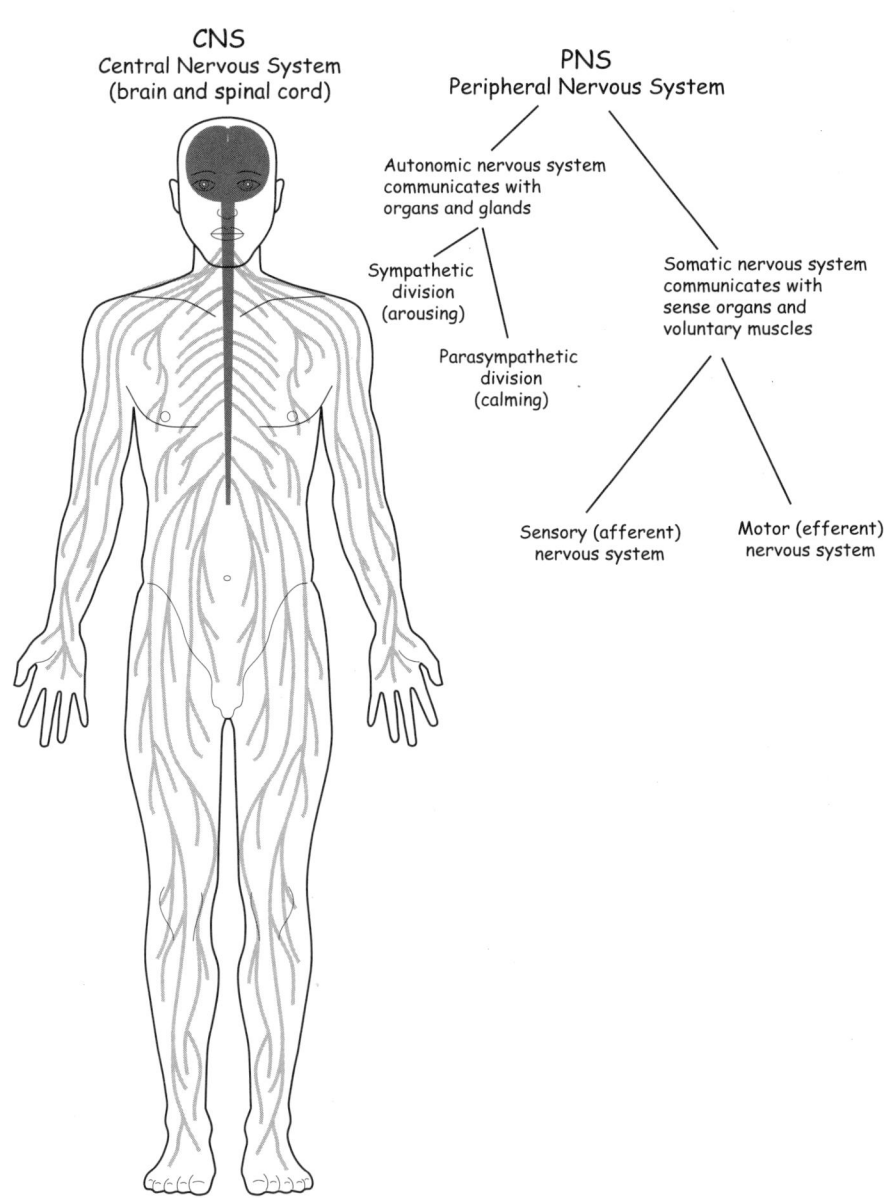

CNS
Central Nervous System
(brain and spinal cord)

PNS
Peripheral Nervous System

Autonomic nervous system
communicates with
organs and glands

Sympathetic
division
(arousing)

Parasympathetic
division
(calming)

Somatic nervous system
communicates with
sense organs and
voluntary muscles

Sensory (afferent)
nervous system

Motor (efferent)
nervous system

NERVOUS TISSUE

The brain is made up of billions of densely packed cells that form the nervous tissue of the body. The tissue of the nervous system is specialized to react to external and internal stimuli and to conduct impulses to and from areas within and outside of the brain. A nerve pathway is formed by a bundle of nerve fibers. Brain tissue is composed of two types of cells: glial cells and neurons.

Glial tissue

Glial tissue is a connective tissue involved in metabolic support, secretion of cerebrospinal fluid, response to injury, and insulation. There are three types of glial tissues.

Astrocytes: star-shaped cells located throughout the system of nerve cells in the brain. These cells have numerous projections that connect to blood capillaries and thereby assist in transporting substances from the blood to the nerve cell.

Oligodendrocytes/Schwann cells: Oligodendrocytes in the CNS and Schwann cells in the PNS form layers of insulation, called myelin, that wrap around the nerve cells.

Microglia: help to keep the nervous system clean by engulfing and destroying harmful organisms.

Neurons

Neurons receive, process, and transmit information to, from, and within the nervous system. There are about 100 billion neurons in the central nervous system. Neurons vary in size and shape, as well as in the total number of their receiving and transmitting processes. The basic structure of a neuron includes:

Soma (cell body): formed by a nucleus surrounded by a mass of cytoplasm containing organelles. Cell bodies make up the "gray matter" of the brain.

Dendrites: projections that branch off the cell body and transmit nerve impulses toward the cell body.

Axon: projection that transmits nerve impulses away from the cell body. Most axons in the central nervous system are wrapped in myelin which insulates and protects the axon. The myelin sheath is not continuous along the axon but is interrupted by breaks called nodes of Ranvier. The nodes are involved in speeding up the rate of nerve transmission, as the nerve impulse traveling along the axon jumps from one node to the next. Axons make up the "white matter" of the brain.

Terminal branches (telodendria): located at the endpoint of the axon.

Terminal buttons: endings of the terminal branches. Vesicles within the terminal buttons contain different types of neurotransmitters.

Synapse: tiny gap between nerve cells. A synapse may occur between the axon of one nerve and the dendrites, cell body, or axon of another nerve or nerves, of a muscle fiber, or of a glandular cell.

Neurons can be classified as:

Motor: convey impulses from the central or peripheral nervous system to muscles and glands.

Sensory: convey impulses from receptors in the muscles, skin, and glands to the nervous system.

Interneurons: connect neurons to each other, either locally within a small area of the CNS or over longer distances (projection neurons). Most neurons in the human NS are interneurons.

Unipolar: have a single process extending from the cell body.

Bipolar: have two processes, one axon and one dendrite. Bipolar cells are specialized sensory neurons for the senses of smell, sight, taste, hearing, and balance.

Multipolar: have multiple dendrites and a single axon. Most neurons in the CNS are multipolar.

Golgi Type I (projection neurons): have long axons that extend to the PNS and synapse with nerves that innervate muscles or glands. Golgi Type I axons are typically myelinated.

Golgi Type II: local circuit neurons with short axons that synapse on nearby neurons within the CNS. Golgi Type II neurons are usually unmyelinated.

Neuron

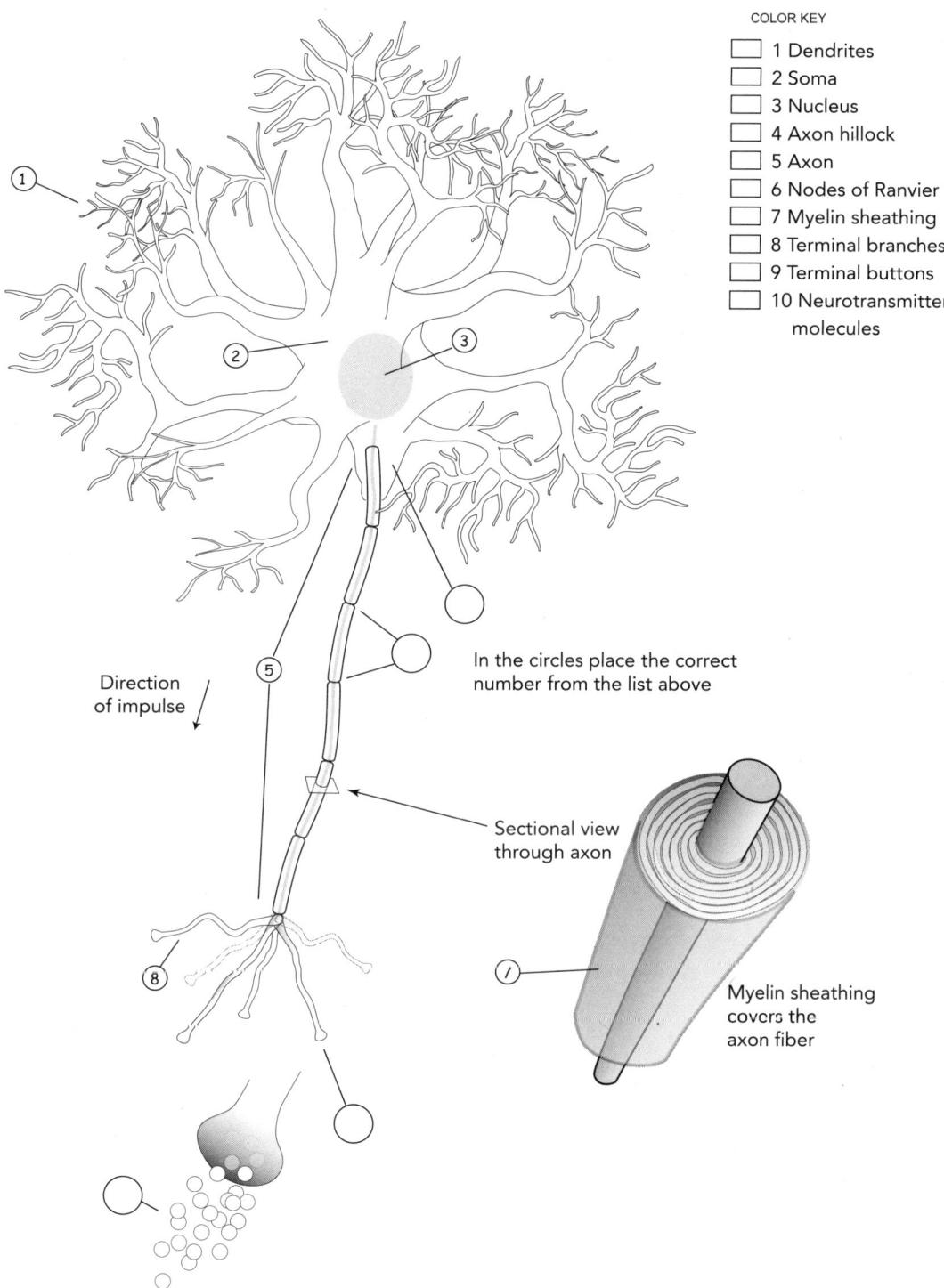

COLOR KEY

☐ 1 Dendrites
☐ 2 Soma
☐ 3 Nucleus
☐ 4 Axon hillock
☐ 5 Axon
☐ 6 Nodes of Ranvier
☐ 7 Myelin sheathing
☐ 8 Terminal branches
☐ 9 Terminal buttons
☐ 10 Neurotransmitter
   molecules

In the circles place the correct number from the list above

Direction of impulse

Sectional view through axon

Myelin sheathing covers the axon fiber

Types of neurons

COLOR KEY

- ☐ 1 Dendrites
- ☐ 2 Somas (cell bodies)
- ☐ 3 Nuclei
- ☐ 4 Axons
- ☐ 5 Terminal branches
- ☐ 6 Terminal buttons

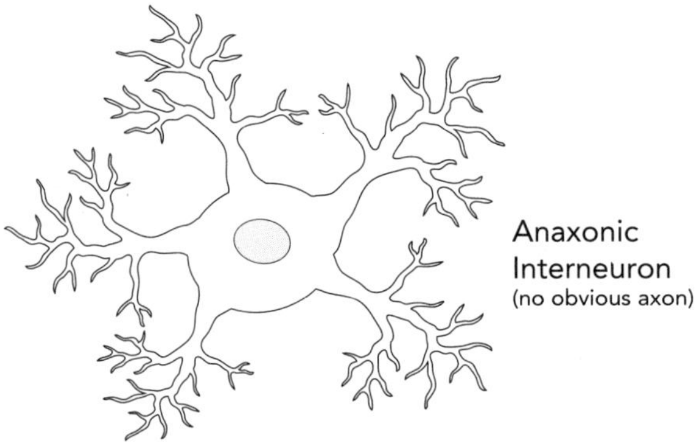

Anaxonic
Interneuron
(no obvious axon)

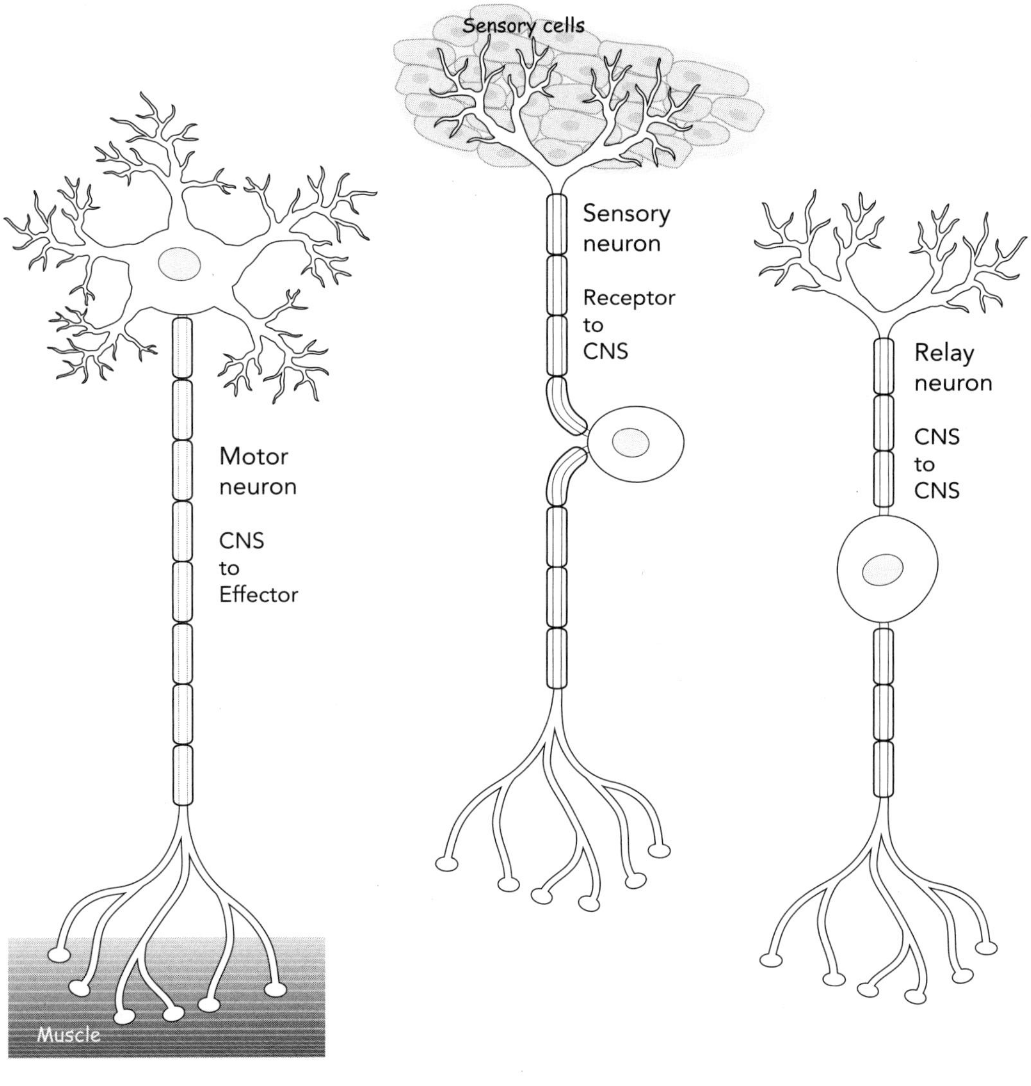

Sensory cells

Sensory
neuron

Receptor
to
CNS

Relay
neuron

CNS
to
CNS

Motor
neuron

CNS
to
Effector

Muscle

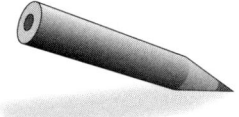

Neurotransmitters

Cells communicate with each other via neurotransmitters. Neurotransmitters are chemicals that are stored within the vesicles located in the terminal buttons of nerve axons. Neurotransmitters act as chemical bridges between neurons. Communication between cells occurs when the vesicles are stimulated to release their neurotransmitter into the synapse between the transmitting neuron (the presynaptic neuron) and the receiving neuron (the post-synaptic neuron).

The neurotransmitter acts like a key to a lock. On the membrane of the post-synaptic neuron are receptors that respond selectively to different neurotransmitters. Much as a specific key will only open a specific lock, receptor sites on the membrane will only respond to specific neurotransmitters.

Neurotransmitters can be excitatory, making it easier for the receiving nerve to react. This is called an excitatory post-synaptic potential (EPSP). Neurotransmitters may be inhibitory, making it harder for the postsynaptic neuron to respond. This is called an inhibitory post-synaptic potential (IPSP).

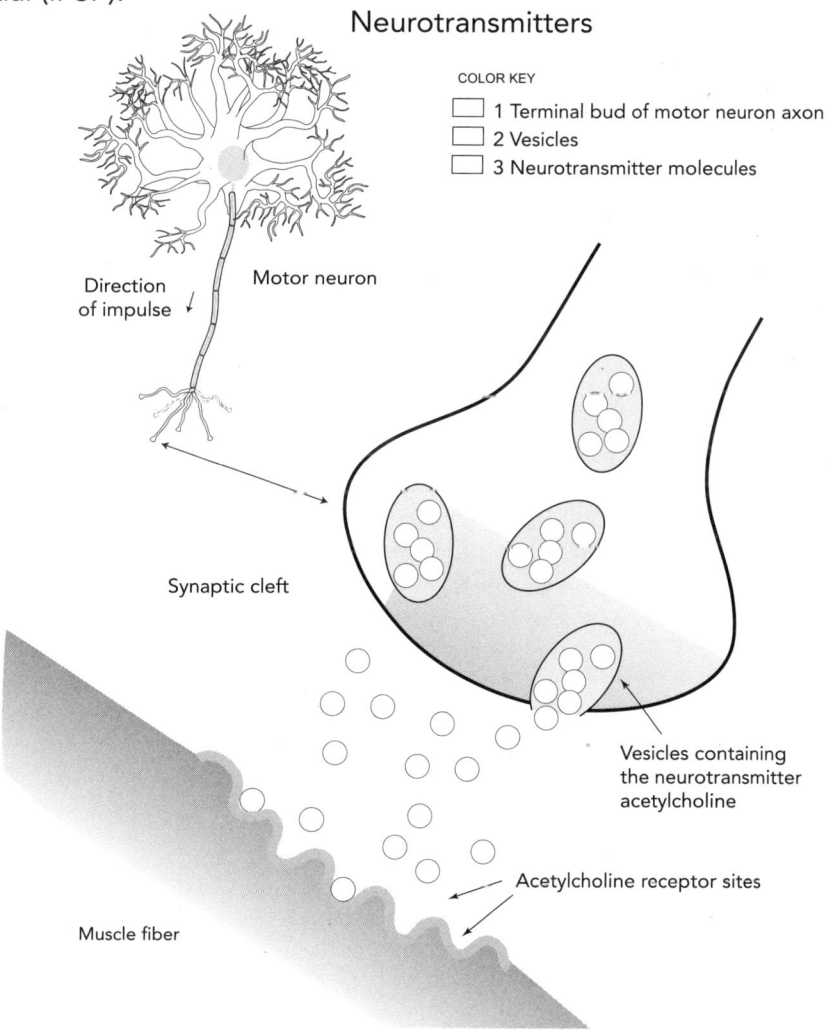

Neurotransmitters

COLOR KEY
1 Terminal bud of motor neuron axon
2 Vesicles
3 Neurotransmitter molecules

Motor neuron

Direction of impulse

Synaptic cleft

Vesicles containing the neurotransmitter acetylcholine

Acetylcholine receptor sites

Muscle fiber

Sensory receptors

In order to make sense of the information from an individual's external and internal environment, the body is richly supplied with different types of receptors. Receptors are specialized nerve cells that respond to changes in the organism or its environment and transmit these responses to the NS. Receptors respond to specific sensory stimuli. For example, receptors in the retina of the eye (rods and cones) respond to light. Receptors of the ear (inner hair cells) respond to sound waves. Receptors in the skin are differentially sensitive to touch, pressure, pain, and temperature.

TYPES OF SENSORY RECEPTORS

Type of receptor	Sensory information	Organ
Teleceptors	Distant environment	Eye, ear
Exteroceptors	Immediate environment	Skin
Proprioceptors	Position of body structures in space	Inner ear, muscles, tendons, joints
Visceroceptors/interoceptors	Visceral structures	Stomach, intestines, liver, etc
Mechanoreceptors	Pressure/deformation	Tissue
Thermoreceptors	Changes in temperature	Various
Nocioreceptors	Tissue damage	Tissue
Photoreceptors	Light	Retina
Chemoreceptors	Taste and smell	Tongue, nose
Baroreceptors	Air pressure	Trachea, bronchi

CENTRAL NERVOUS SYSTEM

The brain and spinal cord are housed within the skull and the spinal column. These bony structures form a layer of protection for nervous tissue. The CNS is additionally protected by three layers of non-nervous tissue, the meninges.

Meninges

Dura mater: outermost layer of the meninges. It is composed of tough, membranous connective tissue. It has two parts: the periosteal layer which attaches to the cranium and the meningeal layer. The dura is well supplied with blood vessels and nerves.

Arachnoid mater: lies immediately deep to the dura mater. It has a delicate web-like appearance with no blood vessels.

Pia mater: innermost layer of the meninges. It is composed of thin, delicate, highly vascular tissue that adheres closely to the grooves and convolutions of the brain.

Subdural space: lies between the dura mater and the arachnoid.

Subarachnoid space: located between the arachnoid and the pia mater.

This space is filled with cerebrospinal fluid (CSF). The CSF circulates around the entire meningeal system, so that the brain and spinal cord are protected by a buoyant fluid shock-absorbing system.

Cerebral cortex

The cortex is the outer covering of the brain which is tissue formed primarily by the cell bodies of neurons. The cortex is commonly known as "gray matter. The cortex is composed of three to six layers of nerve cells. It varies in thickness from about 2 to 4 mm. The cortex is highly convoluted with raised surfaces called gyri (singular: gyrus), shallow depressions called sulci (singular: sulcus), and deeper grooves called fissures. The convolutions serve an important purpose by increasing the surface area of the cortex without increasing the space needed to house it.

Cerebral cortex

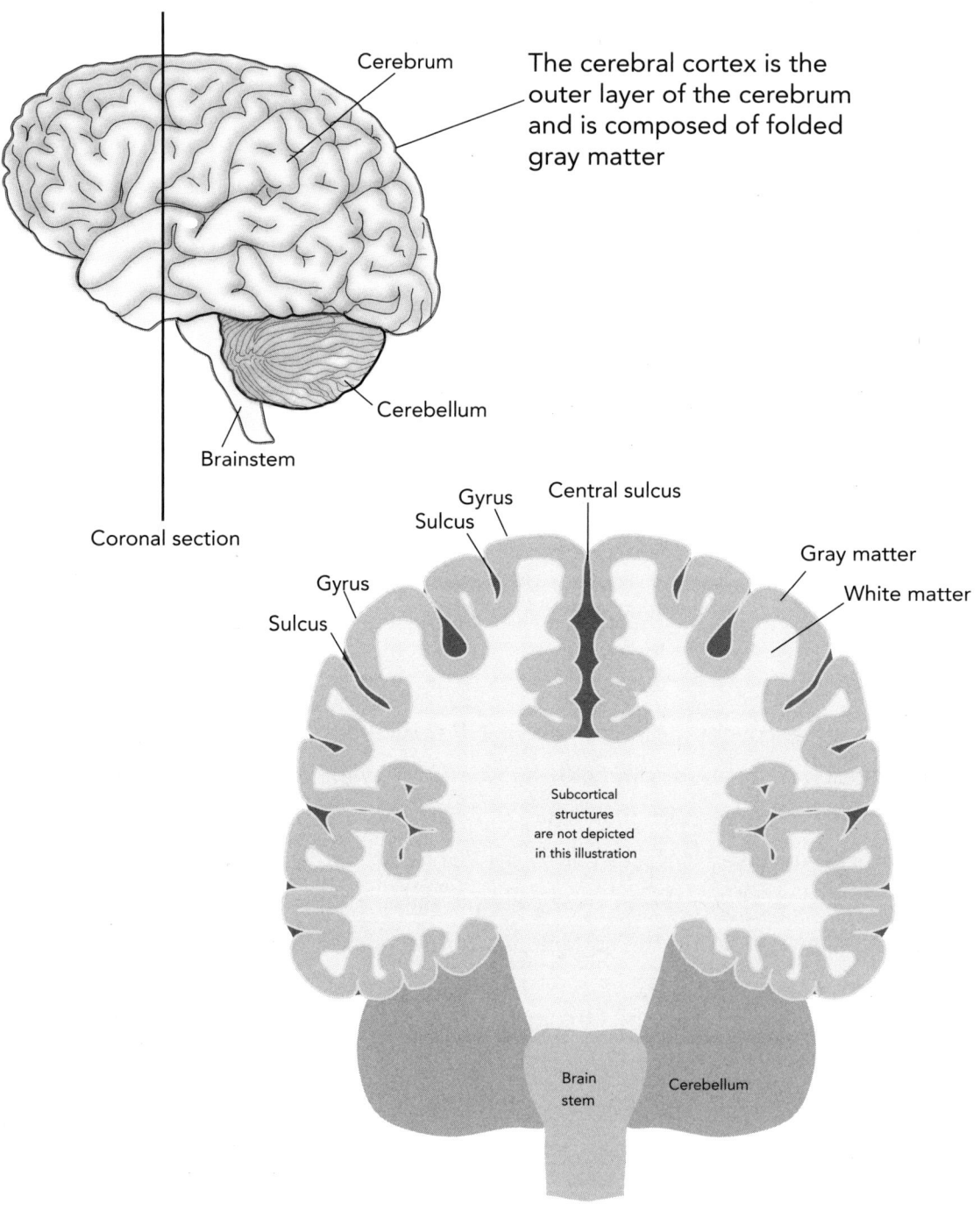

Cerebrum

The cerebral cortex is the outer layer of the cerebrum and is composed of folded gray matter

Cerebellum

Brainstem

Coronal section

Gyrus

Sulcus

Central sulcus

Gyrus

Sulcus

Gray matter

White matter

Subcortical structures are not depicted in this illustration

Brain stem

Cerebellum

Layers of the skull and brain

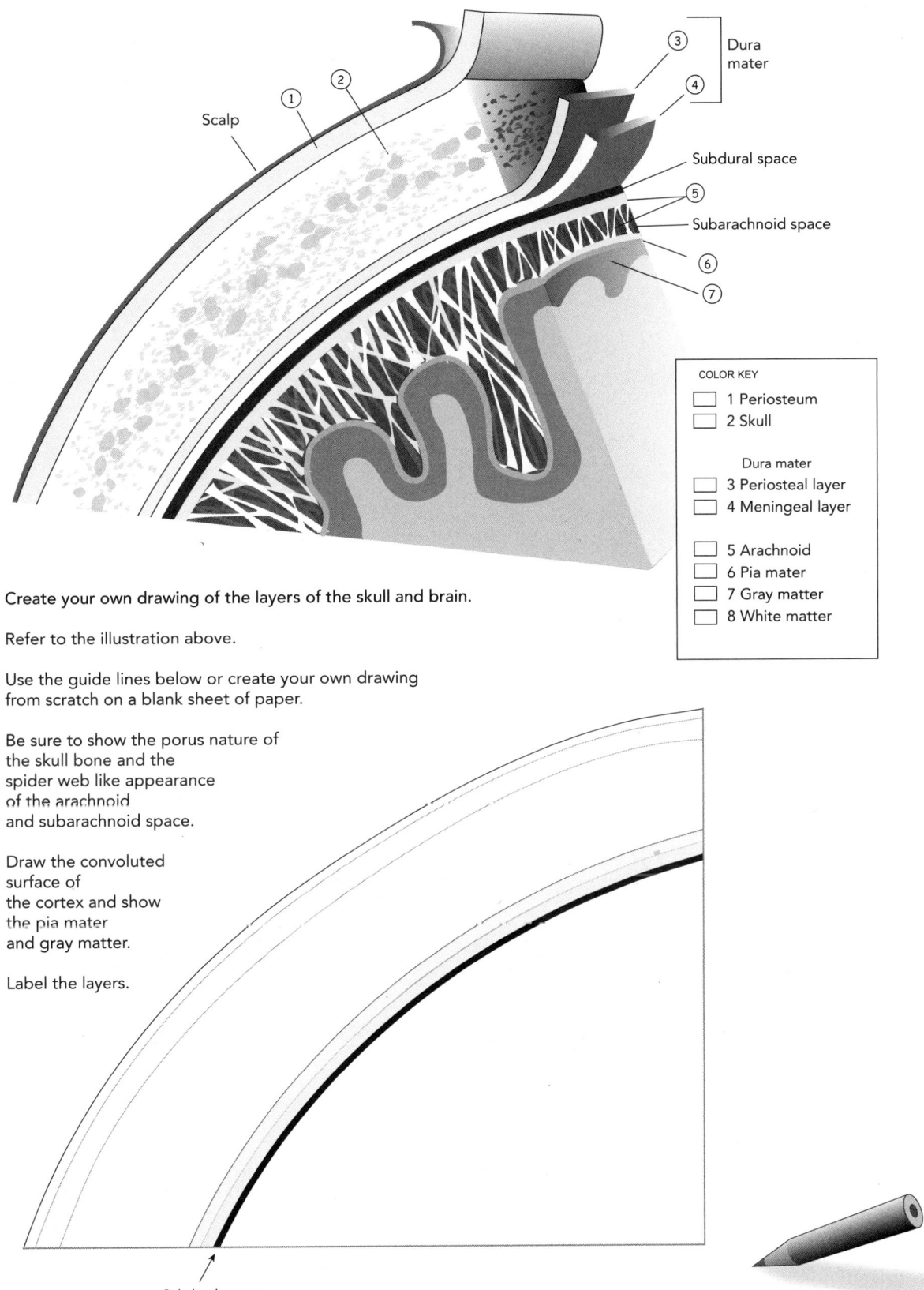

Scalp

Dura mater

Subdural space

Subarachnoid space

COLOR KEY
- [ ] 1 Periosteum
- [ ] 2 Skull

Dura mater
- [ ] 3 Periosteal layer
- [ ] 4 Meningeal layer

- [ ] 5 Arachnoid
- [ ] 6 Pia mater
- [ ] 7 Gray matter
- [ ] 8 White matter

Create your own drawing of the layers of the skull and brain.

Refer to the illustration above.

Use the guide lines below or create your own drawing from scratch on a blank sheet of paper.

Be sure to show the porus nature of the skull bone and the spider web like appearance of the arachnoid and subarachnoid space.

Draw the convoluted surface of the cortex and show the pia mater and gray matter.

Label the layers.

Subdural space

Hemispheres and lobes

The brain is divided into two hemispheres, right and left.

The sulci and fissures separate the brain into four lobes that can be seen on the surface of the brain.

Longitudinal cerebral fissure: divides the brain into left and right hemispheres.

Central sulcus: separates the brain into anterior and posterior portions.

Lateral fissure: separates the brain into superior and inferior regions.

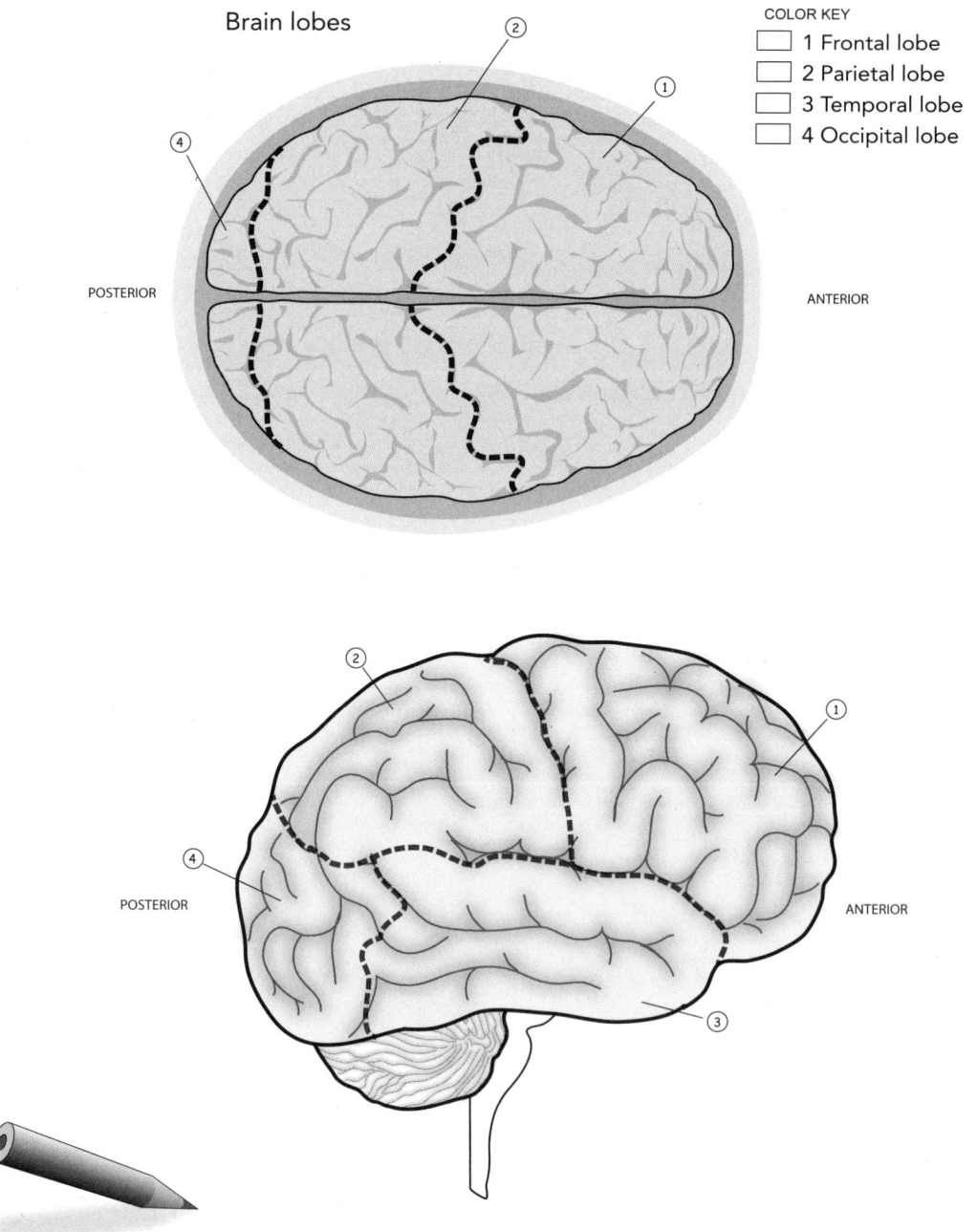

Brain lobes

COLOR KEY
☐ 1 Frontal lobe
☐ 2 Parietal lobe
☐ 3 Temporal lobe
☐ 4 Occipital lobe

POSTERIOR   ANTERIOR

POSTERIOR   ANTERIOR

Cortical connections

Many nerve pathways interconnect various regions of the nervous system to each other. Some of the most important include:

Corpus callosum: connects the right and left hemispheres.

Superior longitudinal fasciculus: links the four major lobes.

Arcuate fasciculus: connects parts of the frontal, parietal, and temporal lobes.

Internal capsule: runs between the cerebral cortex and thalamus.

Corona radiata: continuation of the internal capsule.

Frontal lobe

The frontal lobe is located anterior to the central sulcus and superior to the lateral sulcus. This is the part of the neocortex that contains areas devoted to language and speech, as well as abstract functions including reasoning, problem solving, personality, and symbolic function. Most motor activity is controlled by the frontal lobe.

Important motor areas include the primary motor cortex (M1, also known as the motor strip), premotor area, and supplementary motor area. The primary motor cortex is situated on the precentral gyrus, immediately anterior to the central sulcus. Broca's area is in the lateral portion of the inferior region of the motor strip.

The motor strip is organized somatotopically, so that control of different body structures is located within specific portions of the tissue. Starting at the top of the motor strip and progressing inferiorly toward the lateral fissure are portions of cortex responsible for movement of the hip, trunk (thorax and abdomen), arms, hands, neck, face, and larynx.

Parietal lobes

The parietal lobes are located on the postcentral gyrus, immediately posterior to the central sulcus. These lobes deal with bodily sensation including touch, pressure, pain, proprioception, and temperature. Like the motor cortex, the primary somatosensory areas (S1) are represented somatotopically.

Supramarginal gyrus and angular gyrus: These gyri are located at the bottom portion of the parietal lobe. Both areas are important in integrating sensory modalities including vision, touch, and hearing.

Temporal lobes

The temporal lobes are located immediately inferior to the lateral fissure. They are important for hearing and understanding. The primary auditory cortex (A1) receives information from the ear and auditory nerve. Wernicke's area is essential for the decoding and comprehension of speech.

Arcuate fasciculus: association pathway that connects Broca's area and Wernicke's area. This connection highlights the close neuroanatomical relationship between the understanding and production of speech.

Occipital lobe

The occipital lobe is situated at the posterior of the brain. It is dedicated to the reception and processing of visual information.

Ventricles

There are four ventricles (cavities) located within the brain: two lateral ventricles, one in each hemisphere, the third ventricle, and the fourth ventricle. The two lateral ventricles both connect to the third ventricle by way of the interventricular foramen. The third and fourth ventricles are connected by the cerebral aqueduct. Cerebrospinal fluid (CSF) is manufactured by specialized cells within the ventricles called choroid plexus cells. The fluid flows through the ventricles and their connecting areas to escape through median and lateral apertures into the subarachnoid space. The CSF eventually drains out of the subarachnoid space into the venous portion of the circulatory system. Obstruction within this system that prevents the fluid from flowing freely or draining properly, or any kind of problem that results in an excessive amount of CSF, can cause serious neurological problems.

Ventricles

COLOR KEY
- [ ] Lateral ventricle
- [ ] 3rd ventricle
- [ ] 4th ventricle
- [ ] Interventricular foramen

Interventricular foramen

Lateral Ventricle

Cerebrum →

ANTERIOR

3rd Ventricle

Cerebellum →

Brainstem

4th Ventricle

Brainstem

Cerebellum

3rd Ventricle

ANTERIOR

Cerebral aqueduct

Lateral Ventricle

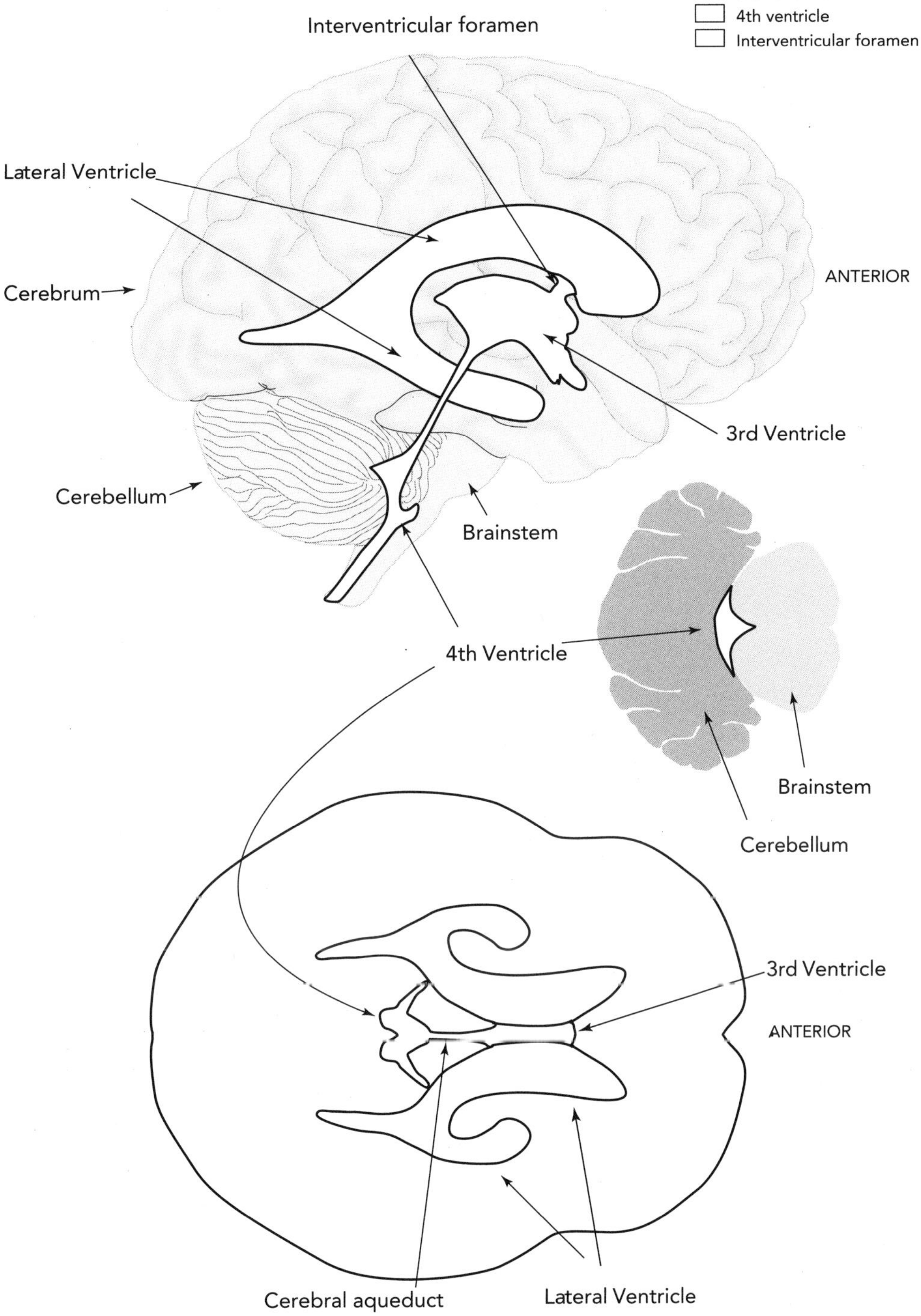

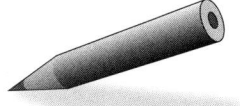

Brodmanns's areas

Areas within each lobe have been associated with specific functions. In 1914 a German neurologist, Brodmann, divided and numbered areas of the brain based on microscopic analyses of the structure and organization of the cells and tissues that comprise the cortex. Brodmann identified 52 functional areas of human cerebral cortex, including areas important for speech and hearing. The numbering system that Brodmann devised is still in use today. Many of the areas that Brodmann identified have been correlated closely to diverse cortical functions using neuropsychological testing and functional brain imaging. The areas listed in the table below are the ones most commonly associated with speech and hearing,

BRODMANN TABLE

On the facing page, locate the following areas and color them and the corresponding color key box in the table below.

Lobe	Brodmann's number	Name(s) of area	COLOR KEY
Frontal	4	Primary motor area, M1	
	6	Premotor area and supplementary motor area	
	44, 45	Broca's area (only in dominant hemisphere)	
Parietal	3, 1, 2	Primary somatosensory area, S1	
	5, 7	Somatosensory association area	
	39	Angular gyrus	
	40	Supramarginal gyrus	
Occipital	17	Primary visual area, V1	
	18, 19	Visual association area	
Temporal	41	Primary auditory area, A1	
	42	Auditory association area	
	22	Wernicke's area	

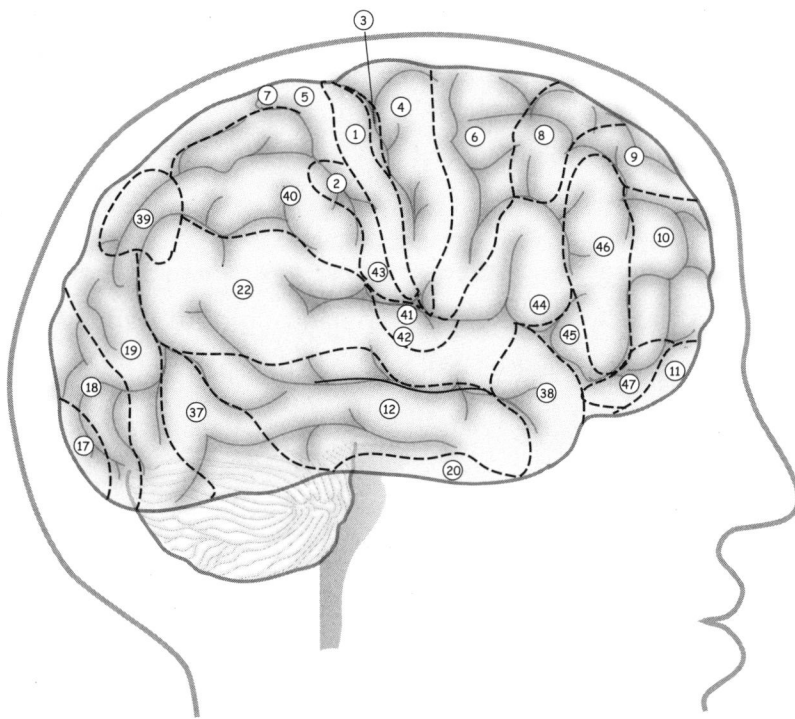

Limbic lobe and limbic system

Unlike the other four lobes of the brain, the limbic lobe is not a separate lobe. Rather, it is made up of the most medial margins of the frontal, parietal, and temporal lobes, and is part of the larger limbic system.

The limbic system comprises several brain structures including the hippocampus, amygdala, septal nuclei, mammillary bodies, and anterior nuclei of the thalamus. The system deals with emotions and memory.

Hippocampus: located in the medial portion of the temporal lobes. It plays an important role in consolidating and coordinating memories, it is also involved in transferring information from short-term to long-term memory.

Amygdala: consists of groups of nuclei located within the medial portion of the temporal lobes. It plays a part in mood and emotional status and is also involved in memory and decision making.

Fornix: large bundle of nerve fibers which serves as the main output of the hypothalamus.

Septal nuclei: formed by groups of nuclei that have reciprocal connections with the hippocampus, amygdala, midbrain, hypothalamus and thalamus. This structure is associated with social behavior, anxiety, fear, and memory-related behaviors.

Mammillary bodies: consist of two groups of nuclei (medial and lateral) and are often included as part of the hypothalamus. They are involved in certain types of memory.

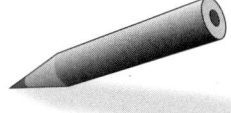

Subcortical Areas of the Brain

Deep within the white matter of the cerebrum are several circumscribed areas of gray matter consisting of collections of nerve cell bodies.

Basal nuclei

The basal nuclei, also called basal ganglia, comprise several areas of gray matter in each hemisphere. The basal nuclei include the caudate nucleus, globus pallidus, putamen and substantia nigra. The putamen and globus pallidus together are called the lenticular nucleus; the caudate and putamen together form the striatum.

The basal nuclei connect with many other structures and pathways. They receive input from the motor and other areas of the cortex and the thalamus. They also make connections with each other and other nuclei. The pathways to, from, and among the components of the basal nuclei form a series of complex circuits. These circuits run between the cerebral cortex, basal nuclei, and thalamus.

One of the primary functions of the basal nuclei is regulating aspects of motor control such as posture, balance, background muscle tone, and coordination of muscle groups. The basal nuclei are also important in the indirect control of precise voluntary movements through a neural mechanism called inhibition.

Thalamus

The thalamus comprises a collection of nuclei, some of which are involved with motor function and some with sensory function.

The thalamus is sometimes called the "gateway to consciousness" because all information traveling to the cerebral cortex, aside from olfaction, passes through the thalamus. The nuclei of the thalamus send information to and receive information from the cerebral cortex via the pathways of the internal capsule. The nuclei of the thalamus participate in motor, sensory, and limbic functions. Each thalamic nucleus projects to a different part of the cerebral cortex (thalamocortical fibers). Likewise, that portion of the cortex reciprocally projects to the originating thalamic nucleus (corticothalamic fibers).

Hypothalamus

The hypothalamus contains nuclei that are involved in sensory and motor control of visceral functions. The hypothalamus regulates hormonal function, body temperature, hunger, sleep–wake cycles, sexual drive, blood pressure, and other functions designed to keep the body's internal environment in a state of equilibrium (homeostasis). The hypothalamus connects with the limbic system, pituitary gland, and brain stem. These connections allow widespread control of the visceral and emotional behavior that influence how individuals react to the internal and external environments. However, hypothalamic functioning is not under conscious control.

Subcortical brain areas

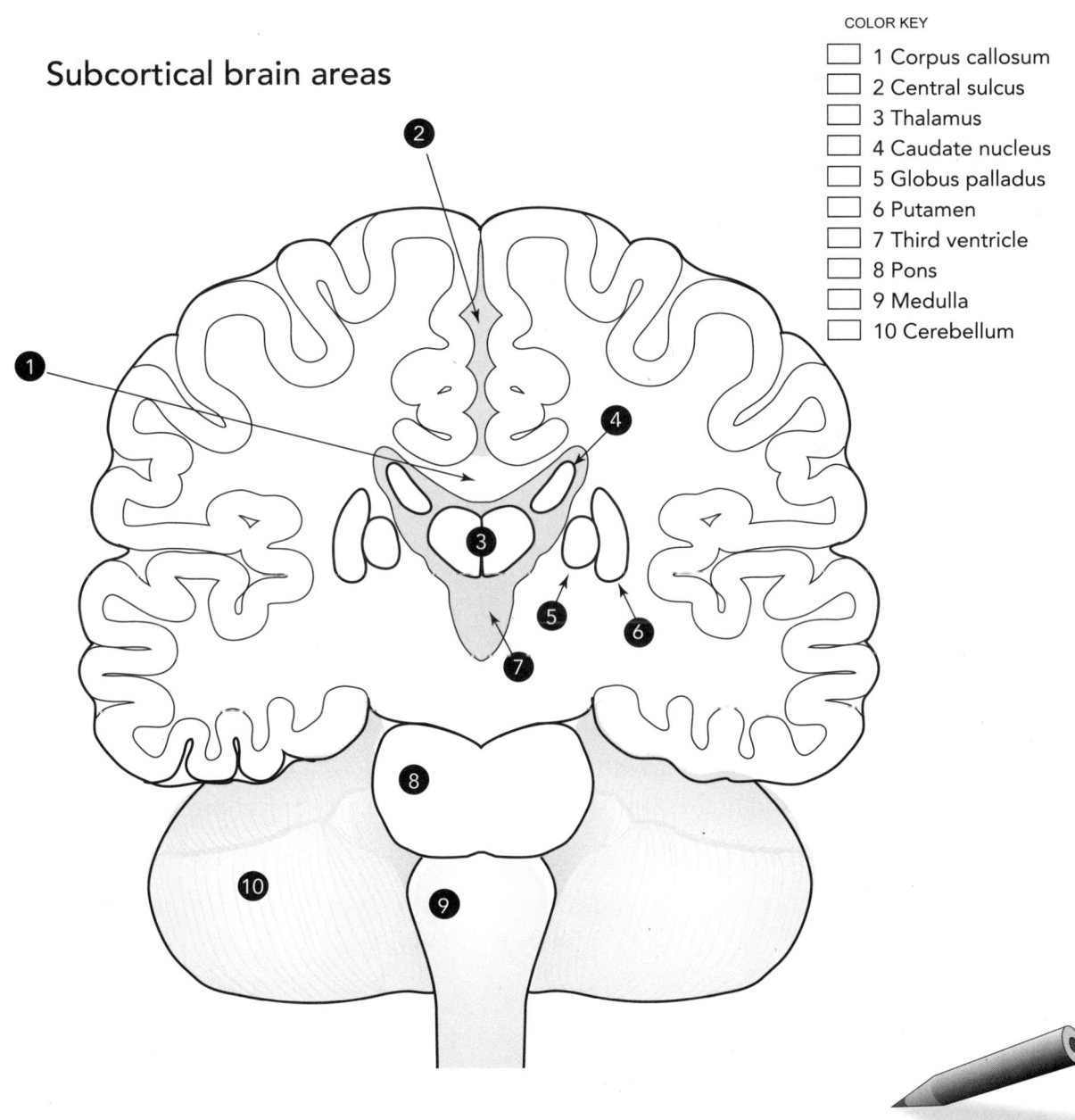

COLOR KEY

- [ ] 1 Corpus callosum
- [ ] 2 Central sulcus
- [ ] 3 Thalamus
- [ ] 4 Caudate nucleus
- [ ] 5 Globus palladus
- [ ] 6 Putamen
- [ ] 7 Third ventricle
- [ ] 8 Pons
- [ ] 9 Medulla
- [ ] 10 Cerebellum

CEREBELLUM

The cerebellum is located posterior to the brain stem and inferior to the cerebrum. It connects to the brain stem by way of the inferior, middle, and superior cerebellar peduncles. (A peduncle is a stem or stalk that attaches a mass of tissue to a body).

The cerebellum is involved in balance, posture, background muscle tone, and the coordination of voluntary movements. With its extensive connections to other motor centers as well as its extensive sensory input, it plays a central role in motor control and coordination. The cerebellum coordinates movements in terms of the direction of the movement, the force and speed with which the movement is executed, and the amount of displacement of the structure that is moving. It also ensures that complex movements are carried out with appropriate timing so that smooth synergistic muscular patterns are maintained.

Structures of the cerebellum

Vermis: thick band of white matter connecting the two hemispheres of the cerebellum.

Lobes: anterior, posterior, and flocculonodular.

Folia: series of ridges on the cerebellar surface.

Arbor vitae (tree of life): inner mass of the cerebellum composed of a branching pattern of white matter.

Deep grey matter: four clusters of grey matter nuclei deep within the inner mass (fastigial, emboliform, globose, and dentate). These nuclei contain most of the efferent neurons of the cerebellum. The nuclei receive input from and project back to specific portions of the cerebellar cortex, and to the brain stem and thalamus via the cerebellar peduncles.

Cerebellum

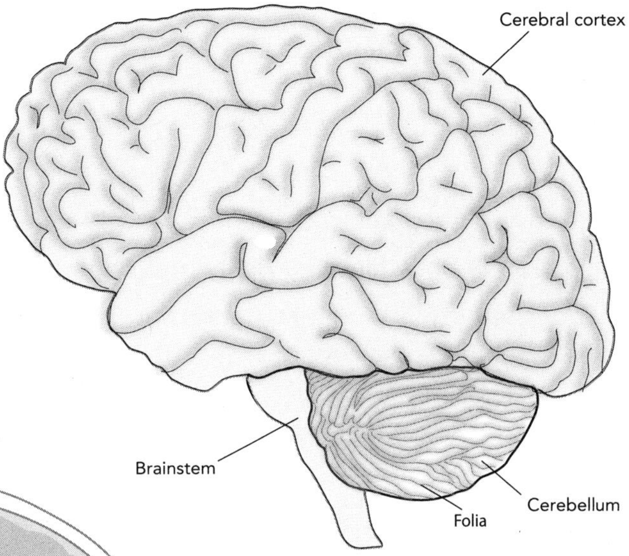
Cerebral cortex
Brainstem
Cerebellum
Folia

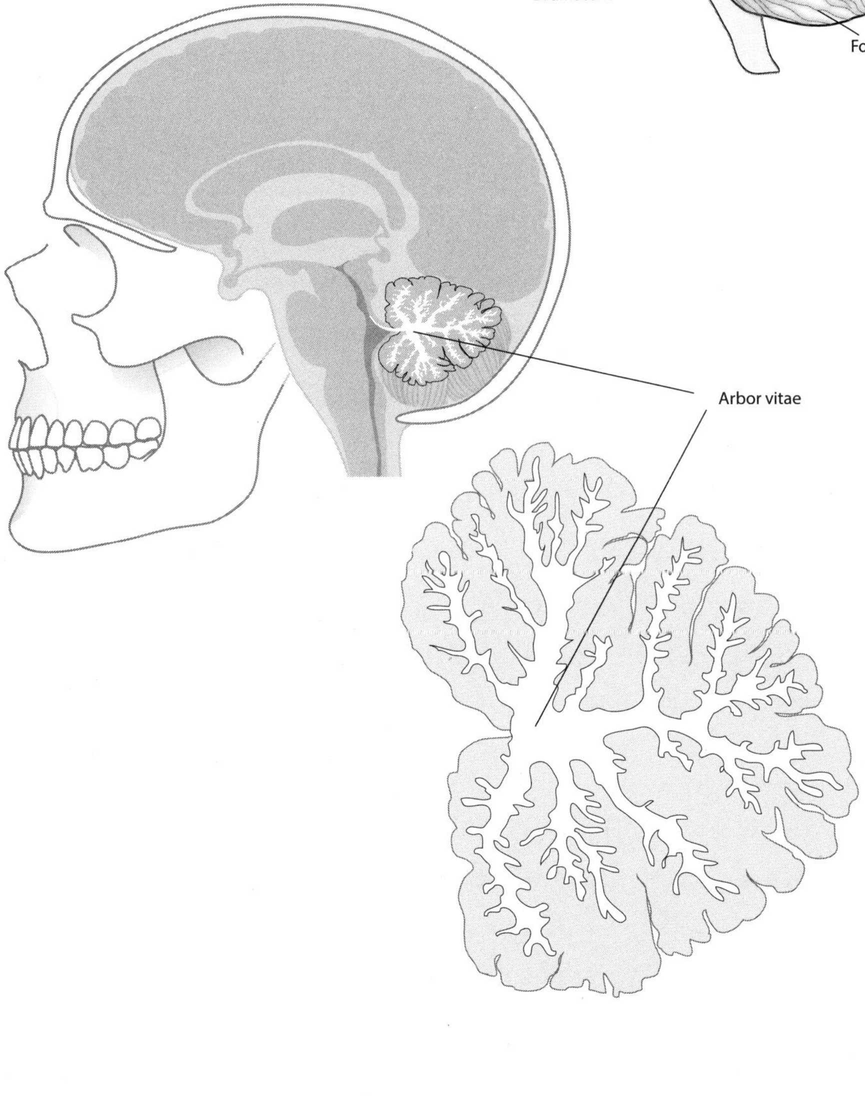
Arbor vitae

BRAIN STEM

The brain stem is a collective term for three separate but tightly linked structures: midbrain, pons, and medulla. The brain stem is the site of many reflexes involved in respiration, body temperature, swallowing, and digestion. It is also the site of origin of the cranial nerves. The topmost portion, the midbrain, is located directly inferior to the cerebrum. The lowermost part, the medulla, connects with the spinal cord. The pons forms a bridge between the midbrain and medulla, and the cerebellum.

Reticular formation: loose and diffuse network of nuclei controlling complex patterns of movement involved in breathing, cardiac function, and swallowing. The reticular activating system is part of the network. The nuclei forming this portion of the brain stem control state of alertness and level of consciousness. Damage to the reticular activating system can result in a coma.

Midbrain

The midbrain is short structure immediately inferior to the cerebrum. It plays an important role in higher level reflexes such as turning one's eyes to the source of a sound and startle responses to unexpected noises.

Cerebral peduncles: two cerebral peduncles are continuations of the internal capsule.

Inferior and superior colliculi: areas of grey matter that have projections to the thalamus. The inferior colliculus is an important auditory center that integrates sound signals from multiple sources. The superior colliculus plays a role in audiovisual integration.

Cerebral aqueduct: links the third and fourth ventricles.

Pons

The pons is located inferior to the midbrain and anterior to the cerebellum. The pons includes nerve pathways (superior and middle cerebellar peduncles) that act as a bridge between the cerebellum and the rest of the nervous system.

Medulla

The medulla is the most inferior part of the brain stem. It is continuous with the pons superiorly and the spinal cord inferiorly. This is where a large percentage of nerve fibers in the cerebral cortex decussate and continue down the contralateral side of the body. The medulla also connects to the cerebellum by way of the inferior cerebellar peduncles. It mediates many reflexes such as coughing, sneezing, and vomiting.

Inferior view of brain

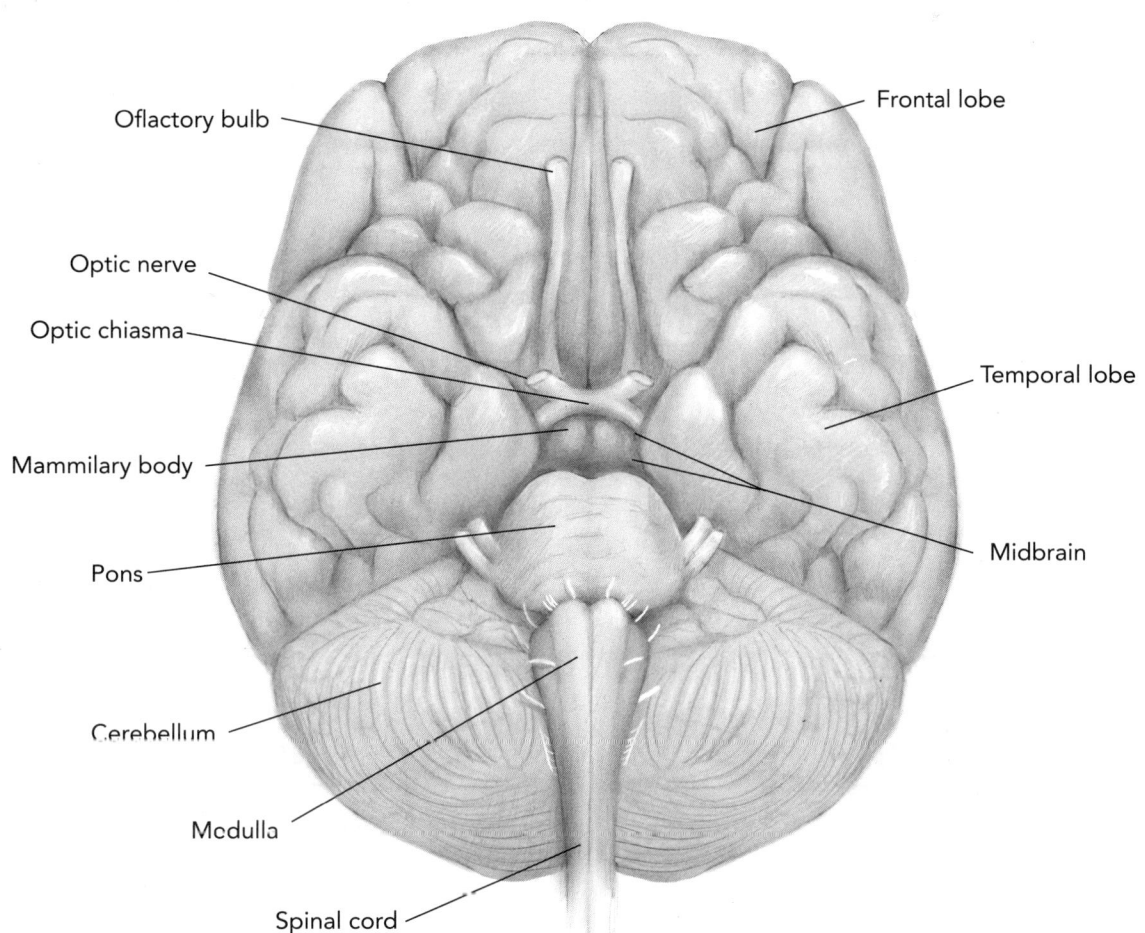

Oflactory bulb

Optic nerve

Optic chiasma

Mammilary body

Pons

Cerebellum

Medulla

Spinal cord

Frontal lobe

Temporal lobe

Midbrain

SPINAL CORD

The spinal cord is the downward continuation of the brain stem and contains the 31 pairs of spinal nerves that run to all the muscles of the body, aside from those of the head and neck. The spinal cord is one continuous structure but is categorized into five sections:

Cervical: neck   Thoracic: chest   Lumbar: lower back   Sacral: pelvis   Coccygeal: tail bone

Spinal nerves

Thirty-one pairs of spinal nerves enter and exit the spinal cord by way of spaces called intervertebral foramina. The intervertebral foramina are located between successive vertebrae. Each spinal nerve has both a sensory and a motor branch. The sensory branch exits the spinal cord via the posterior horn, and the motor branch enters the cord via the anterior horn. The two branches converge outside the spinal cord to form the spinal nerve.

Dorsal (posterior) horns: made up of nerve cell bodies that receive sensory information.

Ventral (anterior) horns: contain the cell bodies that project fibers to skeletal muscles.

Lateral horns: involved in visceral functions.

Intermediate zone: region where the anterior and posterior horns meet.

Peripheral nerves arising from the spinal cord form networks called plexuses.
There are four major plexuses:

Cervical plexus: innervates muscles of the neck.

Brachial plexus: innervates muscles of the shoulder and upper limbs.

Lumbar plexus: innervates muscles of the anterior and medial thigh.

Lumbosacral plexus: innervates the buttocks, pelvis, perineum, and lower limbs.

Reflexes

The spinal cord functions to institute reflexes. A reflex is an involuntary, stereotyped motor response to a sensory input. Simple reflexes are confined to a single cord level (intrasegmental). Complex reflexes involve multiple cord segments (intersegmental) and more than one synapse.

Spinal nerves

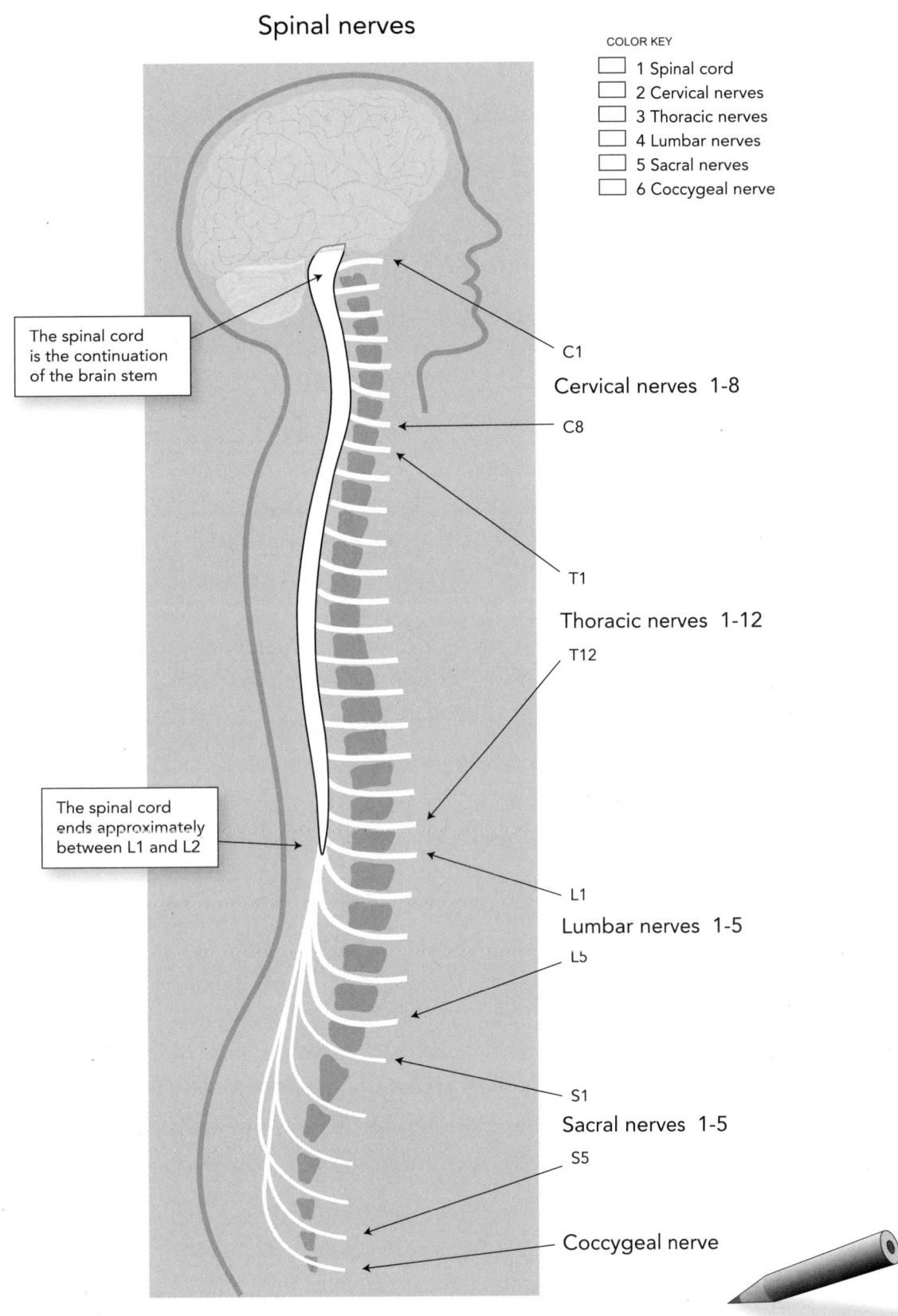

COLOR KEY
- 1 Spinal cord
- 2 Cervical nerves
- 3 Thoracic nerves
- 4 Lumbar nerves
- 5 Sacral nerves
- 6 Coccygeal nerve

The spinal cord is the continuation of the brain stem

The spinal cord ends approximately between L1 and L2

C1

Cervical nerves 1-8

C8

T1

Thoracic nerves 1-12

T12

L1

Lumbar nerves 1-5

L5

S1

Sacral nerves 1-5

S5

Coccygeal nerve

Vertebrae

COLOR KEY

☐ 1 Cervical vertebra	☐ 6 Transverse foramen
☐ 2 Thoracic vertebra	☐ 7 Superior articular facet
☐ 3 Lumbar vertebra	☐ 8 Bifid spinous process
IN THE LOWER ILLUSTRATION	☐ 9 Transverse process
☐ 4 Vertebral foramen	☐ 10 Lamina
☐ 5 Spinal cord	☐ 11 Pedicle

Vertebrae are the individual bones that make up the spinal column.

"Vertebrae" is plural. The singular of vertebrae is "vertebra."

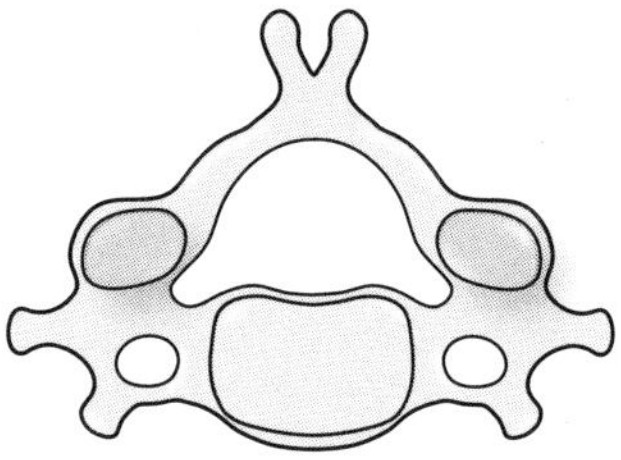

① Cervical vertebra

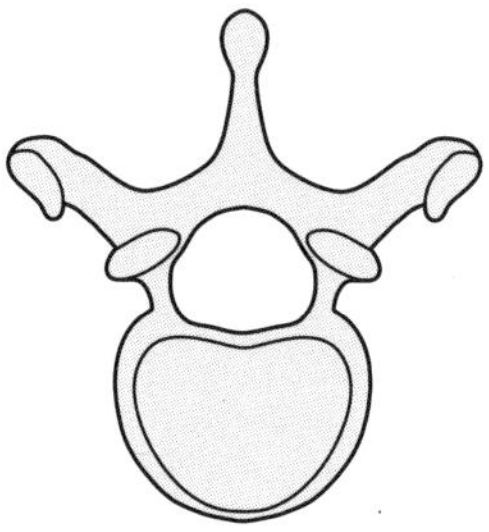

② Thoracic vertebra

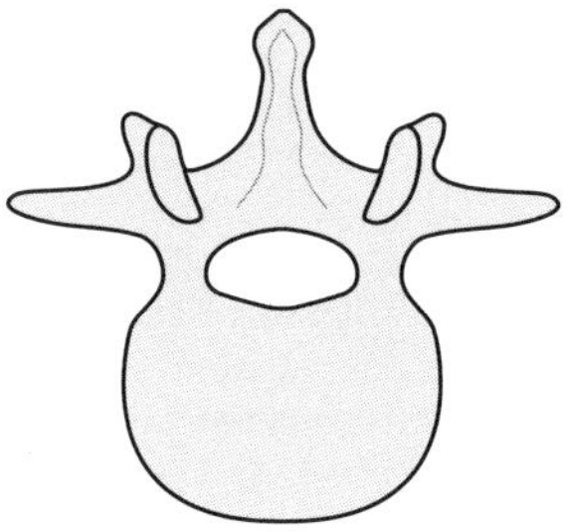

③ Lumbar vertebra

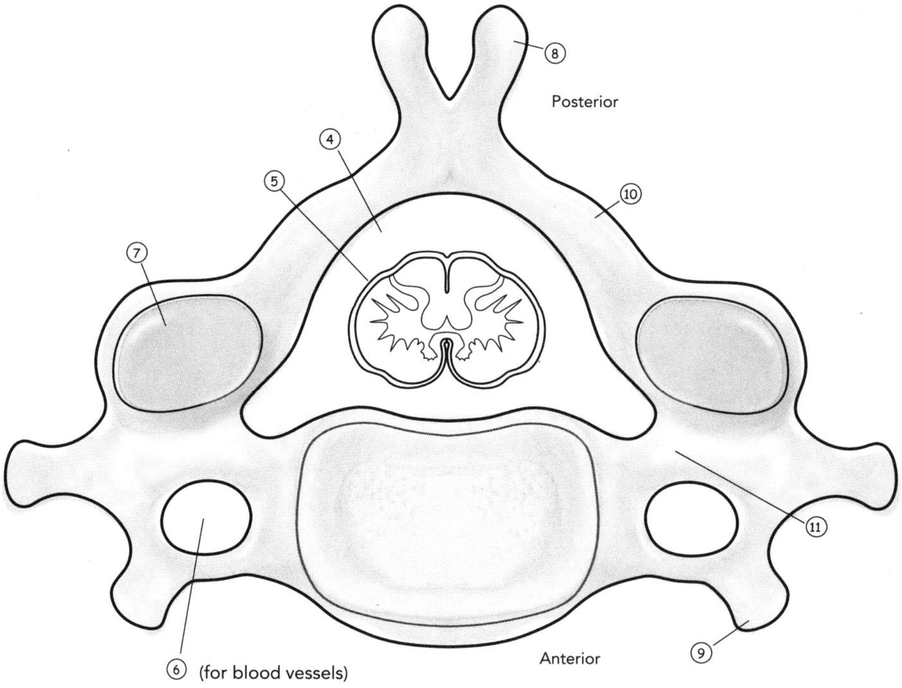

Posterior

Anterior

⑥ (for blood vessels)

Gray and white matter

Like the brain, the spinal cord is made up of areas of gray matter and white matter. In the brain the gray matter forms the outer covering (cortex) and the white matter is located within. This pattern is reversed in the spinal cord, with the white matter on the outside and the gray matter contained within.

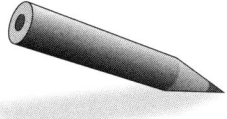

Spinal cord and nerves

COLOR KEY

- ☐ 1 Pia mater
- ☐ 2 White mattter
- ☐ 3 Grey matter
- ☐ 4 Sensory nerve root
- ☐ 5 Motor nerve root
- ☐ 6 Spinal dural sheath (dura mater)
- ☐ 7 Subdural space
- ☐ 8 Arachnoid
- ☐ 9 Subarachnoid space

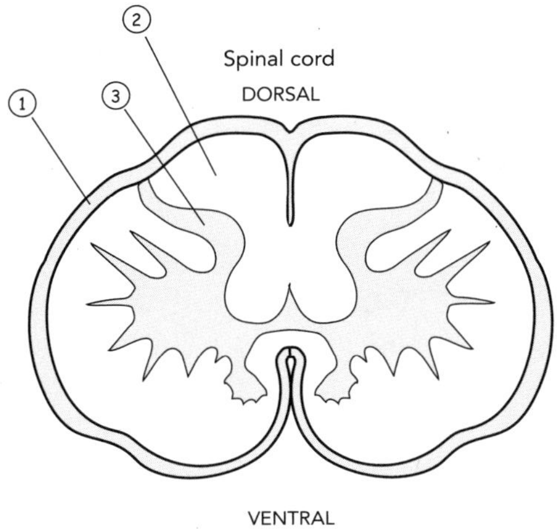
Spinal cord
DORSAL
1
2
3
VENTRAL

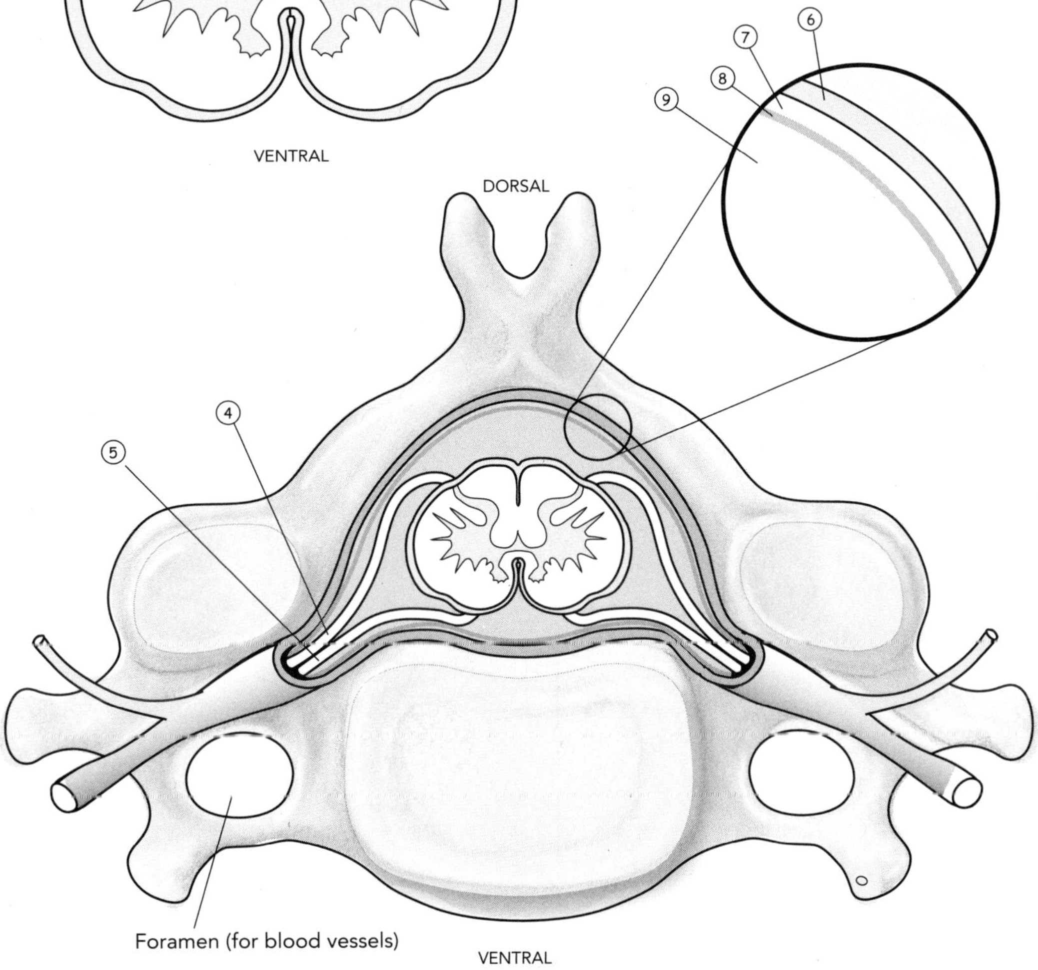
DORSAL
4
5
6
7
8
9
Foramen (for blood vessels)
VENTRAL

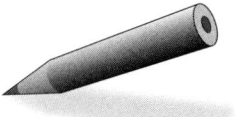

Cranial Nerves

The 12 pairs of cranial nerves transmit information to and from the face and neck regions. The cranial nerves are numbered with Roman numerals from I to XII. Most of the cell bodies of the cranial nerves (III to XII) arise from the brain stem, and the axons project to muscles in the face, head, and ears. The nerves are numbered according to their order of emergence from the brain stem.

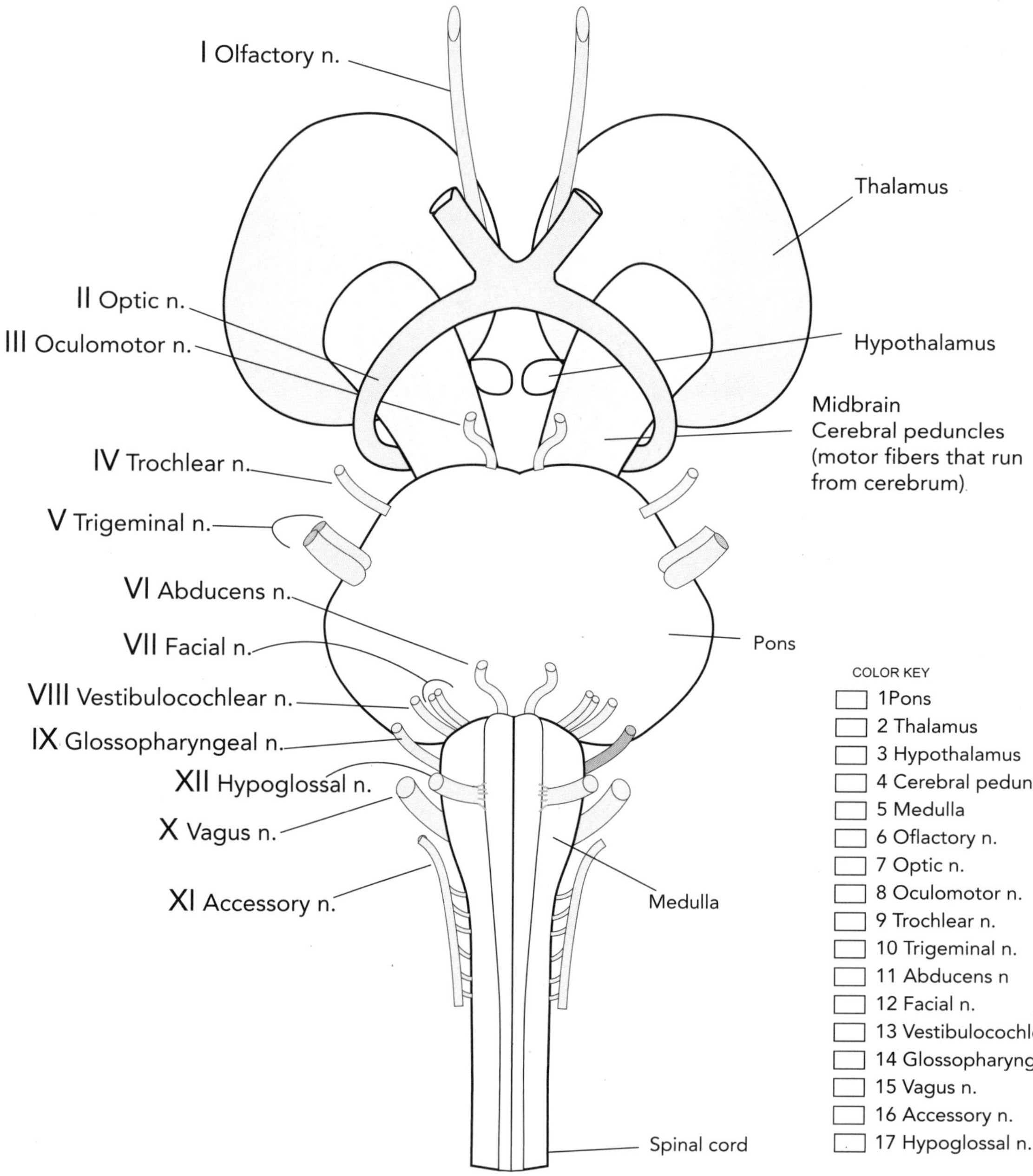

I Olfactory n.

Thalamus

II Optic n.

III Oculomotor n.

Hypothalamus

Midbrain
Cerebral peduncles
(motor fibers that run
from cerebrum)

IV Trochlear n.

V Trigeminal n.

VI Abducens n.

VII Facial n.

Pons

VIII Vestibulocochlear n.

IX Glossopharyngeal n.

XII Hypoglossal n.

X Vagus n.

XI Accessory n.

Medulla

Spinal cord

View is from the front and below

COLOR KEY
- 1 Pons
- 2 Thalamus
- 3 Hypothalamus
- 4 Cerebral peduncles
- 5 Medulla
- 6 Oflactory n.
- 7 Optic n.
- 8 Oculomotor n.
- 9 Trochlear n.
- 10 Trigeminal n.
- 11 Abducens n
- 12 Facial n.
- 13 Vestibulocochlear n.
- 14 Glossopharyngeal n.
- 15 Vagus n.
- 16 Accessory n.
- 17 Hypoglossal n.

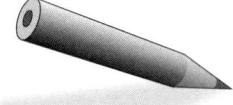

Cranial nerves most involved in speech and swallowing, and hearing.

CN V: Trigeminal

CN V contains three branches: ophthalmic, maxillary, and mandibular. Sensory fibers transmit information about touch, pressure, pain, proprioception, and temperature from various areas of the face—the maxillary branch from the upper lip, teeth, and upper jaw; and the mandibular branch from the lower lip and teeth, lower jaw, and oral cavity. Motor fibers innervate the muscles of mastication, the tensor veli palatini, the tensor tympani, and some of the extrinsic laryngeal muscles.

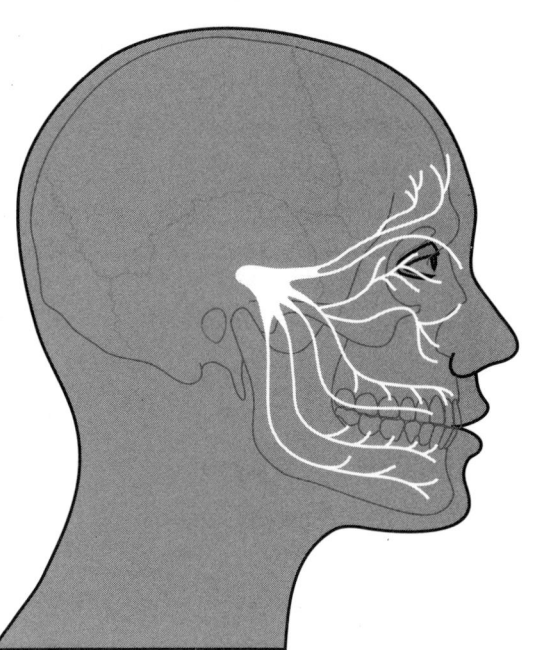

CN V: Trigeminal nerve

CN VII: Facial

Motor fibers from CN VII supply nerve impulses to the muscles of facial expression, the stapedius muscle in the middle ear, and some of the extrinsic laryngeal muscles. Innervation to facial muscles above the eyes is ipsilateral. Innervation to the facial muscles below the eyes is contralateral. Sensory fibers transmit information from the external ear as well as taste information from the anterior two-thirds of the tongue.

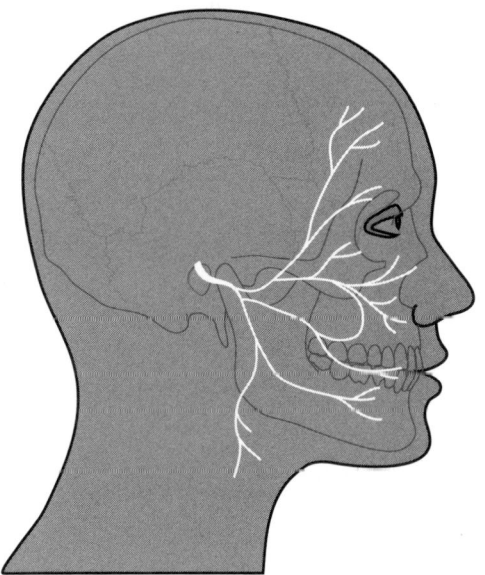

CN VII: Facial nerve

CN VIII: Vestibulocochlear

CN VIII has two branches: vestibular and cochlear. The vestibular fibers arise from the semicircular canals, utricle, and saccule in the inner ear and relay information to the CNS about balance and head position. The cochlear portion arises from the inner hair cells in the cochlea and transmits auditory information.

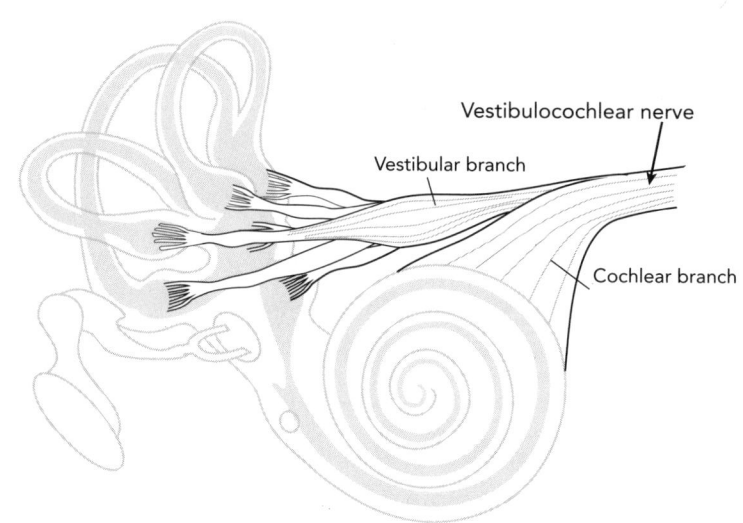

CN VIII: Vestibulocochlear nerve

CN IX: Glossopharyngeal

CN IX transmits sensation from the external ear, Eustachian tube, posterior one-third of the tongue, and pharynx. Motor fibers transmit information to salivary glands in the oral cavity as well as to some of the pharyngeal muscles. In general, the motor fibers are involved in swallowing, and the sensory fibers transmit information about taste, as well as pain, touch, and temperature.

CN X: Vagus

CN X plays a vital role in heart rate, endocrine function, digestion, and phonation. The nerve has many branches which supply visceral organs including the lungs, heart, liver, stomach, pancreas, and others.
Three branches are integral to speech production: the pharyngeal, superior laryngeal, and recurrent laryngeal nerves.

The pharyngeal nerve innervates the muscles of the soft palate (aside from the tensor veli palatini) and the pharynx. The recurrent laryngeal nerve innervates all the intrinsic muscles of the larynx except for the cricothyroid. The cricothyroid muscle is innervated by the superior laryngeal branch. The anatomy of the recurrent laryngeal nerve is not symmetrical on the right and left sides of the body. Before entering the larynx, the recurrent laryngeal nerve descends into the chest and then ascends to enter the larynx. On the right side the nerve loops under the subclavian artery of the heart before ascending; on the left side, the nerve loops under the aorta of the heart, and then travels upward to enter the larynx. The difference in the length of the nerve on the right and left sides helps to explain why the left recurrent laryngeal nerve is more prone to injury than the right. This anatomical configuration also accounts for the fact that certain cardiac problems such as congestive heart failure can affect the recurrent laryngeal nerve, resulting in dysphonia. The vagus also carries afferent fibers from the external ear, a few taste buds around the epiglottis, the thoracic and abdominal viscera as well as from the larynx, pharynx, trachea, and esophagus.

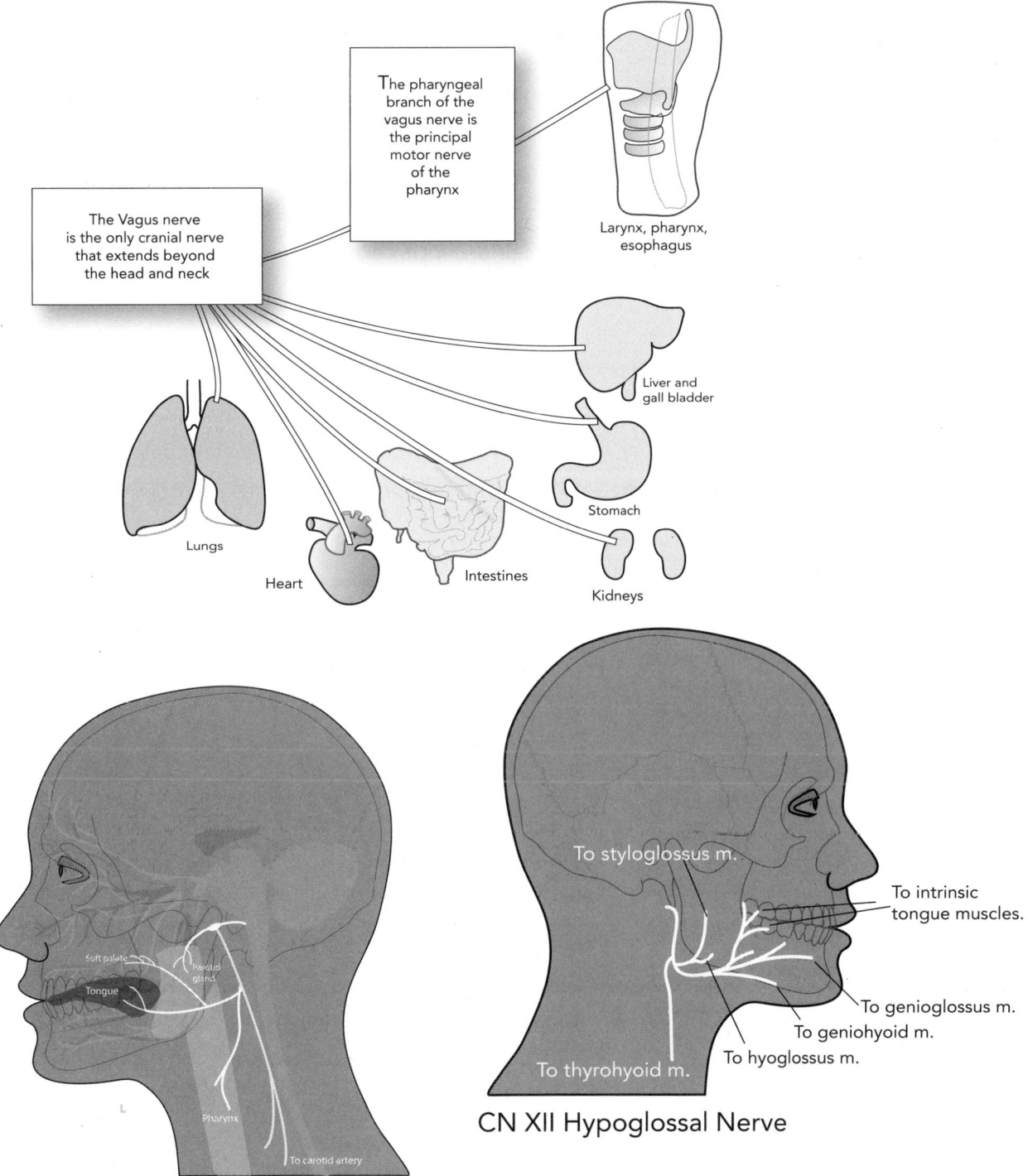

The pharyngeal branch of the vagus nerve is the principal motor nerve of the pharynx

Larynx, pharynx, esophagus

The Vagus nerve is the only cranial nerve that extends beyond the head and neck

Liver and gall bladder

Stomach

Lungs

Heart

Intestines

Kidneys

To styloglossus m.

To intrinsic tongue muscles.

Soft palate

Parotid gland

Tongue

To genioglossus m.

To geniohyoid m.

To hyoglossus m.

To thyrohyoid m.

Pharynx

To carotid artery

CN XII Hypoglossal Nerve

CN IX: Glossopharyngeal Nerve

Upper motor neuron

The upper motor neuron (UMN) comprises the nerve cells and their axons arising from cortical areas and projecting to the brain stem and spinal cord. The two major pathways of the UMN are the corticospinal and corticonuclear (corticobulbar) tracts.

Corticospinal tract: large nerve pathway. About one-third of the fibers arise in the primary motor area, another one-third in premotor and supplementary motor areas, and the remaining one-third in the somatosensory cortex in the parietal lobe. Fibers in this tract synapse directly onto motor nerve cells in the anterior horn of the spinal cord. Most fibers in this tract (85 to 90 percent) decussate in the medulla and continue contralaterally to their spinal targets. A small percentage of fibers continue ipsilaterally. The crossed fibers on either side form the lateral corticospinal pathways. The anterior corticospinal pathways are made up of the uncrossed fibers.

Corticonuclear tract (corticobulbar tract): arises from the face and neck portions of the primary motor cortex and synapses with motor nuclei of CN V, VII, X, and XII. Only striated muscles that are involved in voluntary movement are supplied by the corticonuclear tract. The corticonuclear tract innervates the left and right motor nuclei in the brainstem bilaterally.

Lower motor neuron

The lower motor neuron (LMN) includes nerve cell bodies and axons of cranial and spinal nerves that connect with voluntary muscles. Once motor information from cortical areas has been acted upon by the basal nuclei and cerebellum, the final neuromuscular commands are transmitted by the UMN to the LMN and from there to the target structures for movement execution. Spinal and cranial nerves that make up the LMN are often called the final common pathway, since all cortical and subcortical motor information converges onto these nerves.

Motor units

Lower motor neuron fibers that project from cranial and spinal motor neurons to voluntary muscles have axonic endings that synapse with muscle fibers. The synapse between an axon and the muscle fiber it innervates is called by several names, including neuromuscular junction, myoneural junction, or motor end plate.

Schematic of the lateral corticospinal tract

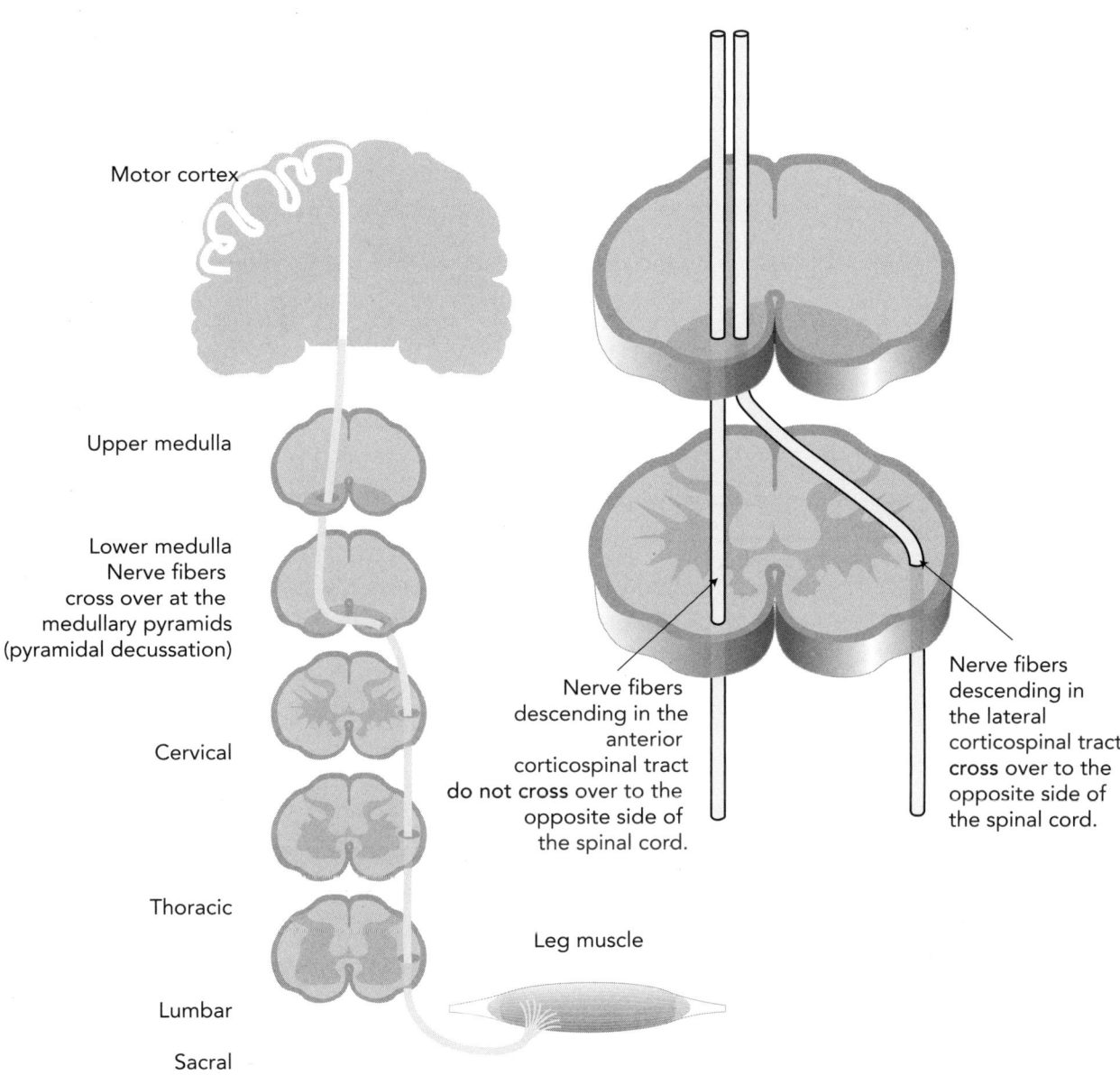

Motor cortex

Upper medulla

Lower medulla
Nerve fibers
cross over at the
medullary pyramids
(pyramidal decussation)

Cervical

Thoracic

Lumbar

Sacral

Nerve fibers
descending in the
anterior
corticospinal tract
do not cross over to the
opposite side of
the spinal cord.

Nerve fibers
descending in
the lateral
corticospinal tract
cross over to the
opposite side of
the spinal cord.

Leg muscle

The myoneural junction functions similarly to a nerve-to-nerve synapse. The vesicles of the presynaptic neuron contain the neurotransmitter acetylcholine (ACh), which acts in an excitatory fashion. When the vesicles are stimulated by a nerve impulse, the acetylcholine is released into the synapse. This generates an excitatory post synaptic potential, which causes the muscle fiber to contract.

One motor neuron can innervate varying numbers of muscle fibers. A motor neuron with its associated muscle fibers is called a motor unit. The ratio of a motor neuron to the number of fibers it innervates is called the innervation ratio. Different structures have motor unit sizes that depend on the function and level of motor control of that structure. How strongly a muscle contracts depends on the number of motor units that are activated.

Blood Supply to the Brain

The brain is dependent on a continuous supply of blood for oxygen and glucose to support the metabolic needs of the nervous tissue. Because the brain does not store these energy-producing elements, the blood supply to the brain cannot be interrupted for more than a few minutes. Longer interruptions can cause permanent brain damage and death as the oxygen supply is cut off and nerve cells start to die. The arteries that supply the brain are patterned in a roughly circular fashion, called the circle of Willis.

Circle of Willis

The Circle of Willis is formed by the internal carotid and the vertebral arteries, as well as branches off these major vessels. Branches include the anterior and posterior communicating arteries. Once it enters the skull, the internal carotid branches into the anterior and middle cerebral arteries (ACA and MCA) on either side of the brain. The ACA supplies portions of the frontal and parietal lobes, the corpus callosum, the basal nuclei, and part of the internal capsule. The MCA provides blood to the temporal lobe, motor strip, and Wernicke's area, among others. The two vertebral arteries, one from each side, join to form the basilar artery, which supplies blood to the brain stem. The basilar artery then branches into the posterior cerebral artery (PCA) and the cerebellar arteries. The PCA provides blood to portions of the temporal and occipital lobes, as well as to the upper midbrain, and the cerebellum. The cerebellar arteries supply the cerebellum.

Blood supply to the brain

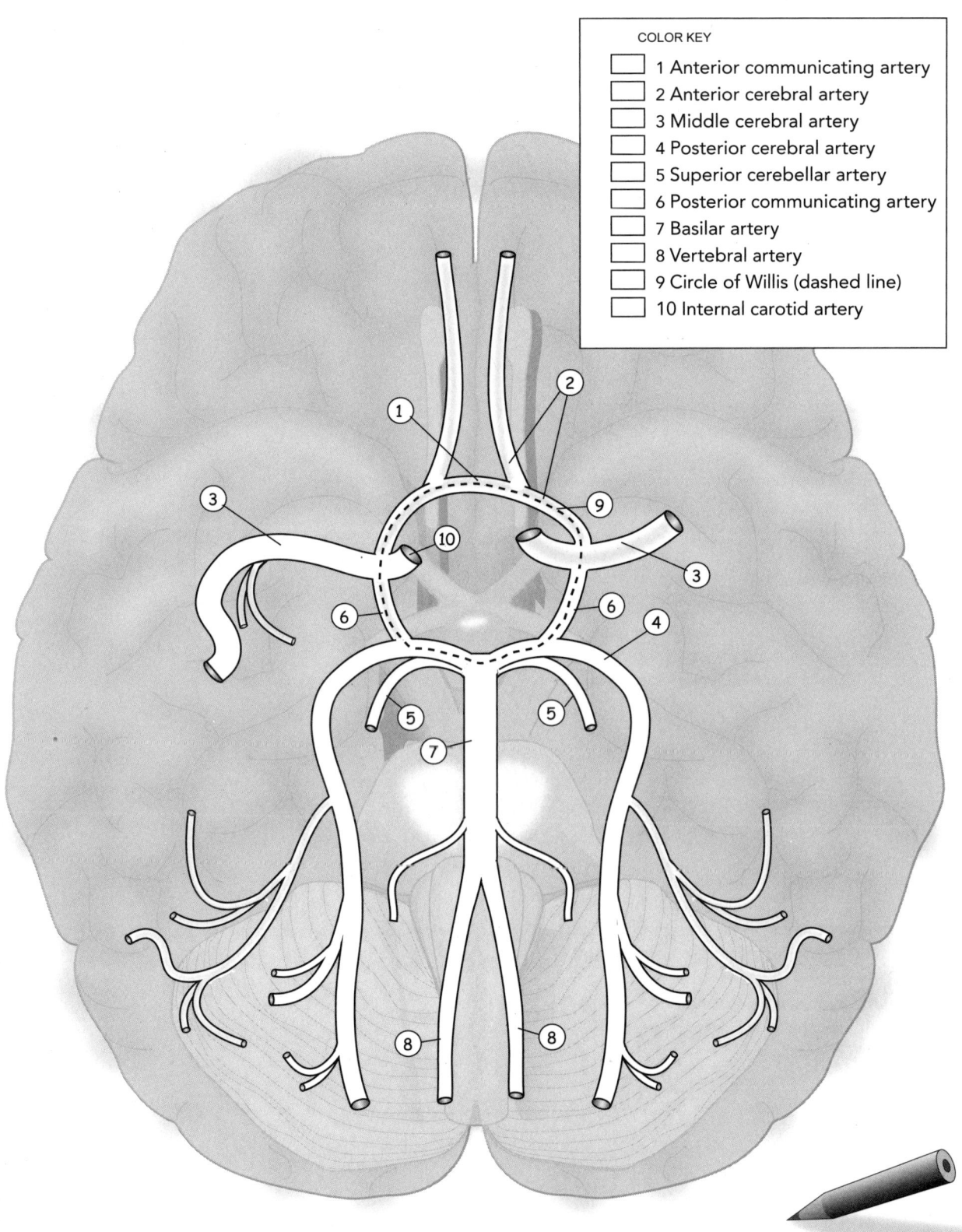

COLOR KEY
1 Anterior communicating artery
2 Anterior cerebral artery
3 Middle cerebral artery
4 Posterior cerebral artery
5 Superior cerebellar artery
6 Posterior communicating artery
7 Basilar artery
8 Vertebral artery
9 Circle of Willis (dashed line)
10 Internal carotid artery

TEST YOURSELF THE NERVOUS SYSTEM

MULTIPLE CHOICE   NERVOUS TISSUE

1 _____   The somatic nervous system
a. Supplies the internal organs of the body
b. Consists of the cranial and spinal nerves
c. Is divided into the central and peripheral nervous systems
d. None of the above

2 _____   The peripheral nervous system
a. Is less important the central nervous system
b. Is divided into somatic and autonomic systems
c. Contains mostly multipolar neurons
d. All the above

3 _____   Neurons
a. Provide metabolic support to brain regions
b. Are a type of specialized glial cell
c. May or may not be present in the central nervous system
d. React to stimuli and conduct impulses to and from areas within and
outside of the brain

4 _____   Which of the following are types of neurons?
a. Sensory
b. Golgi Type 1
c. Unipolar
d. All the above

5 _____   The job of the nervous system is to
a. Receive stimuli as sensory input
b. Integrate a stimulus with a reaction
c. Trigger a motor response
d. All the above

6 _____   Which portion of the nervous system conducts nerve impulses from the CNS to muscles?
a. Afferent
b. Autonomic
c. Somatic
d. Sympathetic

7 _____   Which of the following statements (if any) are NOT true of Golgi Type I neurons?
a. Have long axons that extend to the PNS
b. Synapse with nerves that innervate muscles or glands
c. Are typically unmyelinated
d. All the above statements are true

8 _____   Most neurons in the CNS are
    a. Unipolar
    b. Bipolar
    c. Multipolar
    d. None of the above

9 _____   Most neurons in the CNS are
    a. Motor neurons
    b. Sensory neurons
    c. Interneurons
    d. None of the above

10 _____   Exteroceptors respond to
    a. Distant environment
    b. Immediate environment
    c. Pressure
    d. Tissue damage

11 _____   What type of receptor responds to the position of body structures in space?
    a. Teleceptor
    b. Mechanoreceptor
    c. Thermoreceptor
    d. Proprioceptor

12 _____   The type of receptor that responds to changes in air pressure is a
    a. Baroreceptor
    b. Chemoreceptor
    c. Mechanoreceptor
    d. None of the above

13 _____   Baroreceptors are found in the
    a. Eyes
    b. Ears
    c. Trachea
    d. Skin

14 _____   The type of receptor that responds to tissue damage is a
    a. Nocioreceptor
    h. Chemoreceptor
    c. Exteroceptor
    d. Proprioceptor

15 _____   The types of receptors found in the trachea and bronchi are
    a. Mechanoreceptors
    b. Thermoreceptors
    c. Nocioreceptors
    d. None of the above

16 _____ The types of receptors found in the ear are
    a. Exteroceptors
    b. Proprioceptors
    c. Teleceptors
    d. None of the above

17 _____ Chemoreceptors are found in the
    a. Ears
    b. Tongue
    c. Joints
    d. Eyes

18 _____ The junction between a neuron and its target cell is called a
    a. Neurotransmitter
    b. Node of Ranvier
    c. Synapse
    d. Vesicle

19 _____A synapse may be
    a. Axoaxonal
    b. Axosomatic
    c. Axodendritic
    d. Any of the above

20 _____Neurotransmitters
    a. Act as chemical bridges between neurons
    b. Act like a key to a lock
    c. May be inhibitory or excitatory
    d. All the above

21 _____ Which of the following statements is NOT true of nervous tissue?
    a. Is similar to muscle tissue in its composition
    b. Reacts to stimuli
    c. Conducts impulses toward and away from the brain
    d. Composed of neurons and glial cells

22 _____Cell bodies of neurons
    a. Make up gray matter
    b. Make up white matter
    c. Bring nutrients to glial cells
    d. None of the above

23 _____A nerve pathway is formed through a collection of
    a. Blood vessels
    b. Nerve cell bodies
    c. Glial cells
    d. Nerve fibers

24 ____The junction between two neurons is called the

    a. Node of Ranvier

    b. Synapse

    c. Dendrite

    d. Axon

25 ____Astrocytes

    a. Form layers of myelin that wrap around nerve cells

    b. Engulf and destroy harmful organisms

    c. Transport substances from blood to the nerve cell

    d. All the above

26 ____Which of the following contains the nucleus of a neuron?

    a. Axon

    b. Dendrite

    c. Nodes of Ranvier

    d. Soma

27 ____Which part of a neuron carries impulses away from the cell body?

    a. Axon

    b. Dendrite

    c. Nucleus

    d. None of the above

28 ____Which part of a neuron carries impulses toward the cell body?

    a. Axon

    b. Dendrite

    c. Nucleus

    d. None of the above

29 ____One of the major functions of oligodendrocytes is to

    a. Help to keep the nervous system clean

    b. Transport substances from blood to nerve cells

    c. React to stimuli arriving at the nerve cell

    d. Form layers of myelin around nerve cells

30 ____.Which of the following statements (if any) is NOT true of Nodes of Ranvier?

    a. They are breaks in the myelin sheath around nerves

    b. They help to speed up the rate of nerve transmission

    c. They are part of the gray matter of the brain

    d. All the above are true

31 ____ Terminal branches of axons

    a. End in terminal buttons that contain vesicles of neurotransmitters

    b. Form the junction between nerve cells

    c. Conduct impulses toward the brain

    d. None of the above

32 _____ A synapse can occur between
   a. The axon of one nerve and the dendrites of another
   b. The axon of one nerve and a muscle cell
   c. The axon of one nerve and a glandular cell
   d. All the above

33 _____ The major metabolic activity of the neuron takes place within the
   a. Soma
   b. Dendrites
   c. Axon
   d. Synapse

34 _____ The endpoint of an axon is the
   a. Axon hillock
   b. Synapse
   c. Terminal buttons
   d. Terminal branches

TRUE/FALSE   NERVOUS TISSUE

1 _____   Neurons typically have many short dendrites and a longer axon.

2 _____   Nerve impulses go from sensory neurons in sense organs directly to muscles and glands.

3 _____   Afferent neurons are always sensory.

4 _____   Efferent neurons carry nerve impulses to the CNS.

5 _____   The CNS consists of the brain and spinal cord.

6 _____   Glial cells can divide and reproduce throughout their lives.

7 _____   The somatic system supplies all the internal organs.

8 _____   Golgi Type II neurons have long axons that extend to the PNS.

9 _____   Most neurons in the nervous system are interneurons.

10 _____   Receptors are specialized nerve cells that respond to specific sensory stimuli.

11 _____   Nocioreceptors respond to changes in the distant environment.

12 _____   The retina contains photoreceptors that respond to light.

13 _____   Baroreceptors respond to changes in temperature.

14 _____   Proprioceptors are found in muscles, tendons, and joints.

15 _____   Neurotransmitters may be excitatory or inhibitory.

16 _____ Glial tissue is involved in metabolic support, secretion of
         cerebrospinal fluid, response to injury, and insulation.

17 _____ The basic structure of a glial cell includes the soma, dendrites,
         and axon.

18 _____ Astrocytes form layers of insulation that wrap around the nerve cells.

19____ Microglia engulf and destroy harmful organisms in the nervous system.

20 ____ The grey matter in the brain is composed of cell bodies of neurons.

21 ____ Dendrites conduct impulses toward the cell body while axons

conduct impulses away from the cell body.

22____ Most axons in the central NS are wrapped in a continuous

sheath of myelin.

23 ____ Nodes of Ranvier make up the white matter of the brain.

24 ____ Terminal branches end in terminal buttons that contain vesicles.

25____ Different types of neurotransmitters are located in the synapse.

26____ A synapse may occur between the axon of one nerve and the

dendrites, cell body, or axon of another nerve or nerves.

27 ____ Interneurons convey impulses between sensory and motor neurons.

MATCHING   NERVOUS TISSUE

	Visceroceptor	1 Respond to changes in temperature
	Golgi type I neuron	2 Receive information from the distant environment
	Mechanoreceptor	3 Receive information from visceral structures
	Exteroceptor	4 Found in the tongue and nose
	Thermoreceptor	5 Responds to tissue damage
	Nocioreceptor	6 Have a single process extending from the cell body
	Proprioceptor	7 Have two processes and are involved with special senses
	Golgi type II neuron	8 Respond to light
	Excitatory post-synaptic potential	9 Chemical substance in axon vesicles
	Bipolar neuron	10 Have multiple dendrites and a single axon
	Teleceptor	11 Long myelinated axons extending to the peripheral nervous system
	Photoreceptor	12 Receive information from the skin
	Unipolar neuron	13 Provide information about the position of the body in space
	Chemoreceptor	14 Post-synaptic neuron is stimulated to fire more easily
	Neurotransmitter	15 Local circuit neurons that are usually unmyelinated
	Multipolar neuron	16 Receive information regarding pressure from tissues
	Terminal branches	17 Has numerous projections that connect to blood capillaries
	Interneurons	18 Convey impulses from the CNS or PNS to muscles and glands
	Dendrites	19 Engulf and destroy harmful organisms
	Motor	20 Gap between nerve cells
	Astrocytes	21 End point of an axon
	Synapse	22 Convey impulses from receptors in muscles, skin, glands to the nervous system
	Axon	23 Nucleus surrounded by cytoplasm
	Oligodendrocytes	24 Convey impulses between motor and sensory neurons
	Sensory	25 Branch off cell body and transmit impulses toward the cell body
	Soma	26 Projection that transmits nerve impulses away from the cell body
	Microglia	27 Form layers of insulation around axons

FILL IN THE BLANK   NERVOUS TISSUE

1   A _____ refers to the gap between nerve cells.

2   Local circuit neurons are called _____ .

3   Neurons that carry information toward the CNS are _____ .

4   The _____ system supplies the internal organs.

5   The _____ division of the PNS consists of the cranial and spinal nerves.

6   _____ cells can divide and reproduce throughout their lives.

7   _____ neurons have long axons that extend to the PNS.

8   _____ respond to pressure and deformation of tissues.

9   Taste and smell are sensed by _____ .

10   Most neurons in the nervous system are _____ .

11   The position of body structures in space is sensed by _____ .

12   _____ respond to changes in air pressure.

13   Cells in the retina that respond to light are _____ .

14   Thermoreceptors respond to changes in _____ .

15   Damage to tissues is sensed by _____ .

16   The _____ is the site of communication between neurons.

17   _____ act as a chemical bridge between neurons.

18   _____ are star-shaped cells located throughout the system of nerve cells in the brain.

19   _____ and _____

      form layers of insulation called _____ .

20   Harmful organisms are engulfed and destroyed by _____ .

21   _____ are breaks along the myelin sheath.

22   _____ are located at the endpoint of the axon.

MULTIPLE CHOICE   CENTRAL NERVOUS SYSTEM

1 _____   The meninges are composed of
a. Nerve tissue
b. Glial tissue
c. Connective tissue
d. Muscle tissue

2 _____   The innermost layer of the meninges is the
a. Dura mater
b. Pia mater
c. Arachnoid
d. Subdural space

3 _____   The outermost layer of the meninges is the
a. Dura mater
b. Pia mater
c. Arachnoid
d. Subdural space

4 _____   Which layer of the meninges contains no blood vessels?
a. Dura mater
b. Pia mater
c. Arachnoid
d. Subdural space

5 _____   Which part of the meninges is filled with cerebrospinal fluid?
a. Subarachnoid space
b. Subdural space
c. Subpial space
d. None of the above

6 _____   Cerebrospinal fluid is manufactured within the
a. Subarachnoid space
b. Subdural space
c. Subpial space
d. Ventricles

7 _____   The interventricular foramen connects the
a. Lateral ventricles to each other
b. Lateral ventricles to the third ventricle
c. Lateral ventricles to the fourth ventricle
d. Third ventricle to the fourth ventricle

8 _____   The cerebral aqueduct connects the
    a. Lateral ventricles to each other
    b. Lateral ventricles to the third ventricle
    c. Lateral ventricles to the fourth ventricle
    d. Third ventricle to the fourth ventricle

9 _____   The longitudinal cerebral fissure
    a. Divides the brain into two hemispheres
    b. Separates the brain into superior and inferior regions
    c. Divides the brain into anterior and posterior portions
    d. Divides the brain into four lobes

10 _____   The central sulcus
    a. Divides the brain into two hemispheres
    b. Separates the brain into superior and inferior regions
    c. Divides the brain into anterior and posterior portions
    d. Divides the brain into four lobes

11 _____   The lateral fissure
    a. Divides the brain into two hemispheres
    b. Separates the brain into superior and inferior regions
    c. Divides the brain into anterior and posterior portions
    d. Divides the brain into four lobes

12 _____   The cerebellum is located
    a. Immediately posterior to the cerebrum
    b. Immediately anterior to the cerebrum
    c. Immediately superior to the cerebrum
    d. None of the above

13 _____   The brain stem consists of the
    a. Cerebellum, cerebrum, and midbrain
    b. Cerebellum, pons, and midbrain
    c. Midbrain, pons, and medulla
    d. Midbrain, pons, and cerebrum

14 _____   Cranial nerves originate in the
    a. Brain stem
    b. Cerebellum
    c. Spinal cord
    d. Cerebrum

15 _____   The cortex
    a. Is convoluted due to sulci, gyri, and fissures
    b. Is composed of 3-6 layers of nerve cells
    c. Is mostly composed of neocortex
    d. All the above

16 _____   The cortex is involved with all EXCEPT
    a. Abstract reasoning
    b. Speech and language
    c. Olfaction and visceral and emotional reactions
    d. Understanding

17 _____   The lobe that is located anterior to the central sulcus and superior to the lateral sulcus is the
    a. Parietal
    b. Temporal
    c. Limbic
    d. Frontal

18 _____   The primary motor cortex
    a. Is also known as the motor strip
    b. Is situated on the precentral gyrus
    c. Is somatotopically organized
    d. All the above

19 _____   The lobe that is important for understanding is the
    a. Parietal
    b. Temporal
    c. Occipital
    d. Frontal

20 _____Which statement (if any) is NOT true of the parietal lobes?
    a. Situated on the postcentral gyrus
    b. Deal with bodily sensation
    c. Is connected to Broca's area via the arcuate fasciculus
    d. Areas are represented somatotopically

21 _____   Brodmann area 4 is the
    a. Primary motor area
    b. Premotor area
    c. Broca's area
    d. Wernicke's area

22 ____The supramarginal gyrus and angular gyrus
     a. Connect Broca's and Wernicke's areas
     b. Are involved in visual processing
     c. Integrate sensory modalities including vision, touch, and hearing
     d. All the above

23 ____ Wernicke's area is located in
     a. Area 4
     b. Areas 44 and 45
     c. Area 41
     d. Area 22

24 ____The only lobe that is not part of the limbic lobe is
     a. Occipital
     b. Frontal
     c. Parietal
     d. Temporal

25 ____The brain structure important in transferring information from short-term to long-term memory is the
     a. Septal nuclei
     b. Amygdala
     c. Hypothalamus
     d. Hippocampus

26 ____The septal nuclei are associated with
     a. Memory
     b. Social behavior
     c. Understanding
     d. Motor function

27 ____The nerve tract that links the two hemispheres is the
     a. Arcuate fasciculus
     b. Superior longitudinal fasciculus
     c. Corpus callosum
     d. Internal capsule

28 ____The nerve tract that links the four major lobes is the
     a. Arcuate fasciculus
     b. Superior longitudinal fasciculus
     c. Corpus callosum
     d. Internal capsule

29 _____ The internal capsule

    a. Is formed by a large mass of myelinated fibers

    b. Runs mainly between the thalamus and the cerebral cortex

    c. Transmits neural information from the cortex to the brain stem

    d. All the above

30 _____ The limbic system is involved in

    a. Emotional and sexual function

    b. Feeding behavior

    c. Temperature regulation

    d. All the above

TRUE/FALSE   CENTRAL NERVOUS SYSTEM

1 _____ The dura mater is the innermost layer of the meninges.

2 _____ The pia mater adheres closely to the grooves and convolutions of the brain.

3 _____ The dura mater and pia mater contain blood vessels but the arachnoid does not.

4 _____ The subdural space is filled with cerebrospinal fluid.

5 _____ The ventricles are important in the manufacture of cerebrospinal fluid.

6 _____ The third and fourth ventricles are connected by the cerebral aqueduct.

7 _____ The cerebrum is primarily made of nerve axons bundled into pathways and covered with myelin.

8 _____ The cerebellum is located immediately inferior to the cerebrum.

9 _____ The brainstem consists of the midbrain, pons, and medulla.

10 _____ The cranial and spinal nerves originate in the brainstem.

11 _____ The central sulcus separates the brain into superior and inferior portions.

12 _____ The longitudinal cerebral fissure divides the brain into right and left hemispheres.

13 _____ The convolutions increase the surface area of the cortex.

14 _____ Abstract processing occurs in the cortex.

15 _____ Most motor activity is controlled by the primary motor cortex, premotor area,

    and supplementary motor area.

16 _____ Somatotopic organization represents control of different body structures by different areas

    of the motor cortex.

17 _____ The primary motor cortex is situated on the postcentral gyrus.

18 _____ The parietal lobes are connected to each other by the arcuate fasciculus.

19 _____ The parietal lobes are located immediately posterior to the central sulcus

    and deal with bodily sensation.

20 _____ Wernicke's area is in the temporal lobe.

21 ____ The arcuate fasciculus connects the temporal and occipital lobes.

22 ____ Brodmann's area 6 corresponds to the primary motor cortex.

23 ____ Wernicke's area corresponds to Brodmann area 42.

24 ____ Broca's area corresponds to Brodmann areas 44 and 45.

25 ____The primary somatosensory area corresponds to Brodmann areas 3, 1, and 2.

26 ____The limbic lobe is made up of the most medial margins of the frontal, parietal,

and temporal lobes.

27 ____The amygdala is involved in transferring information from short-term to long-term memory.

28 ____The septal nuclei are associated with social behavior, anxiety, and fear.

29 ____The hippocampus, amygdala, septal nuclei, and mammillary bodies are all involved

with aspects of memory.

30 ____The corpus callosum connects the superior and inferior portions of the brain.

31 ____ The superior longitudinal fasciculus links the four major lobes.

32 ____The internal capsule and the corona radiata are formed by myelinated axons that

reach many areas in the cortex and the cerebrum.

FILL-IN THE BLANK   CENTRAL NERVOUS SYSTEM

1   The _____ layer of the meninges attaches to the cranium and the meningeal layer.

2   The _____ of the meninges has a delicate web-like appearance with no blood vessels.

3   Between the dura mater and the arachnoid is the _____.

4   The third and fourth ventricles are connected by the _____.

5   Cerebrospinal fluid is manufactured by _____.

6   The _____   _____ consists of the midbrain, pons, and medulla.

7   The _   _____ divides the brain into two hemispheres.

8   The brain is separated into anterior and posterior portions by the _____ .

9   The _____ separates the brain into superior and inferior regions.

10   The _____ lobe is involved with symbolic function.

11   Understanding is mediated by the _____ lobe.

12   The _____ lobe is responsible for somatosensory function.

13   The area in the lateral portion of the inferior region of the motor strip is known

       as _____.

14   The primary motor cortex is situated on the _____ gyrus.

15   The supramarginal gyrus and the angular gyrus are on the _____ lobe.

16   The _____ connects Broca's and Wernicke's areas.

17   Differing amount of neural tissue allocated to control of different bodily

       structures is called _____.

18   The _____ lobes are located immediately inferior to the lateral fissure.

19   The parietal lobes are located on the _____ gyrus.

20   Area 17 is the _____.

21   Area 4 is the _____.

22   The angular gyrus is area _____.

23   Area 6 contains the _____ and _____.

24   Wernicke's area is in area _____.

25   The _____ consolidates and coordinates memories.

26   The _____ are often included as part of the hypothalamus.

27   The _____ plays a part in mood and emotional status.

28   The _____ links the four major lobes.

29   The right and left hemispheres are connected by the _____.

30   The large mass of fibers running mainly between the thalamus and the cerebral

       cortex is the _____.

MATCHING   CENTRAL NERVOUS SYSTEM

	Lateral fissure	1 Separates the brain into superior and inferior regions
	Primary motor cortex	2 Made up of the most medial margins of the frontal, parietal, and temporal lobes
	Cerebrospinal fluid	3 Manufactured by specialized cells within the ventricles
	Brainstem	4 Transfers information from short to long term memory
	Wernicke's area	5 Connects Broca's and Wernicke's areas
	Limbic system	6 Innermost layer of the meninges
	Pia mater	7 Integrates sensory modalities of vision, touch, and hearing
	Longitudinal cerebral fissure	8 Comprises hippocampus, amygdala, septal nuclei, mammillary bodies
	Arcuate fasciculus	9 Divides the brain into anterior and posterior portions
	Cerebral aqueduct	10 Connects the third and fourth ventricles
	Subdural space	11 Situated on the precentral gyrus
	Limbic lobe	12 Located between the dura mater and arachnoid
	Central sulcus	13 Consists of the midbrain, pons, and medulla
	Supramarginal and angular gyri	14 Divides the brain into two hemispheres
	Corpus callosum	15 Filled with cerebrospinal fluid
	Subarachnoid space	16 Part of the receptive speech association cortex
	Hippocampus	17 Connects the right and left hemispheres

MULTIPLE CHOICE   CNS AND PNS

1 _____   The basal nuclei include the
a. Lenticular nucleus
b. Striatum
c. Substantia nigra
d. All the above

2 _____   The outflow from the basal nuclei to the thalamus and back to the motor cortex is
a. Excitatory
b. Inhibitory
c. Neutral
d. Indeterminate

3_____   The basal nuclei regulate aspects of motor control including
a. Posture and balance
b. Background muscle tone
c. Coordination of muscle groups
d. All the above

4 _____   All sensory information travels through the thalamus expect for
a. Vision
b. Hearing
c. Taste
d. Olfaction

5 _____   The hypothalamus is involved with all the following except
a. Hormonal function
b. Body temperature
c. Voluntary chewing motions
d. Hunger

6_____   The brainstem
a. Consists of the midbrain, pons, and cerebellum
b. Connects with the limbic system and pituitary gland
c. Is designed to keep the body's internal environment in a state of equilibrium
d. Contains the reticular formation

7 _____   The cerebral peduncles are
a. Found within the thalamus
b. Continuations of the internal capsule
c. Involved with olfaction
d. Part of the reticular activating system

8 ____   The superior and middle cerebellar peduncles
      a. Connect the midbrain to the cerebellum
      c. Connect the midbrain to the pons
      c. Connect the pons to the cerebellum
      d. None of the above

9 ____   Most nerve fibers that originate at the cerebral cortex decussate at the
      a. Midbrain
      b. Pons
      c. Medulla
      d. Spinal cord

10 ____   The medulla connects to the cerebellum by way of the
      a. Inferior cerebellar peduncles
      b. Middle cerebellar peduncles
      c. Superior cerebellar peduncles
      d. None of the above

11 ____   Which of the following statements (if any) is NOT true of the cerebellum?
      a. Is composed of a mass of white matter overlaid by an outer cortex
      b. Contains concentrations of subcortical cell bodies deep within the white matter
      c. Has two hemispheres connected by a thick nerve fiber bundle
      d. All the above statements are true

12 ____   The vermis refers to
      a. The ridged appearance of the cerebellar cortex
      b. The nerve fiber bundle that connects the two hemispheres of the cerebellum
      c. The smallest lobe of the cerebellum
      d. The inner mass of the cerebellum

13 ____The cerebellar folia refer to
      a. The ridged appearance of the cerebellar cortex
      b. The nerve fiber bundle that connects the two hemispheres of the cerebellum
      c. The smallest lobe of the cerebellum
      d. The inner mass of the cerebellum

14 ____   The deep nuclei contain mostly
      a. Afferent neurons
      b. Interneurons
      c. Efferent neurons
      d. All the above

15 ____The cerebellum plays an important role in
      a. Balance, posture, and background muscle tone
      b. Coordination of voluntary movements
      c. Timing, force, and speed of voluntary movements
      d. All the above

16 ____The spinal cord
   a. Is divided into five sections
   b. Is enveloped by the meninges
   c. Is made up of grey and white matter
   d. All the above

17 ____The dorsal posterior horns are
   a. Motor
   b. Sensory
   c. Both motor and sensory
   d. Visceral

18 ____The anterior corticospinal tract
   a. Is formed by 10 to 15 percent of descending fibers from the cortical motor areas
      that do not decussate
   b. Originates in the midbrain
   c. Originates in the vestibular nuclei in the medulla
   d. Transmits information about pain, temperature, touch, and proprioception

19 ____The tract that decussates at the level of the medulla is the
   a. Spinocerebellar
   b. Lateral corticospinal
   c. Anterior corticospinal
   d. Rubrospinal

20 ____The spinal nerves
   a. Enter and exit the spinal cord by way of intervertebral foramina
   b. Have both sensory and motor branches which converge outside the
      spinal cord to form the spinal nerve
   c. Exit and enter the spinal cord via the posterior and anterior horns
   d. All the above

21 ____The brachial plexus innervates muscles of the
   a. Neck
   b. Shoulder and upper limbs
   c. Anterior and medial thigh
   d. Buttocks, pelvis, perineum, and lower limbs

22 ____The lumbar plexus innervates muscles of the
   a. Neck
   b. Shoulder and upper limbs
   c. Anterior and medial thigh
   d. Buttocks, pelvis, perineum, and lower limbs

23 ____ Cranial nerve (CN) V
   a. Contains ophthalmic, maxillary, and mandibular fibers
   b. Transmits information about touch, pressure, pain, proprioception, and
      temperature
   c. Innervates the muscles of mastication, tensor veli palatini, tensor tympani, and some
      extrinsic laryngeal muscles
   d. All the above

24 ____The facial nerve
    a. Contains vestibular and cochlear branches
    b. Transmits sensation from the external ear, Eustachian tube, posterior
       one-third of the tongue, and pharynx
    c. Receives both ipsilateral and contralateral innervation
    d. Is important in heart rate, endocrine function, digestion, and phonation

25 ____The nerve that transmits auditory information is the
    a. Facial
    b. Hypoglossal
    c. Vestibulocochlear
    d. Trigeminal

26 ____Which of the following muscles is NOT innervated by the recurrent laryngeal nerve?
    a. Cricothyroid
    b. Lateral cricoarytenoid
    c. Posterior cricoarytenoid
    d. Interarytenoid

27 ____CN IX is involved in
    a. Audition
    b. Facial expression
    c. Swallowing
    d. Endocrine function

28 ____The superior laryngeal branch of CN X innervates the
    a. Cricothyroid muscle
    b. Intrinsic and extrinsic muscles of the tongue
    c. Velum
    d. Pharyngeal constrictors

29 ____Which of the following statements (if any) is NOT true of the corticospinal tract?
    a. Arises from the face and neck portions of the primary motor cortex
    b. Fibers synapse directly onto motor nerve cells in the spinal cord
    c. Around 80 to 90% of fibers decussate in the medulla
    d. All the above statements are true

30 ____The corticonuclear tract
    a. Synapses with motor nuclei of CN V, VII, X, and XII
    b. Innervates voluntary muscles
    c. Has bilateral innervation
    d. All the above

31 ____The lower motor neuron (LMN)
    a. Is made up of nerve cells and their axons arising from cortical areas and
       projecting to the brain stem and spinal cord
    b. Is comprised of the corticospinal and corticonuclear tracts
    c. Includes nerve cell bodies and axons of cranial and spinal nerves that
       connect with voluntary muscles
    d. None of the above

32 ____The myoneural junction refers to the
   a. Nerve cell bodies and axons of cranial and spinal nerves that connect
      with voluntary muscles
   b. The synapse between an axon and the muscle fiber it innervates
   c. Fibers of the corticonuclear tract
   d. Final common pathway

33 ____ A muscle fiber contracts when
   a. The vesicles of the presynaptic neuron are stimulated by a nerve impulse
   b. Acetylcholine is released into the synapse
   c. An excitatory post-synaptic potential is generated
   d. All the above

34 ____The middle cerebral artery provides blood to the
   a. Temporal lobe, motor strip, and Wernicke's area
   b. Corpus callosum and basal nuclei
   c. Brainstem
   d. Cerebellum

TRUE/FALSE   CNS AND PNS

1 _____   The basal nuclei include the thalamus, hypothalamus, and amygdala.

2 _____   The lenticular nucleus comprises the caudate and putamen.

3 _____   The basal nuclei are involved in the control of precise voluntary movements through neural excitation.

4 _____   The basal nuclei regulate posture, balance, background muscle tone, and coordination of muscle groups.

5 _____   All information aside from pain and pressure passes through the thalamus on the way to

the cerebral cortex.

6 _____   The thalamic nuclei send and receive information via the internal capsule.

7 _____   The thalamus is important in maintaining the body's homeostasis.

8 _____   The hypothalamus connects with the limbic system, pituitary gland, and brain stem.

9 _____   The brain stem controls many reflexes involved in respiration, body temperature, swallowing, and digestion.

10_____   The reticular activating system is located within the brainstem and controls alertness and consciousness.

11 _____   The midbrain consists of two cerebral peduncles and the superior and inferior colliculi.

12 _____   The cerebral peduncles are continuations of the internal capsule.

13 _____   The superior and middle cerebellar peduncles act as a bridge between the pons and the cerebellum.

14 _____   Decussation of nerve fibers occurs mostly at the pontine level.

15 _____The medulla connects to the cerebellum by way of the superior cerebellar peduncles.

16 _____The cerebellum is composed of a mass of white matter overlaid by an outer cortex.

17 _____The cerebellum has two hemispheres that are connected by the corpus callosum.

18 _____Like the cerebral cortex, the cerebellum is divided into lobes.

19 _____The inner mass of the cerebellum has a branching pattern.

20 _____The deep nuclei within the cerebellum contain most of the sensory neurons.

21_____The cerebellum plays an integral role in motor control and coordination.

22 _____The spinal cord is divided into cervical, thoracic, lumbar, sacral, and coccygeal sections.

23 _____The gray matter in the spinal cord forms the outer covering and the white matter is located within.

24 _____The lateral corticospinal tract is formed by the 10 to 15 percent of descending fibers

   from the cortical motor areas that do not decussate.

25_____The four spinal plexuses include the cervical, brachial, lumbar, and lumbosacral.

26 _____CN V contains ophthalmic, maxillary, and mandibular branches.

27 _____The facial nerve receives both ipsilateral and contralateral innervation.

28 _____The facial nerve is the only cranial nerve that contains only motor fibers.

29 _____The vestibular fibers in CN XIII relay information to the CNS about balance and head position.

30 _____The pharyngeal branch of the vagus nerve innervates the muscles of the soft palate.

31 _____The cricothyroid muscle is innervated by the superior laryngeal branch of CN X.

32_____The recurrent laryngeal nerve loops under the subclavian artery on the right side,

   and under the aorta on the left side.

33 _____The corticonuclear tract arises from the face and neck portions of the primary motor cortex and

   synapses with motor nuclei of CN V, VII, X, and XII.

34 _____Fibers of the corticospinal tract arise from both motor and sensory portions of the cortex.

35 _____The corticonuclear tracts innervates only striated muscles that are involved in voluntary movement.

36 _____The lower motor neuron includes nerve cell bodies and axons of cranial and spinal nerves.

37 _____Acetylcholine is an inhibitory neurotransmitter located in the vesicles of a presynaptic neuron

   in a myoneural junction.

38 _____The circle of Willis is formed by the internal carotid and the vertebral arteries.

39 _____The anterior cerebral artery provides blood to the temporal lobe, motor strip, and Wernicke's area.

MATCHING   CNS AND PNS

	Facial nerve	1 Blood supply to temporal lobe, motor strip and Wernicke's area
	Corticonuclear tract	2 Includes caudate nucleus, globus pallidus, putamen, substantia nigra
	Hypoglossal nerve	3 Innervates muscles of the buttocks, pelvis, perineum, lower limbs
	Middle cerebral artery	4 Innervates muscles of the shoulder and upper limbs
	Recurrent laryngeal nerve	5 Integrates sound signals from multiple sources
	Basal nuclei	6 Blood supply to the brain stem
	Inferior colliculi	7 Regulates hormonal function, body temperature, hunger, sexual function
	Reticular formation	8 Network of nuclei involved in breathing, cardiac function, swallowing
	Circle of Willis	9 Made up of corticospinal fibers that do not decussate at the medulla
	Arbor vitae	10 Innervates muscles of the tongue and some extrinsic laryngeal muscles
	Striatum	11 Blood to frontal, parietal lobes, corpus callosum, basal nuclei, internal capsule
	Glossopharyngeal nerve	12 Structure where decussation of nerve fibers occurs
	Lumbosacral plexus	13 Includes the caudate and putamen
	Vermis	14 Region where anterior and posterior horns of the spinal nerves meet
	Medulla	15 Nerve fibers connecting the two hemispheres of the cerebellum
	Corticospinal tract	16 Inner mass of the cerebellum composed of white matter
	Neuromuscular junction	17 Innervates muscles of the neck
	Trigeminal nerve	18 Contains opthalmic, maxillary, and mandibular branches
	Cervical plexus	19 Cranial nerve providing both ipsilateral and contralateral innervation
	Superior laryngeal nerve	20 Has fibers arising from the semicircular canals and inner hair cells
	Motor unit	21 Transmits sensation from external ear, Eustachian tube, tongue, and pharynx
	Basilar artery	22 Innervates most muscles of the soft palate and the pharynx
	Hypothalamus	23 Fibers from frontal and parietal lobes synapse directly with spinal cord
	Vestibulocochlear nerve	24 Innervates muscles of the anterior and medial thigh
	Anterior cerebral artery	25 Synapse between an axon and the muscle fiber it innervates
	Intermediate zone	26 Fibers from face and neck motor cortex synapse with CN V, VII, X, and XII
	Brachial plexus	27 Blood supply to the brain formed by internal carotid and vertebral arteries
	Lumbar plexus	28 Ratio of a motor neuron to the number of fibers it innervates
	Anterior corticospinal tract	29 Innervates the cricothyroid muscle
	Innervation ratio	30 Motor neuron with its associated muscle fibers
	Pharyngeal nerve	31 Innervates all the intrinsic muscles of the larynx except cricothyroid

FILL IN THE BLANK   CNS AND PNS

1   The basal nuclei include the _____, _____,

_____ and _____ .

2   The _____ is formed by the caudate and putamen.

3   Cranial nerves originate in the _____.

4   The _____ controls alertness and consciousness.

5   The _____ acts as a bridge between the cerebellum and the

rest of the nervous system.

6   Decussation of nerve fibers occurs at the _____.

7   The cerebellum has two hemispheres that are connected by the _____.

8   The deep nuclei contain most of the _____ neurons of the cerebellum.

9   The _____ horns of the spinal cord receive sensory information.

10   Motor information is processed by the _____ horns.

11   The _____ is formed by the 10 to 15 percent of descending

fibers from the cortical motor areas that do not decussate.

12   Most of the descending fibers of the _____

decussate at the medulla.

13   The _____ plexus innervates muscles of the neck.

14   The muscles of the shoulder and upper limbs are innervated by the _____ plexus.

15   The muscles of the anterior and medial thigh are supplied by the _____ plexus.

16   The _____ plexus innervates the buttocks, pelvis, perineum, and lower limbs.

17   Some of the extrinsic laryngeal muscles are innervated by CN _____,

CN _____, and CN _____.

18   The _____ nerve transmits sensation from the external ear,

19   Intrinsic and extrinsic muscles of the tongue are supplied by CN _____.

20   The trigeminal nerve has _____, _____,

and _____ branches.

21   Muscles of facial expression are innervated by CN _____.

22   The only nerve that transmits both ipsilateral and contralateral innervation is CN_____.

23   The _____ nerve: pharyngeal, superior laryngeal, and recurrent laryngeal branches.

24   The superior laryngeal branch innervates the _____ muscle.

25   Aside from the cricothyroid, the intrinsic muscles of the larynx are supplied by

the _____ nerve.

26   The nerve cells and their axons arising from cortical areas and projecting to the

brain stem and spinal cord make up the _____ pathway.

27   The corticonuclear tract synapses with motor nuclei of CN _____, _____,

_____, and _____.

28   The synapse between an axon and the muscle fiber it innervates is called _____,

or _____, or _____ .

29   The _____ refers to a motor neuron with its associated muscle fibers.

30   The roughly circular system of arteries that supply the brain is called the _____ _____.

31   The _____ artery provides blood to the temporal lobe,

motor strip, and Wernicke's area.

32   The _____ artery supplies blood to the brainstem.

Neurology

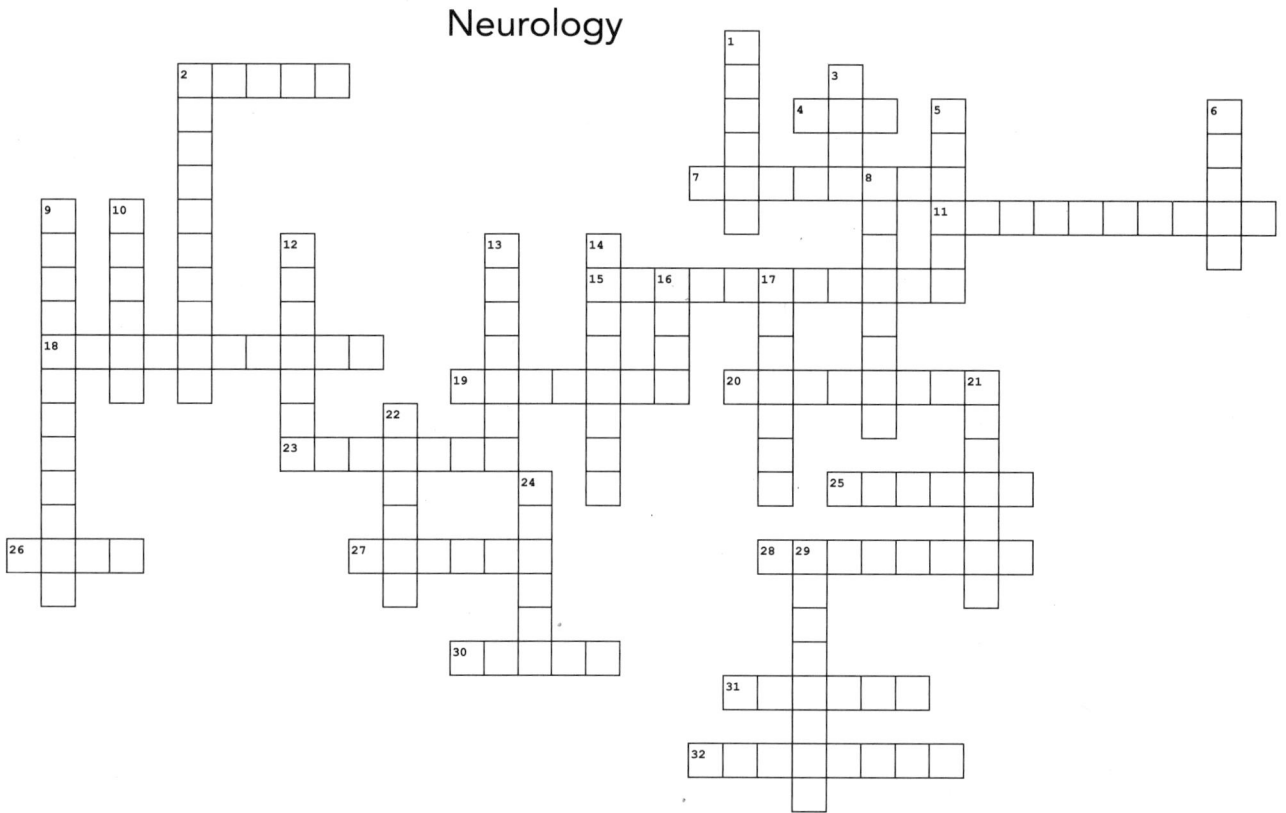

Across

2. Recurrent laryngeal nerve is a branch of this cranial nerve

4. Layer of the meninges closest to the brain

7. Lobes that deal with bodily sensation

11. Important in balance, posture, and coordination

15. Helps to coordinate and consolidate memories

18. Cranial nerve that contains three branches

19. Area involved with speech production

20. Caudate and putamen

23. Fissure that separates the brain into superior and inferior parts

25. Network of peripheral nerves

26. Outermost layer of the meninges

27. This lobe comprises portions of other lobes

28. Involved in mood and emotional status

30. Series of ridges on the cerebellar surface

31. Outer covering of the brain

32. These structures protect the brain and spinal cord

Down

1. Horns that receive sensory information

2. Spaces within the brain

3. The spinal cord has this many sections

5. Shallow depression

6. Raised surface

8. Necessary lobe for understanding

9. Involved with visceral functions

10. Circle

12. Lobe that controls most motor activity

13. Horns that project to skeletal muscles

14. Gateway to consciousness

16. Bridge to the cerebellum

17. This sulcus divides the brain into anterior and posterior sections

21. Nerve decussation occurs here

22. Connects the two hemispheres of the cerebellum

24. CN VII

29. Structure immediately inferior to the cerebrum

Neurology 2

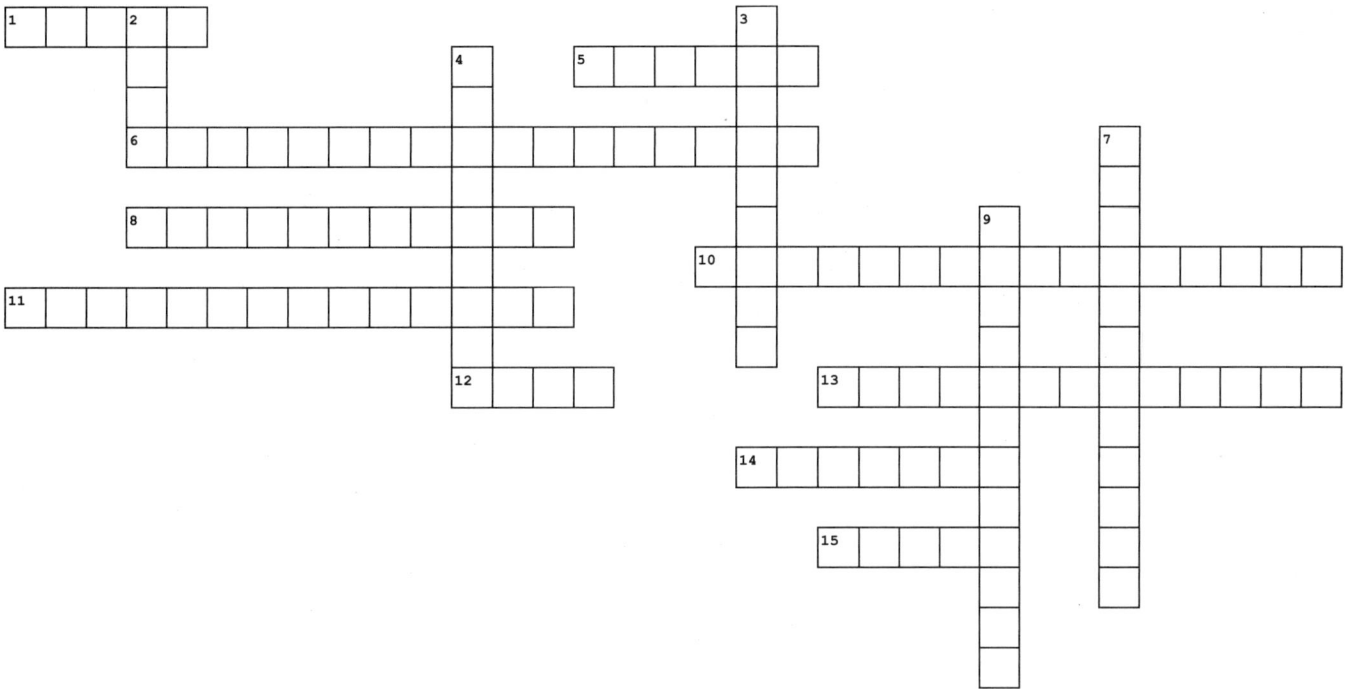

Across

1. Type of connective tissue in the brain
5. Layer of insulation around nerve cells
6. Chemical bridges between neurons
8. The axon ends here
10. These glial cells wrap around nerve cells
11. Helps you to sense changes in temperature
12. Synonym for cell body
13. Tells you where you are in space
14. Gap between nerve cells
15. These nerves send impulses to muscles and glands

Down

2. Transmit nerve impulses away from the cell body
3. Cleaners of the nervous system
4. Transmit nerve impulses toward the cell body
7. Responds to air pressure
9. Connect neurons to each other

Glossary

A

Abdominal muscles   Compress the contents of the abdominal cavity; decrease the volume of the thoracic cavity

Abduction   Movements are directed laterally; bone is moved away from the midline of the body or structure

Accessory muscles of respiration   Participate in respiration as needed

Acetylcholine   Excitatory neurotransmitter

Adipocytes   Cells that store and release triglycerides and produce hormones and growth factors

Adipose tissue   Composed primarily of fat cells (adipocytes)

Adduction   Movements are directed medially; bone is moved toward the midline of the body or structure

Afferent neurons   Convey impulses from receptors in the muscles, skin, and glands to the nervous system (see also Sensory neurons)

Agranular leukocytes   White blood cells that do not contain digestive enzymes

Allocortex   More primitive area of cerebral cortex involved with olfaction and visceral and emotional reactions

Alveolar ridge   Raised area behind the upper front teeth formed by the alveolar processes of the maxilla

Alveolar sacs   Microscopic, thin-walled air-filled structures surrounded by microscopic blood capillaries; location of gas exchange between oxygen and carbon dioxide

Amphiarthrodial joints   Are partly movable

Ampulla   Enlargement of each semicircular canal within the inner ear

Amygdala   Consists of groups of nuclei within the medial portion of the temporal lobes; involved in mood and emotional status and memory and decision making

Anaphase   Phase of mitosis during which sister chromatids are pulled apart

Angular gyrus   Located at the bottom portion of the parietal lobe; important in integrating sensory modalities including vision, touch, and hearing

Anterior   Toward the front of the body (see also Ventral)

Anterior commissure   Point at which the vocal folds attach anteriorly to the thyroid cartilage

Anterior corticospinal nerve tract   Formed by the 10 to 15 percent of descending fibers from the cortical motor areas that do not decussate

Anterior horns of the spinal cord   Contain the cell bodies that project fibers to skeletal muscles (see also Ventral horns)

Antihelix   Fold of tissue on the pinna anterior to the helix

Antitragus   Cartilaginous protrusion that is smaller and opposite to the tragus; forms the inferior boundary of the concha

Apex of tongue   Anterior-most portion of the tongue

Arachnoid mater   Meningeal layer immediately deep to the dura mater

Arbor vitae (tree of life)   Inner mass of the cerebellum composed of a branching pattern of white matter

Arcuate fasciculus   Pathway connecting Broca's and Wernicke's areas

Areolar tissue   Loosely organized array of collagen and elastic fibers and many blood vessels

Arytenoid cartilages   Paired small cone shaped cartilages; located on the superior surface of the quadrate lamina

Aryepiglottic folds   Bundles of connective tissue and muscle; run from the superior and lateral margins of the epiglottis to the apex of each arytenoid

Astrocytes   Star-shaped glial cells in the brain with numerous projections that connect to blood capillaries

Auricularis anterior   Muscle that surrounds the outer ear and draws it forward and upward

Auricularis posterior   Muscle that surrounds the outer ear and draws it backward

Auricularis superior   Muscle that surrounds the outer ear and slightly raises it

Axon   Projection off a neuron that transmits nerve impulses away from the cell body

B

Back of tongue   Part of tongue situated inferior to the soft palate

Ball and socket joints   Ball-shaped head fits into the concave socket

Basal ganglia   Include the caudate nucleus, globus pallidus, putamen and substantia nigra (see also Basal nuclei)

Basal nuclei   Include the caudate nucleus, globus pallidus, putamen and substantia nigra (see also Basal ganglia)

Base of tongue   Portion of the tongue lying in the pharynx

Basilar membrane   Forms the base of the cochlear duct

Basophils   Function in immune, allergic, and inflammatory reactions

Bipolar neurons   Have one axon and one dendrite; specialized sensory neurons for smell, sight, taste, hearing, and balance

Blade of tongue   Part of the tongue that lies below the alveolar ridge when it is at rest

Body of tongue   Major mass of the tongue

Body of vocal folds   Innermost layer of the vocal folds made up of the thyroarytenoid muscle; least compliant layer of the vocal folds

Bone   Connective tissue with rigid matrix

Brachial plexus   Innervates muscles of the shoulder and upper limbs

Brain stem   Includes midbrain, pons, and medulla; site of many reflexes involved in respiration, body temperature, swallowing, and digestion; site of origin of the cranial nerves

Broca's area   Located in the lateral portion of the inferior region of the motor strip

Bronchi   Trachea divides into two primary bronchi; primary bronchi subdivide into secondary and tertiary bronchi

Bronchioles   Subdivisions of the tertiary bronchi

Buccinator   Facial muscle that draws cheeks inwards to keep food between the molars while chewing

C

Cancellous bone   Porous interior of bone; allows space for blood vessels and marrow (see also Spongy bone/ Trabecular bone)

Cardiac muscle   Striated and possesses myofilaments but is involuntary

Cartilage   Connective tissue characterized by a firm, gel-like extracellular matrix

Cartilaginous joints   Permit some movement between adjoining bones

Caudal   Away from the head; lower (see also Inferior)

Cell membrane   Separates the interior of the cell from the outside environment (see also Plasma membrane)

Central   Toward the center

Central nervous system   Consists of the brain and spinal cord

Central sulcus   Separates the brain into anterior and posterior portions

Centriole   Bundles of microtubules involved in cell division

Cerebellum   Located posterior to the brain stem and inferior to the cerebrum; involved in balance, posture, background muscle tone, and the coordination of voluntary movements

Cerebral aqueduct   Channel in the midbrain that links the third and fourth ventricles

Cerebral cortex   Highly convoluted outer covering of the brain

Cerebral peduncles   Continuations of the internal capsule; located in the midbrain

Cerumen   Waxy substance that lubricates the external auditory meatus

Cervical plexus   Innervates muscles of the neck

Choroid plexus cells   Specialized cells within the ventricles that manufacture cerebrospinal fluid

Chromatin   Diffuse network of fine fibrils and proteins in the DNA in the nucleus

Chromosome   Located in the cell nucleus; made up of DNA and proteins

Circle of Willis   Circular system of blood vessels to the brain formed by the internal carotid and the vertebral arteries, as well as branches off these major vessels

Circular muscle   Fibers form a sphincter that closes off tubes

Circumduction   Circular movement resulting from the movements of flexion, abduction, extension, and adduction performed in sequence

Class I occlusion   Normal occlusal relationship; first permanent molar of the upper jaw is positioned one half-tooth behind the first permanent molar of the lower jaw (see also Neutroclusion)

Class II occlusion   First molar of the lower jaw is posterior to the normal position; mandible is retracted (see also Distoclusion, Overjet)

Class III occlusion   First molar of the lower jaw is anterior to the normal position; mandible protrudes too far forward (see also Mesioclusion, Prognathic jaw)

Clavicle   Collar bones

Cochlea   Snail-shaped, bony spiral canal housed in the petrous portion of the temporal bone

Cochlear duct   Membranous canal that lies inside the bony canal of the cochlea

Columnar epithelium   Cells are slender and taller than they are wide

Compact bone   Dense outer layer of bone (see also Cortical bone)

Cranial   Toward the head of the body; upper (see also Superior, Rostral)

Cranial nerves   Transmit information to and from the face and neck regions

Cricoarytenoid joint   Connects the base of each arytenoid cartilage and the superior surface of the quadrate lamina of the cricoid; involved in vocal fold adduction and abduction

Cricoid cartilage   Complete ring of hyaline cartilage; narrow in the front (the arch), broader and wider in the back (quadrate lamina)

Cricopharyngeus muscle   Forms a ring around the top opening of the esophagus; remains contracted during rest and relaxes during swallowing

Cricothyroid joint   Located between the inferior horns of the thyroid cartilage and the sides of the cricoid cartilage; involved in pitch regulation

Cricothyroid membrane   Attaches thyroid and cricoid cartilages

Cricothyroid muscle   Intrinsic laryngeal muscle composed of pars recta and pars oblique fibers; contraction increases the distance between the thyroid and arytenoid cartilages to stretch and tense the vocal folds

Cuboidal epithelium   Cells are about as tall as they are wide

Cuneiform cartilages   Small elastic cartilages embedded within the aryepiglottic folds

Cytoplasm   Gel-like fluid substance that makes up the main mass of a cell within the cell membrane

D

Deep   Away from the body surface

Deep layer of the lamina propria   Consists mostly of collagen fibers; less flexible and compliant than the intermediate layer

Dendrites   Projections that branch off the cell body of a neuron and transmit nerve impulses toward the cell body

Dental occlusion   Relationship between the upper and lower dental arches and the positioning of individual teeth

Depressor anguli oris   Muscle that pulls the corner of the mouth downward

Depressor labii inferioris   Muscle that pulls the lower lip downward

Diaphragm   Large muscle that attaches to the bottom six ribs on either side of the ribcage; forms the floor of the thoracic cavity

Diaphysis   Long shaft of a bone

Diarthrodial joints   Are freely movable

Distal   Away from or farthest from the trunk or the point or origin of a part

Distoclusion   First molar of the lower jaw is posterior to the normal position; mandible is retracted (see also Class II occlusion, Overjet)

Dorsal   Toward the back of the body (see also Posterior)

Dorsal horns of the spinal cord   Made up of nerve cell bodies that receive sensory information from all areas of the body (see also Posterior horns)

Dorsum of tongue   Broad superior surface of the tongue

Dura mater   Outermost layer of the meninges

E

Efferent neurons   Convey impulses from the central or peripheral nervous system to muscles and glands (see also Motor neurons)

Elastic cartilage Contains numerous elastic fibers in its matrix; extremely flexible

Elastic dense connective tissue   Consists of branching elastic fibers and densely packed collagen fibers; provides resilience and flexibility

Ellipsoidal joints   Formed by the oval tip of one bone moving within an elliptical cavity formed by the other bone

End-expiratory level (EEL)   Endpoint of a quiet expiration (see also Resting expiratory level)

Endomysium   Thin sheet of connective tissue separating individual muscle fibers

Eosinophils Cells that respond to allergens and parasitic infections

Epiglottis   Leaf shaped, elastic cartilage attached to the thyroid cartilage and hyoid bone

Epimysium   Connective tissue surrounding multiple fascicles to form a complete muscle "belly"

Epiphysis   Expanded end of a long bone covered by a thin layer of articular cartilage

Epithelial tissue: Characterized by cells which are packed very closely together

Erythrocytes   Deliver oxygen to every cell in the body through the circulatory system (see also Red blood cells)

Ethmoid bone   Unpaired cranial bone that separates the nasal cavity from the brain; main parts are the perpendicular plate, crista galli, labyrinths, and cribriform plate

Eustachian tube   Runs from the nasopharynx to the middle ear; ventilates and drains the middle ear

Eversion   Turns the sole of the foot outward

Excitatory post-synaptic potential   Threshold of the cell membrane is lowered making it easier for the neuron to fire

Expiratory reserve volume (ERV)   Amount of air that can be exhaled below tidal volume

Extension   Movements are directed in the sagittal plane; angle between the bones is increased

External   On the outer surface

External auditory meatus   Canal leading from the pinna to the tympanic membrane; resonates and boosts the amplitude of high-frequency sounds entering the ear

External intercostal muscles   11 pairs that run between the ribs; elevate the rib cage

F

Facial muscles   Group of flat subcutaneous muscles; connect either on to other facial muscles or directly into the connective tissue of the skin

False vocal folds   Located inferior to the aryepiglottic folds and superior to the true vocal folds (see also Ventricular folds)

Fascicle   Bundle of skeletal muscle cells

Fibroblasts   Cells within connective tissue that produce the fibers and other substances that make up the extracellular matrix

Fibrocartilage   Contains numerous coarse fibers in its extracellular matrix

Fibrous joints   Seam of tough connective tissue that fuses adjoining bones (see also Suture)

Final common pathway   Term for the spinal and cranial nerves that make up the lower motor neuron

Fissures   Deep grooves on the cerebral cortex

Flat muscle   Fibers are arranged in parallel

Flexion   Movements are directed in the sagittal plane; angle between the bones is decreased

Folia   Series of ridges on the cerebellar surface

Frontal bone   Unpaired cranial bone that forms the front portion of the skull above the eyes

Frontal lobe   Anterior to the central sulcus and superior to the lateral sulcus; deals with abstract functions and motor activity

Frontalis muscle   Elevates the eyebrows and forehead and wrinkles the forehead

Frontal plane   Vertical plane that divides the body or any of its parts into front and back portions (see also Coronal plane)

Front of tongue   Part of the tongue lying just below the hard palate

Functional residual capacity (FRC)   Amount of air in the lungs and airways at the end-expiratory level; combines expiratory reserve volume and residual volume

Fusiform muscle   Thick in the center and tapered at the ends

G

Gene   Basic unit of heredity; made of DNA

Genioglossus muscle   Forms the main body of the tongue; contraction of anterior fibers retracts the tongue; contraction of posterior fibers pulls the tongue forward

Glial tissue   Connective tissue in the brain

Gliding joints   Connect flat bones (see also Plane joints)

Glottis   Space between the vocal folds; divided into membranous and cartilaginous portions

Golgi apparatus   Series of flattened sacs that modifies, sorts, and packages proteins for use in the cell or for export

Golgi Type I neurons   Have long myelinated axons that extend to the peripheral nervous system

Golgi Type II neurons   Have short unmyelinated axons that synapse on nearby neurons within the central nervous system

Granular leukocytes   Have granules in their cells that contain digestive enzymes

Gyri   Raised surfaces on the cerebral cortex

H

Hamulus   Hook-like process at the end of the medial pterygoid plate of the sphenoid bone

Helicotrema   Point of communication in the cochlea where the vestibular and tympanic canals meet each other at the end of the cochlear duct

Helix   Fold of tissue that forms the outer margin of the pinna

Hinge joints   Have a spool-shaped surface that fits into a concave surface

Hippocampus   Located in the medial portion of the temporal lobes; involved in consolidating and coordinating memories, and transferring information from short-term to long-term memory

Horizontal plane   Divides the body or any of its parts into upper and lower sections (see also Transverse plane)

Hyaline cartilage Most common type of cartilage

Hyoepiglottic ligaments   Attach epiglottis to the hyoid bone

Hyoglossus muscle   Pulls the sides of the tongue downward

Hyoid bone   Point of attachment for the tongue; larynx is suspended from the hyoid bone by a sheet of membrane

Hypothalamus   Subcortical grey matter that contains nuclei involved in sensory and motor control of visceral functions

I

Inferior   Away from the head; lower (see also Caudal)

Inferior colliculus   Auditory center in the midbrain that integrates sound signals from multiple sources

Inferior labial frenulum   Small flap of tissue connecting the lower lip to the midline of the mandible

Inferior longitudinal muscle   Pulls down the tip of the tongue; retracts tongue

Infrahyoid muscles   Group of extrinsic laryngeal muscles attaching below the hyoid; contraction lowers the larynx

Inhibitory post-synaptic potential   Threshold of the cell membrane is raised making it harder for the neuron to fire

Innervation ratio   Ratio of a motor neuron to the number of fibers it innervates

Intermaxillary suture   Immovable joint between two irregularly shaped bones of the maxilla

Intermediate zone of the spinal cord   Region where the anterior and posterior horns meet

Internal   On the inner surface

Internal intercostal muscles   11 pairs that run between the ribs; contraction lowers the rib cage

Interphase   Time in a cell's life between cell divisions; cell carries out its normal metabolic activities

Intervertebral foramina   Spaces located between successive vertebrae

Insertion   More mobile attachment of a skeletal muscle

Inspiratory capacity   Amount of air that can be inhaled from end-expiratory level; combines tidal volume plus inspiratory reserve volume

Inspiratory reserve volume   Amount of air that can be inhaled above tidal volume

Interarytenoid muscle   Intrinsic laryngeal muscle composed of oblique and transverse fibers; contraction adducts the vocal folds to close the cartilaginous glottis

Intermediate layer of the lamina propria   Composed of densely organized elastin fibers; less compliant than the superficial layer

Internal capsule   Nerve pathway formed by a large mass of myelinated fibers that runs mainly between the thalamus and the cerebral cortex

Interneurons   Connect neurons to each other

L

Lacrimal bones   Smallest and most fragile bones of the face

Lamina propria   Three-part layer of mucous membrane that lies deep to the vocal fold epithelium

Laryngopharynx   Part of the pharynx located behind the larynx

Lateral   Away from the midline of the body; toward the side

Lateral corticospinal tract   Nerve tract that originates at sensorimotor areas of the cerebral cortex; most of the fibers decussate at the medulla

Lateral cricoarytenoid muscle   Intrinsic laryngeal muscle that adducts the vocal folds and closes the membranous glottis

Lateral fissure   Separates the brain into superior and inferior regions

Lateral horns of the spinal cord   Involved in visceral functions

Lateral pterygoid muscle   Muscle of mastication, bilateral contraction depresses the chin to open the jaw; unilateral contraction produces side-to-side movements of the jaw

Lenticular nucleus   Formed by the putamen and globus pallidus of the basal nuclei

Leukocytes   Cells of the immune system involved in defending the body against infectious diseases and foreign materials (see also White blood cells)

Levator anguli oris   Muscle that pulls the corner of the mouth upward

Levator labii superioris   Muscle that elevates the upper lip

Levator labii superioris alaeque nasi   Muscle that elevates the upper lip and flares the nostrils

Levator veli palatini muscle   Elevates the velum

Limbic lobe   Made up of the most medial margins of the frontal, parietal, and temporal lobes

Limbic system   Comprises brain structures including the hippocampus, amygdala, septal nuclei, mammillary bodies, and anterior nuclei of the thalamus; involved in emotional and sexual function, feeding behavior, and temperature regulation

Lingual frenulum (frenum)   Band of connective tissue joining the inferior tongue and the mandible

Lips   Composed of muscle, mucous membrane, glandular tissues, and fat; covered by a layer of epithelium

Lobule   Non-cartilaginous inferior portion of the pinna

Longitudinal cerebral fissure   Divides the brain into two hemispheres

Longitudinal phase difference   Slight time lag between the horizontal opening and closing of the vocal folds during vocal fold vibration

Lower motor neuron   Includes nerve cell bodies and axons of cranial and spinal nerves that connect with voluntary muscles

Lumbar plexus   Innervates muscles of the anterior and medial thigh

Lumbosacral plexus   Innervates muscles of the buttocks, pelvis, perineum, and lower limbs

Lung capacities   Combination of two or more lung volumes

Lungs   Cone shaped elastic structures housed within the thoracic cavity

Lung volumes   Single non-overlapping quantities of air inhaled/exhaled

Lymphocytes   Main cells of the immune system; produce circulating antibodies, and can kill virus-infected cells

Lysosomes Contain enzymes that break down unwanted material in a cell and recycle useful substances

M

Macrophages Cells that eliminate damaged cells or pathogens by engulfing them

Mamillary bodies   Part of the limbic system; involved in certain types of memory

Mandible   Large bone that forms the lower jaw

Marrow cavity   Hollow cylindrical space within the diaphysis of a long bone containing yellow marrow and stem cells

Masseter muscle   Muscle of mastication; elevates and protrudes the mandible

Mast cells   Involved in immune responses

Maxilla   Large, immovable bone that forms the anterior three quarters of the hard palate

Medial   Toward the midline of the body

Medial compression   Force exerted by the lateral cricoarytenoid and interarytenoid muscles that adducts the vocal folds during vibration

Medial pterygoid muscle   Muscle of mastication: elevates the mandible and produces a grinding motion when fibers act alternately

Median palatine suture   Immovable joint where the two horizontal plates of the palatine bones articulate with each other

Median sulcus   Divides tongue into right and left sides

Medulla   Most inferior portion of the brain stem

Meninges   Three layers of non-nervous tissue surrounding the brain and spinal cord

Mentalis   Facial muscle that protrudes the lower lip and elevates the skin of the chin

Mesioclusion   First molar of the lower jaw is anterior to the normal position; mandible protrudes too far forward (see also Class III occlusion, Prognathic jaw)

Metaphase   Phase of mitosis during which sister chromatids line up in the center of the cell, with half (46) on one side and half (46) on the other side

Metaphysis   Region in a long bone between the diaphysis and epiphysis

Microglia   Glial cells in the nervous system that engulf and destroy harmful organisms

Microtubules and microfilaments   Networks of protein fibers that provide structural support to the cell and allow internal cell parts to be transported within and outside of the cell

Midbrain   Short structure immediately inferior to the cerebrum; site of higher level reflexes

Midsagittal plane   Vertical plane that divides the body or structure into right and left parts; cut is at midline

Middle ear   Air-filled cavity divided into the tympanic cavity and the epitympanic recess

Mitochondria Convert carbohydrates, lipids, and protein molecules into adenosine triphosphate (ATP)

Mitosis   Process of cell division composed of four stages: prophase, metaphase, anaphase, and telophase

Modiolus   Bony core of the cochlea

Monocytes   Agranular leukocyte involved in immune function

Motor end plate   Synapse between an axon and the muscle fiber it innervates (see also Myoneural junction; Neuromuscular junction)

Motor neurons   Convey impulses from the central or peripheral nervous system to muscles and glands (see also Efferent neurons)

Mucosal wave   Describes the wave-like motion of vocal fold opening and closing during vibration

Multipolar neurons   Have multiple dendrites and a single axon

Muscle   Composed of many fascicles

Muscle tissue   Composed of myofibers that respond to stimulation by contracting and becoming shorter

Muscular process   Posterolateral projection of arytenoid cartilage; point of attachment for intrinsic laryngeal muscles

Musculus uvuli   Located on the nasal surface of the velum; bunches up the velum and helps to raise it

Myelin   Insulation around nerve cells formed by oligodendrocytes in the central nervous system and Schwann cells in the peripheral nervous system

Myocytes   Smooth muscle cells

Myoelastic-aerodynamic theory   Describes one cycle of vocal fold vibration as an interaction of muscle forces, elastic recoil forces, and aerodynamic forces

Myofibroblasts   Cells in connective tissue that function like fibroblasts and are also capable of contraction

Myofilaments   Contractile proteins (actin and myosin) in skeletal muscles

Myoneural junction   Synapse between an axon and the muscle fiber it innervates (see also Motor end plate; Neuromuscular junction)

N

Nasal bones   Two small fused bones that form the bridge of the nose

Nasal conchae   Small bones that divide the nasal cavity into four groove-like passages (see also Nasal turbinates)

Nasalis   Facial muscle that narrows the nose

Nasal cavities   Formed by the fusion of many of the bones of the skull

Nasal septum   Divides the nose into left and right cavities

Nasal turbinates   Small bones that divide the nasal cavity into four groove-like passages (see also Nasal conchae)

Nasopharynx   Portion of the pharynx located behind the nasal cavities

Neocortex   Part of the cerebral cortex where abstract processing occurs

Neural inhibition   Inhibitory outflow from the basal nuclei to the thalamus and back to the motor cortex

Neuromuscular junction   Synapse between an axon and the muscle fiber it innervates (see also Motor end plate; Myoneural junction)

Neurons   Receive, process, and transmit information to, from, and within the nervous system

Neurotransmitters   Chemicals stored within the vesicles of the terminal buttons of nerve axons; can be inhibitory or excitatory

Neutroclusion   Normal occlusal relationship; first permanent molar of the upper jaw is positioned one half-tooth behind the first permanent molar of the lower jaw (see also Class I occlusion)

Neutrophils Type of white blood cell that responds to injury at sites of inflammation

Nodes of Ranvier   Small breaks along the myelin sheath of an axon

Nucleolus   Mass of ribonucleic acid (RNA) with some DNA and proteins within the nucleus

Nucleus   Area of the cell containing deoxyribonucleic acid (DNA) and proteins

O

Oblique line   Slight ridge along the side of the thyroid lamina; point of attachment for two extrinsic laryngeal muscles

Occipital bone   Unpaired cranial bone situated at the back and lower part of the cranium; contains the foramen magnum

Occipital lobe   Situated at the posterior of the brain; deals with the reception and processing of visual information

Oligodendrocytes   Glial cells in the central nervous system that form layers of insulation that wrap around the nerve cells

Oral cavity   Space bounded by the lips anteriorly, the cheeks laterally, and the palate superiorly; tongue makes up the movable floor; back opens into the oropharynx

Oral tongue   Portion of the tongue surface within the oral cavity

Orbicularis oculi   Muscle that closes the eyelids and produces winking, blinking, and squinting

Orbicularis oris   Circular muscle surrounding the upper and lower lips; closes and protrudes the lips

Organ of Corti   Situated within the cochlear duct; contains the sensory cells for hearing

Origin   Less mobile attachment of a muscle

Oropharynx   Section of the pharynx located behind the oral cavity

Osseous spiral lamina   Bony shelf that projects from the modiolus in the cochlea

Ossicles   Three bones in the middle ear; include malleus, incus, and stapes

Osteoblast Type of fibroblast which forms bone

Osteoclast Type of fibroblast which breaks down bone

Oval window   Membrane-covered opening between the middle and inner ears

Overjet   First molar of the lower jaw is posterior to the normal position; mandible is retracted (see also Class II occlusion, Distoclusion)

P

Palatal aponeurosis   Large flat tendon that attaches the velum to the posterior portion of the hard palate

Palatine bones   Paired bones situated at the posterior edge of the nasal cavity; horizontal plates of the bones form the posterior one quarter of the hard palate and the floor of the nasal cavity

Palatoglossus muscle   Elevates the dorsum and back of the tongue and depresses the soft palate; forms the anterior faucial pillar

Palatopharyngeus muscle   Helps to elevate and open the pharynx during swallowing; forms the posterior faucial pillar

Parasagittal   Vertical plane that divides the body or structure into right and left parts; cut is away from midline

Parietal bones   Paired cranial bones that form the sides and roof of the cranium

Parietal lobes   Located on the postcentral gyrus immediately posterior to the central sulcus; deal with bodily sensation

Parietal pleura   Membrane that lines the inside surface of the thoracic cavity

Pars flaccida   Small superior section of the tympanic membrane

Pars tensa   Larger section of the tympanic membrane

Pennate muscle   Looks feathered; may be unipennate, bipennate, or multipennate

Perimysium   Sheet of connective tissue between muscle fascicles

Periosteum   Tough sheath of connective tissue covering the outer surface of a long bone

Peripheral   Toward the periphery

Peripheral nervous system   Consists of the cranial and spinal nerves; divided into somatic and autonomic systems

Peroxisomes   Small vesicles that absorb nutrients and digest fatty acids

Petiole   Narrow base of the epiglottis

Pharyngeal constrictor muscles   Include inferior, middle, and superior bundles; constrict the pharynx during swallowing

Pharyngeal nerve   Innervates the muscles of the soft palate (aside from the tensor veli palatini) and the pharynx

Pharyngoesophageal segment (PE segment)   Ring of muscle formed by the cricopharyngeus muscle around the top opening of the esophagus

Pharynx   Long hollow tube made of muscle, connective tissue, and mucous lining; runs behind the nasal cavities, oral cavity, and larynx

Pia mater   Innermost layer of the meninges

Pinna   Made of flexible elastic cartilage; helps to channel sound waves into the ear canal and in sound localization

Pinocytic vesicles   Membrane-lined sacs that transport cellular material (see also Vacuoles)

Pivot joints   Formed by a ring of bone rotating about an axle of bone

Plane joints   Connect flat bones (see also Gliding joints)

Planes   Used to show structures from different views

Plasma   Liquid portion of blood comprising about 55% of the blood volume; composed primarily of water

Plasma cells   Synthesize antibodies

Plasma membrane   Separates the interior of a cell from the outside environment (see also Cell membrane)

Platelets   Cell fragments that can bind together to form clots and stop bleeding

Platysma   Primarily a muscle of the neck but contributes to facial expression

Pleural fluid   Located within the pleural space; has a permanent negative pressure

Pleural linkage   Negative pressure that allows the thorax and lungs to act as an integrated unit

Pleural space   Space between the parietal and visceral pleurae

Plexus   Network of peripheral nerves arising from the spinal cord

Pons   Portion of the brainstem inferior to the midbrain and anterior to the cerebellum; has nerve pathways that connect to the cerebellum

Posterior   Toward the back of the body (see also Dorsal)

Posterior cricoarytenoid muscle   Intrinsic laryngeal muscle that abducts the vocal folds and opens the glottis

Posterior horns of the spinal cord   Made up of nerve cell bodies that receive sensory information from all areas of the body (see also Dorsal horns)

Primary motor cortex   Situated on the precentral gyrus immediately anterior to the central sulcus

Procerus   Muscle that wrinkles the root of the nose

Prognathic jaw   First molar of the lower jaw is anterior to the normal position; mandible protrudes too far forward (see also Class III occlusion, Mesioclusion)

Pronation   Combines movements of eversion and abduction around a vertical axis (in the foot)

Prone   Body lying face down

Prophase   Phase of mitosis when fibrils of chromatin become condensed into short, thick, coiled chromosomes; each chromosome contains two copies of its DNA

Proteins   Composed of one or more chains of small molecules called amino acids; major structural components of skin, hair, fingernails, muscle, and organs

Proximal   Toward or nearest the trunk or the point of origin of a part

Pseudostratified epithelium   Cells' nuclei are distributed at different levels

Q

Quadrate lamina   Posterior portion of cricoid cartilage

Quadrate muscle   Four-sided

R

Ramus   Perpendicular portion of the mandible that extends superiorly from the mandibular body

Recurrent laryngeal nerve   Innervates all the intrinsic muscles of the larynx except for the cricothyroid

Red blood cells   Deliver oxygen to every cell in the body through the circulatory system (see also Erythrocytes)

Reflex   Involuntary stereotyped motor response to a sensory input; may be simple or complex

Regular dense connective tissue   Composed of tightly packed collagen fibers arranged in parallel, e.g., tendons and ligaments

Reinke's space   Consists mostly of loosely organized elastin fibers as well as small amounts of collagen; very compliant (see also Superficial layer of the lamina propria)

Remodeling   Process by which bones are remodeled as osteoblasts lay down bone tissue and osteoclasts selectively remove it

Residual volume (RV)   Volume of air remaining in the lungs even after a maximum exhalation

Respiratory bronchioles   Terminations of bronchioles; open into alveolar ducts which end in alveolar sacs

Resting expiratory level (REL)   State of equilibrium in the respiratory system in which alveolar pressure and atmospheric pressure are equalized (see also end-expiratory level)

Reticular activating system   Part of the reticular formation in the brainstem; controls state of alertness and level of consciousness

Reticular formation   Loose and diffuse network of nuclei in the brain stem controlling complex patterns of movement involved in breathing, cardiac function, and swallowing

Ribosomes   Organelles in a cell that synthesize proteins by assembling amino acids into specific sequences

Risorius   Facial muscle located around the mouth area; stretches the mouth laterally

Rostral   Toward the head end of the body; upper (see also Superior, Cranial)

Rotation   Moving bone is turned about its axis; can be medial (internal) or lateral (external)

Rough endoplasmic reticulum   Series of membranes studded with ribosomes; transports proteins synthesized at the ribosomes

Round window   Membrane-covered opening between the middle and inner ears

S

Saccule   Adjacent to the cochlea in the inner ear; senses acceleration in the vertical plane

Saddle joints   Formed between a roughly U-shaped end of one bone into which the end of the other fits

Sagittal plane   Vertical plane running from front to back that divides the body or any of its parts into right and left sides

Salpingopharyngeus muscle   Helps to elevate and open the pharynx during swallowing

Scapha   Groove between the helix and the antihelix

Scapulae   Shoulder blades

Schwann cells   Glial cells in the peripheral nervous system that form layers of insulation that wrap around the nerve cells

Semicircular canals   Organ of balance within the inner ear

Sensory neurons   Convey impulses from receptors in the muscles, skin, and glands to the nervous system (see also Afferent neurons)

Septal nuclei   Part of the limbic system formed by a group of nuclei that have reciprocal connections with the hippocampus, amygdala, midbrain, hypothalamus and thalamus; associated with social behavior, anxiety, fear, and memory-related behaviors

Simple epithelium   Single layer of cells

Simple reflex   Confined to a single spinal cord level

Skeletal muscle fibers   Contain contractile proteins (myofilaments)

Smooth endoplasmic reticulum   Series of membranes in a cell without attached ribosomes; synthesizes lipids, stores calcium in muscle, and breaks down toxins in the liver

Smooth muscle   Lacks striation and is involuntary

Soft palate   Soft muscular portion of the palate posterior to the hard palate (see also Velum)

Soma   Cell body of a neuron formed by a nucleus surrounded by a mass of cytoplasm containing organelles

Somatic division of the peripheral nervous system   Consists of the cranial and spinal nerves that transmit and receive nerve impulses to and from all the muscles and glands of the body

Somatotopic organization   Motor control of different body structures is located within specific portions of cortical tissue

Sphenoid bone   Unpaired cranial bone located at the base of the skull anterior to the temporal bone and basal portion of the occipital bone; divided into a body, two great and two small wings, and two pterygoid processes

Spinal cord   Downward continuation of the brain stem

Spongy bone   Porous interior of bone; allows space for blood vessels and marrow (see also Cancellous bone/ Trabecular bone)

Squamous epithelium   Cells are thin and flat

Standard anatomical position   Point of reference in which body is erect, feet together, palms face forward, thumbs point away from the body

Stapedius muscle   Muscle of the middle ear involved in the acoustic reflex

Sternum   Breastbone

Stratified epithelium   More than one layer of cells

Striatum   Formed by the caudate and putamen nuclei of the basal nuclei

Styloglossus muscle   Elevates and retracts the tongue

Stylopharyngeus muscle   Helps to elevate and open the pharynx during swallowing

Subarachnoid space   Space between the arachnoid and the pia mater; filled with cerebrospinal fluid

Subdural space   Space between the dura mater and the arachnoid

Sulci   Shallow depressions on the cerebral cortex

Superficial   Toward the body surface

Superficial layer of the lamina propria   Consists mostly of loosely organized elastin fibers as well as small amounts of collagen; very compliant (see also Reinke's space)

Superior   Toward the head of the body; upper (see also Cranial, Rostral)

Superior colliculus   Area in the midbrain that plays a role in audiovisual integration

Superior labial frenulum   Connects the inner surface of the upper lip to the midline of the alveolar region

Superior laryngeal nerve   Innervates the cricothyroid muscle

Superior longitudinal fasciculus   Nerve pathway that links the four major lobes of the brain

Superior longitudinal muscle   Elevates the tongue tip

Supination   Combines movements of inversion and adduction around a vertical axis (in the foot)

Supine   Body lying face up

Suprahyoid muscles   Group of extrinsic laryngeal muscles attaching above the level of the hyoid; contraction raises the larynx

Supramarginal gyrus   Located at the bottom portion of the parietal lobe; important in integrating sensory modalities including vision, touch, and hearing

Suture   Seam of tough connective tissue that fuses adjoining bones together (see also Fibrous joints)

Synapse   Tiny gap between adjacent nerve cells; may be axoaxonic, axosomatic, or axodendritic

Synarthrodial joints   Are immovable

Synovial joints   Permit a wide range of movements

T

Tectorial membrane   Gelatinous structure that forms the roof of the organ of Corti in the cochlea

Telodendria   Located at the endpoint of the axon (see also Terminal branches)

Telophase   Phase of cell division during which the cell pinches off in the center, forming two daughter cells

Temporal bones   Paired cranial bones located at the base and sides of the skull directly inferior to the temple

Temporalis muscle   Muscle of mastication; elevates mandible to close the jaw; posterior fibers retract the mandible

Temporal lobes   Located immediately inferior to the lateral fissure; important for hearing and understanding

Temporomandibular joint   Joint between the condylar process of the mandible and the temporal bone

Tensor tympani muscle   Muscle of the middle ear that connects with the manubrium of the malleus; contraction pulls the malleus inward

Tensor veli palatini muscle   Opens the Eustachian tube

Terminal branches   Located at the endpoint of the axon (see also Telodendria)

Terminal buttons   Endpoint of terminal branches; contain vesicles

Thalamocortical nerve fibers   Send impulses from the thalamus to the cerebral cortex

Thalamus   Comprises a collection of nuclei involved with motor and sensory function

Thyroarytenoid muscle   Intrinsic laryngeal muscle composed of thyrovocalis and thyromuscularis fibers; extends from the anterior commissure to the vocal processes of the arytenoid cartilages; innermost layer of the vocal folds; less compliant than the other layers

Thyroepiglottic ligaments   Attach the epiglottis to the thyroid cartilage

Thyrohyoid ligament   Connects the thyroid cartilage to the hyoid bone

Thyroid cartilage   Largest cartilage of the larynx; formed by two sheets of hyaline cartilage which are fused in the front and open in the back

Tidal volume (TV)   Volume of air inhaled and exhaled during a cycle of respiration

Total lung capacity (TLC)   Total amount of air that the lungs can hold; combines tidal volume, inspiratory reserve volume, expiratory reserve volume, and residual volume

Trabecular bone   Porous interior of bone; allows space for blood vessels and marrow (see also Cancellous bone/ Spongy bone)

Trachea   Hollow tube lined with pseudostratified ciliated columnar epithelium

Tracheobronchial tree   Air conducting system formed by the trachea, bronchi, bronchioles, and alveolar sacs

Tragus   Slight protrusion of cartilage anterior to the external auditory meatus

Transverse muscle   Pulls the edges of the tongue toward midline to narrow the tongue

Transverse palatine suture   Immovable joint between the palatine bones and maxilla

Transverse plane   Divides the body or any of its parts into upper and lower sections (see also Horizontal plane)

Triangular fossa   Concave space between the antihelix and the ascending portion of the helix

True vocal folds   Five layered structure; attaches anteriorly at the anterior commissure of the thyroid cartilage, and posteriorly to the vocal process of each arytenoid cartilage

Tunnel of Corti   Formed by two rows of pillar cells; separate the inner and outer hair cells

Tympanic canal   Space below the basilar membrane in the cochlea; terminates at the round window

Tympanic membrane   Semi-transparent oval-shaped sheet of membrane that forms the interface between the outer and middle ears; primary function is to vibrate when acoustic pressure waves impinge on it

U

Umbo   Tip of the cone of the tympanic membrane

Unipolar neurons   Have a single process extending from the cell body

Upper motor neuron   Comprises the nerve cells and their axons arising from cortical areas and projecting to the brain stem and spinal cord

Utricle   Adjacent to the semi-circular canals in the inner ear; senses acceleration in the horizontal plane

V

Vacuoles   Membrane-lined sacs that transport cellular material (see also Pinocytic vesicles)

Vallecula   Space between the base of the tongue and the epiglottis

Velopharyngeal passage (port)   Passageway between the velum and the posterior pharyngeal wall; can be opened and closed

Velum   Soft muscular portion of the palate posterior to the hard palate (see also Soft palate)

Ventral   Toward the front of the body (see also Anterior)

Ventral horns of the spinal cord   Contain the cell bodies that project fibers to skeletal muscles (see also Anterior horns)

Ventricles   Four interconnected cavities located within the brain; manufacture cerebrospinal fluid

Ventricular folds   Located inferior to the aryepiglottic folds and superior to the true folds (see also False vocal folds)

Vermis   Thick band of white matter connecting the two hemispheres of the cerebellum

Vertical muscle   Pulls the tongue downward

Vertical phase difference   Slight time lag between the closing and opening of the lower and upper edges of the vocal folds

Vestibular canal   Space above the vestibular membrane in the cochlea; terminates at the oval window

Vestibular duct   Cavity in the cochlea filled with perilymph; separated from the cochlear duct by the vestibular membrane

Vestibular membrane   Membrane inside the cochlea that separates the cochlear duct and the vestibular duct (also called Reissner's membrane)

Visceral pleura   Airtight membrane enclosing each lung

Vital capacity (VC)   Maximum amount of air that can be exhaled after a maximum inhalation; combination of tidal volume, inspiratory reserve volume, and expiratory reserve volume

Vocal ligament   Formed by the intermediate and deep layers of the lamina propria; less compliant than the cover

Vocal process   Anterior projection of arytenoid cartilage; attaches to the vocal folds

Vocal tract   Hollow muscular tube consisting of the pharynx, oral cavity, and nasal cavities

Vomer   Thin, quadrilateral-shaped bone; forms the posterior part of the nasal septum

W

Wernicke's area   Located in the temporal lobe; essential for decoding and comprehension of speech

White blood cells   Cells of the immune system involved in defending the body against infectious diseases and foreign materials (see also Leukocytes)

Z

Zygomatic bones   Paired bones that form the prominences of the cheek

Zygomaticus major   Muscle that extends from each zygomatic arch to the corners of the mouth; pulls the angle of the mouth upward and outward

Zygomaticus minor   Muscle that runs from the zygomatic arch to the outer part of the upper lip; moves the upper lip backward, upward, and outward

PLANES AND TERMINOLOGY

Page 4 Multiple choice

1 B
2 A
3 C
4 C
5 B
6 A

Page 5 True or False

1 T
2 F
3 F
4 T
5 T
6 F
7 T

Page 5 Matching

1. 2
2. 8
3. 7
4. 6
5. 4
6. 11
7. 1
8. 3
9. 14
10. 17
11. 5
12. 15
13. 9
14. 16
15. 13
16. 18
17. 10
18. 12

Page 6 Fill in the blank

1 Coronal/Frontal
2 Transverse
3 Sagittal
4 Front
5 Distal
6 Prone
7 Side
8 Proximal
9 Superior/cranial/rostral
10 Inferior/Caudal
11 Away
12 Contralateral

Page 7 Fill in the blank

Midsagittal
Transverse
Coronal

SECTION 1
CELLS AND TISSUES

Page 34 Multiple choice

1 C
2 B
3 D
4 C
5 A
6 D
7 D
8 A
9 C
10 C

Page 35 True or False

1 T
2 F
3 T
4 T
5 T
6 T
7 F
8 F
9 F
10 T
11 T
12 T

Page 36 Fill in the blank

1 Stem cells
2 Inclusions
3 Cell membrane
4 Ribosomes
5 Cytoplasm
6 Golgi apparatus
7 Peroxysomes
8 Rough endoplasmic reticulum
9 Mitochondria
10 Nucleus
11 Nucleolus
12 Smooth endoplasmic reticulum
13 Lysosomes
14 Centrioles
15 Chromatin
16 Microtubules and microfilaments

Page 37 Matching

1. 3
2. 4
3. 1
4. 5
5. 8
6. 2
7. 9
8. 10
9. 12
10. 14
11. 6
12. 11
13. 15

14. 16
15. 13
16. 7

Page 38 Multiple choice

1 D
2 C
3 A
4 D
5 A
6 D
7 A
8 D
9 B
10 B
11 B
12 A

Page 39 Fill in the blank

1 Mitosis
2 Meiosis
3 Interphase
4 Telophase
5 Interphase
6 Interphase
7 Anaphase
8 Metaphase
9 Prophase
10 Telophase
11 Prophase
12 Interphase

Page 40 Matching

1. 3
2. 1
3. 4
4. 5
5. 2

Page 40 True or False

1 F
2 T
3 F
4 T
5 T
6 T
7 F
8 F
9 T
10 T

Page 41 Multiple choice

1 A
2 A
3 C
4 D
5 A
6 B
7 C
8 D
9 B
10 B
11 A

12 D
13 D
14 C
15 D
16 B
17 B

Page 43 True or False

1 T	9 F
2 T	10 T
3 T	11 F
4 T	12 T
5 F	13 T
6 T	14 F
7 T	15 T
8 F	
9 F	

Page 44 Fill in the blank

1 Columnar
2 Squamous
3 Ciliated columnar epithelium
4 Keratinized
5 Squamous
6 Basement
7 Extracellular matrix
8 Macrophages
9 Adipocytes
10 Fibroblasts
11 Myofibroblasts
12 Areolar
13 Collagen
14 Elastic
15 Irregular

Page 45 Matching

1. 5
2. 9
3. 2
4. 12
5. 13
6. 10
7. 7
8. 8
9. 4
10. 14
11. 1
12. 6
13. 11
14. 3

Page 45 Multiple choice

1 B
2 A
3 D
4 D

5 C
6 C
7 C
8 A
9 C
10 B
11 C
12 D
13 B
14 A
15 A
16 C
17 A

Page 50 True or false
1 T
2 T
3 F
4 T
5 F
6 T
7 F
8 T
9 T
10 T
11 F
12 F
13 T
14 T
15 F
16 F
17 T
18 F
19 T
20 T
21 T

Page 51 Fill in the blank
2 Hyaline
3 Fibrocartilage
4 Elastic
5 Hyaline
6 Calcium and phosphate
7 Osteoblasts, osteoclasts
8 D
9 Compact/dense/cortical
10 Trabecular/cancellous/spongy
11 Flat
12 Diaphysis
13 Epiphysis
14 Diaphysis, epiphysis, metaphysis
15 Platelets
16 Leukocytes
17 Lymphocytes
18 Eosinophils
19 Red
20 Plasma
21 Hemoglobin
22 Granular

Page 52 Matching
1. 4
2. 6
3. 2
4. 7
5. 1
6. 3
7. 9
8. 11
9. 13
10. 12
11. 10
12. 5
13. 8

Page 52 Multiple choice
1 B
2 D
3 C
4 A
5 B
6 C
7 C
8 A
9 B
10 A
11 C
12 A
13 C

Page 54 Matching
1. 7
2. 11
3. 9
4. 2
5. 5
6. 8
7. 12
8. 14
9. 10
10. 6
11. 3
12. 1
13. 4
14. 13
15. 16
16. 15

Page 55 True and false
1 F
2 F
3 T
4 T
5 T
6 F
7 T
8 T
9 T
10 F
11 F
12 T

Page 55 Fill in the blank
1 Fibrous
2 Synovial/diarthrodial
3 Synovial

4 Pivot
5 Plane
6 Ball and socket
7 Hinge
8 Ellipsoidal
9 Circumduction
10 Flexion
11 Toward
12 Inversion
13 Extension
14 Abduction

Page 56 Multiple choice
1 D
2 D
3 B
4 C
5 B
6 A
7 C
8 A
9 A
10 C
11 D
12 A

Page 57 True or false
1 F
2 T
3 T
4 F
5 F
6 T
7 F
8
9 T
10 F
11 T
12 F
13 T

Page 58 Fill in the blank
1 Myofibers
2 Myofilament
3 Origin, insertion
4 Sarcolemma
5 Fascicles
6 Tendons
7 Perimysium
8 Epimysium
9 Myosin, actin
10 Flat
11 Pennate
12 Fusiform
13 Circular

Page 59 Matching
1. 6
2. 9
3. 2
4. 8
5. 4

6. 3
7. 12
8. 7
9. 10
10. 11
11. 5
12. 1

SECTION 2 RESPIRATION

Page 80 Multiple choice
1 C
2 C
3 D
4 B
5 A
6 B
7 C
8 D
9 C
10 A
11 D
12 B
13 B
14 D
15 A
16 A

Page 82 True or false
1 F
2 T
3 F
4 F
5 T
6 T
7 T
8 F
9 T
10 T
11 T
12 F
13 T
14 F

Page 82 Fill in the blank
1 Pseudostratified ciliated columnar epithelium
2 Bronchi
3 2,8,3,10
4 Bronchioles
5 Alveolar ducts
6 Alveoli
7 Visceral pleura, parietal pleura
8 Negative
9 Depress
10 External intercostal
11 Diaphragm
12 Decreases
13 Decreases
14 Increases

Page 83 Matching

1. 5
2. 4
3. 11
4. 2
5. 3
6. 12
7. 8
8. 13
9. 9
10. 1
11. 14
12. 10
13. 6
14. 7

Page 84 Multiple choice

1 D
2 A
3 A
4 D
5 C
6 B
7 B
8 B
9 B
10 A
11 C
12 B
13 A

Page 86 True or false

1 T
2 F
3 T
4 T
5 T
6 F
7 F
8 T
9 T
10 T
11 T
12 T

Page 86 Fill in the blank

1 Resting expiratory level
2 End expiratory level
3 Capacities
4 Tidal volume
5 Residual volume
6 Expiratory reserve volume
7 Vital capacity
8 35-40
9 5000
10 500
11 Functional residual capacity
12 10
13 20
14 Inspiratory capacity
15 Passive, active

Page 87 Matching

1. 8
2. 5
3. 2
4. 3
5. 6
6. 9
7. 1
8. 4
9. 7

SECTION 3 PHONATION

Page 134 Multiple choice

1 C
2 D
3 B
4 D
5 A
6 A
7 A
8 C
9 B
10 D
11 B
12 C

Page 135 True or false

1 F
2 F
3 F
4 T
5 T
6 F
7 F
8 T
9 F
10 T
11 F
12 T
13 F
14 T

Page 136 Matching

1. 4
2. 7
3. 11
4. 2
5. 8
6. 12
7. 10
8. 5
9. 1
10. 9
11. 3
12. 6

Page 136 Fill in the blank

1 Thyroid
2 Hyoid bone
3 Hyoid bone
4 Thyroid cartilage
5 Anterior commissure
6 Quadrate lamina
7 Cricothyroid
8 Petiole
9 Vallecula
10 Vocal process
11 Oblique line
12 Corniculate
13 Cuneiform
14 Cricoarytenoid
15 Cricothyroid

Page 137 Multiple choice

1 D
2 A
3 D
4 B
5 D
6 B
7 A
8 B
9 B
10 B
11 A
12 C
13 D
14 D
15 B
16 C
17 A
18 D
19 A

Page 140 True or false

1 T
2 T
3 F
4 T
5 F
6 T
7 T
8 F
9 F
10 F
11 T
12 T
13 F
14 T
15 F
16 T
17 T
18 F
19 T
20 T

Page 141 Matching

1. 8
2. 10
3. 7
4. 4
5. 2
6. 9
7. 11
8. 1
9. 5
10. 6
11. 12
12. 13
13. 3

Page 141 Fill in the blank

1 Aryepiglottic folds
2 False vocal folds
3 Thyroarytenoid
4 Non keratinizing stratified squamous epithelium
5 Deep
6 Superficial
7 Dense elastic fibers
8 Body/thyroarytenoid muscle
9 Cover
10 Intermediate, deep
11 Epithelium, superficial layer of the lamina propria
12 Open
13 Membranous, cartilaginous
14 Transverse interarytenoid
15 Posterior cricoarytenoid
16 Cricothyroid
17 Aryepiglottic
18 Lateral cricoarytenoid
19 Interarytenoids
20 Vocalis
21 Lateral cricoarytenoid, interarytenoid
22 Elasticity, negative pressure
23 Mucosal wave
24 Vertical phase difference

Page 143 Fill in the names

1 Hyoid bone
2 Thyroid cartilage
3 Cricoid cartilage
4 Mastoid process
5 Anterior belly of digastric
6 Posterior belly of digastric
7 Stylohyoid muscle
8 Sternohyoid muscle
9 Omohyoid muscle
10 Sternocleidomastoid muscle
11 Mylohyoid muscle

Page 144 Laryngeal jumble

1 Cricoid cartilage
2 Arytenoid cartilage
3 Thyroid cartilage
4 Epiglottic cartilage
5 Corniculate cartilage
6 Hyoid bone
7 Thyroid cartilage
8 Cricoid cartilage
9 Corniculate cartilage
10 Arytenoid cartilage
11 Hyoid bone
12 Thyroid cartilage
13 Hyoid bone
14 Thyroid cartilage
15 Tracheal rings

Page 145 Fill in the names

A Epitglottis
B Hyoid bone
C Triticeal cartilage
D Thyrohyoid membrane
E Thyroid cartilage
F False vocal folds
G True vocal folds
H Trachea
I Cricoid cartilage
J Tracheal cartilage rings
K Foramen
L Arytenoid cartilage
M Corniculate cartilage
N Middle thryohyoid ligament
O Middle cricothyroid ligament

SECTION 4 ARTICULATION

Page 194 Multiple choice

1 C
2 C
3 B
4 A
5 B
6 C
7 D
8 B
9 C
10 B
11 D
12 D
13 C
14 A

Page 196 True or false

1 F
2 F
3 T
4 T
5 T
6 T
7 T
8 F
9 F
10 T
11 T
12 T
13 F
14 T
15 T
16 T
17 F
18 T
19 T
20 F
21 F
22 T

Page 197 Matching

1. 6
2. 7
3. 12
4. 13
5. 9
6. 8
7. 10
8. 2
9. 1
10. 14
11. 11
12. 4
13. 5
14. 3

Page 197 Fill in the blank

1 Zygomatic
2 Maxilla
3 Sphenoid
4 Parietal
5 Vomer
6 Crista galli
7 Palatine
8 Ethmoid
9 Nasal concha
10 Petrous portion of temporal bone

Page 198 Multiple choice

1 B
2 C
3 D
4 A
5 C
6 B
7 C
8 A
9 C
10 D

Page 199 True or false

1 T
2 F
3 F
4 T
5 T
6 F
7 T
8 F
9 T
10 T
11 F
12 T
13 F

Page 200 Fill in the blank

1 Auricularis anterior
2 Temporalis
3 Levator labii superioris
4 Depressor labii inferioris
5 Risorius
6 Orbicularis oris
7 Temporalis
8 Lateral pterygoid
9 Auricularis posterior
10 Mentalis
11 Buccinator
12 Levator labii superioris
13 Lateral pterygoid
14 Temporalis

Page 200 Name the structures

1 Philtrum
2 Philtral ridges
3 Cupid's bow
4 Oral commissure
5 Tubercles

Page 201 Match the numbers and structures

8 Levator anguli oris
4 Levator labii superioris
1 Buccinator
10 Masseter
3 Depressor angui oris
5 Levator labii superioris alaeque nasi
7 Zygomaticus minor
2 Orbicularis oris
6 Zygomaticus major
9 Mentalis
11 Temporalis
12 Depressor labii inferioris

Page 202 Multiple choice

1 B
2 C
3 D
4 D

Page 202 True or false

1 F
2 T
3 F
4 T
5 T
6 F
7 F
8 T

Page 203 Fill in the blank

1 Palatopharyngeus
2 Inferior
3 Superior constrictor
4 Cricopharyngeus
5 Stylopharyngeus
6 Sapingopharyngeus
7 Palatopharyngeus

Page 203 Matching

1. 3
2. 6
3. 1
4. 5

5. 2
6. 7
7. 4

Page 204 Multiple choice
1 B
2 C
3 A
4 B
5 C
6 B
7 C
8 D
9 C
10 A
11 C
12 B
13 D
14 A
15 B
16 D
17 D
18 B
19 A
20 D

Page 207 True or false
1 T
2 F
3 T
4 T
5 F
6 T
7 F
8 F
9 F
10 T
11 T
12 T
13 F
14 F
15 T
16 F
17 F
18 T
19 T
20 F

Page 208 Fill in the blank
1 Mesioclusion
2 Distoclusion
3 Intermaxillary suture
4 Palatine bones
5 Musculus uvuli
6 Tesnor veli palatini
7 Levator veli palatini
8 Palatoglossus, palatopharyngeus
9 Palatoglossus
10 Blade
11 Dorsum
12 Hyoid bone

13 Median sulcus
14 Inferior longitudinal
15 Palatoglossus
16 Transverse
17 Vertical
18 Styloglossus
19 Hyoglossus
20 Genioglossus

Page 209 Matching
1. 4
2. 6
3. 7
4. 8
5. 3
6. 12
7. 9
8. 11
9. 2
10. 1
11. 14
12. 15
13. 13
14. 17
15. 5
16. 10
17. 16
18. 18

SECTION 4 AUDITORY
Page 232 Multiple choice
1 D
2 A
3 D
4 A
5 B
6 D
7 C
8 C
9 A
10 C
11 D
12 D
13 B
14 D
15 B
16 B

Page 234 True or false
1 F
2 T
3 F
4 F
5 T
6 T
7 T
8 F
9 T
10 F
11 T
12 F

13 T
14 F
15 T
16 F

Page 235 Fill in the blank
1 Concha
2 Helix
3 Lobule
4 2.5-3.5 cm, 6 mm
5 Epidermis
6 Meatus
7 Umbo
8 Tesnor veli palatini
9 Stapes
10 Stapedius
11 Triangular fossa
12 Scapha
13 Antitragus

Page 236 Match the letters and numbers
1 W
2 E
3 Q
4 L
5 M
6 N
7 S
8 B
9 P
10 V
11 X
12 J
13 D
14 G
15 K
16 A
17 I
18 O
19 R
20 U
21 T
22 C
23 H

Page 237 Matching
1. 11
2. 8
3. 9
3. 10
5. 2
6. 7
7. 3
8. 6
9. 1
10. 4
11. 5
12. 12
13. 13

Page 237 Match the letters and numbers
1 A
2 H
3 E
4 K
5 C
6 G
7 D
8 J
9 F
10 I
11 B
12 L

Page 238 Multiple choice
1 A
2 A
3 D
4 B
5 B
6 D
7 D
8 A
9 C
10 A
11 D
12 B
13 D
14 C
15 B
16 C
17 C
18 C
19 B
20 A

Page 241 Matching
1. 11
2. 12
3. 2
4. 6
5. 8
6. 13
7. 9
8. 10
9. 3
10. 1
11. 4
12. 5
13. 7
14. 15
15. 14

Page 241 True or false
1 T
2 F
3 T
4 F
5 F
6 T

7 F
8 T
9 T
10 T
11 F
12 F
13 F
14 T
15 T
16 T
17 F
18 T

Page 242 Fill in the blank

1 Petrous portion of the temporal bone
2 Modiolus
3 Cochlear duct
4 Perilymph
5 Basilar membrane
6 Tectorial membrane
7 Vestibular membrane
8 Helicotrema
9 Basilar membrane
10 Ampulla, cupola
11 Horizontal
12 Vertical
13 Tunnel of Corti
14 Inner hair cells

SECTION 5 NERVOUS

Page 280 Multiple choice

1 B
2 B
3 D
4 D
5 D
6 C
7 C
8 C
9 C
10 B
11 D
12 A
13 C
14 A
15 D
16 C
17 B
18 C
19 D
20 D
21 A
22 A
23 D
24 B
25 C
26 D
27 A
28 B

29 D
30 C
31 A
32 D
33 A
34 D

Page 284 True or false

1 T
2 F
3 T
4 F
5 T
6 T
7 F
8 F
9 T
10 T
11 F
12 T
13 F
14 T
15 T
16 T
17 F
18 F
19 T
20 T
21 T
22 F
23 F
24 T
25 F
26 T
27 T

Page 286 Matching

1. 3
2. 11
3. 16
4. 12
5. 1
6. 5
7. 13
8. 15
9. 14
10. 7
11. 2
12. 8
13. 6
14. 4
15. 9
16. 10
17. 21
18. 24
19. 25
20. 18
21. 17
22. 20
23. 26

24. 27
25. 22
26. 23
27. 19

Page 287 Fill in the blank

1 Synapse
2 Golgi Type II
3 Sensory/afferent
4 Autonomic
5 Somatic
6 Glial
7 Golgi Type I
8 Mechanoreceptors
9 Chemoreceptors
10 Interneurons/multipolar
11 Proprioceptors
12 Baroreceptors
13 Photoreceptors
14 Temperature
15 Nocioreceptors
16 Synapse
17 Neurotransmitters
18 Astrocytes
19 Oligodendrocytes, Schwann cells, myelin
20 Microglia
21 Nodes of Ranvier
22 Terminal branches

Page 288 Multiple choice

1 C
2 B
3 A
4 C
5 A
6 D
7 B
8 D
9 A
10 C
11 B
12 A
13 C
14 A
15 D
16 C
17 D
18 D
19 B
20 C
21 A
22 C
23 D
24 A
25 D
26 C
27 C
28 B
29 B

30 D

Page 292 True or false

1 F
2 T
3 T
4 F
5 T
6 T
7 T
8 F
9 T
10 F
11 F
12 T
13 T
14 T
15 T
16 T
17 F
18 F
19 T
20 T
21 F
22 F
23 F
24 T
25 T
26 T
27 F
28 T
29 T
30 F
31 T
32 T

Page 293 Fill in the blank

1 Periosteal
2 Arachnoid
3 Subdural space
4 Cerebral aqueduct
5 Choroid plexus cells
6 Brain stem
7 Longitudinal cerebral fissure
8 Central sulcus
9 Lateral fissure
10 Frontal
11 Temporal
12 Parietal
13 Broca's area
14 Precentral
15 Parietal
16 Arcuate fasciculus
17 Somatotopic
18 Temporal
19 Post central
20 Primary visual area
21 Primary motor area
22 39

23 Premotor area, supplementary motor area
24 22
25 Hippocampus
26 Maxillary bodies
27 Amygdala
28 Superior longitudinal fasciculus
29 Corpus callosum
30 Internal capsule

Page 295 Matching
1. 1
2. 11
3. 3
4. 13
5. 16
6. 8
7. 6
8. 14
9. 5
10. 10
11. 12
12. 2
13. 9
14. 7
15. 17
16. 15
17. 4

Page 296 Multiple choice
1 D
2 B
3 D
4 D
5 C
6 D
7 B
8 C
9 C
10 A
11 D
12 B
13 A
14 C
15 D
16 D
17 B
18 A
19 B
20 D
21 B
22 C
23 D
24 C
25 C
26 A
27 C
28 A
29 D
30 D

31 C
32 B
33 D
34 A

Page 301 True or false
1 F
2 F
3 F
4 T
5 F
6 T
7 F
8 T
9 T
10 T
11 T
12 T
13 T
14 F
15 F
16 T
17 F
18 T
19 T
20 F
21 T
22 T
23 F
24 F
25 T
26 T
27 T
28 F
29 T
30 T
31 T
32 T
33 T
34 T
35 T
36 T
37 F
38 T
39 F

Page 303 Matching
1. 19
2. 26
3. 10
4. 1
5. 31
6. 2
7. 5
8. 8
9. 27
10 16
11. 13
12. 21
13. 3

14. 15
15. 12
16. 23
17. 25
18. 18
19. 17
20 29
21. 30
22. 6
23. 7
24. 20
25. 11
26. 14
27. 4
28. 24
29. 9
30. 28
31. 22

Page 304 Fill in the blank
1 Caudate, globus pallidus, putamen, substantia nigra
2 Striatum
3 Brain stem
4 Reticular activating system
5 Pons
6 Medulla
7 Vermis
8 Efferent/motor
9 Dorsal/posterior
10 Ventral/anterior
11 Anterior corticospinal
12 Corticospinal
13 Cervical
14 Brachial
15 Lumbar
16 Lumbosacral
17 XII, VII, V
18 Facial
19 XII
20 Opthalmic, maxillary, mandibular
21 VII
22 VII
23 Vagus
24 Cricothyroid
25 Recurrrent laryngeal
26 Upper motor neuron
27 V, VII, X, XII
28 Neuromuscular junction, myoneural junction, motor end plate
29 Motor unit
30 Circle of Willis
31 Middle cerebral artery
32 Basilar

Planes and Terminology

Tissues and Joints

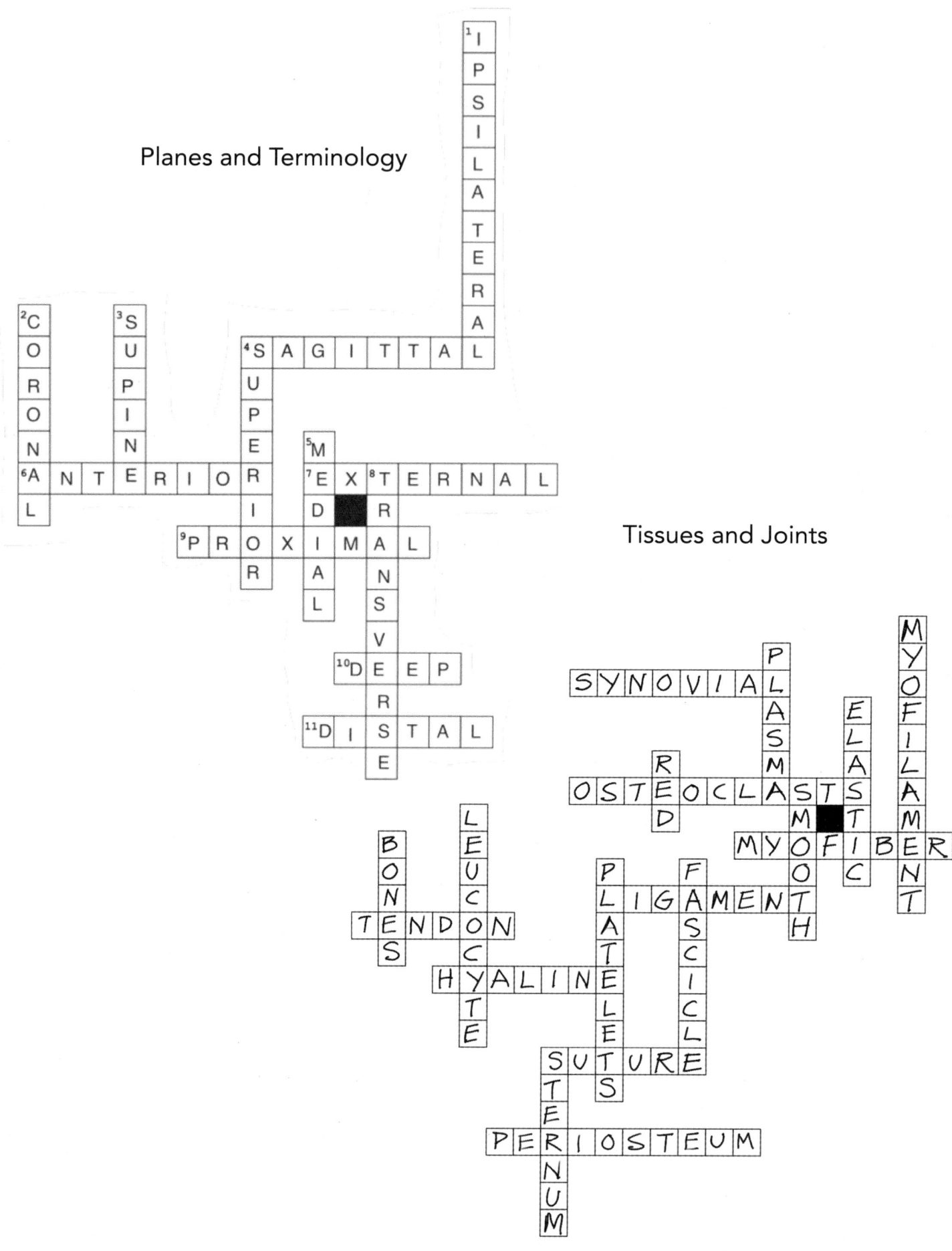

Cells

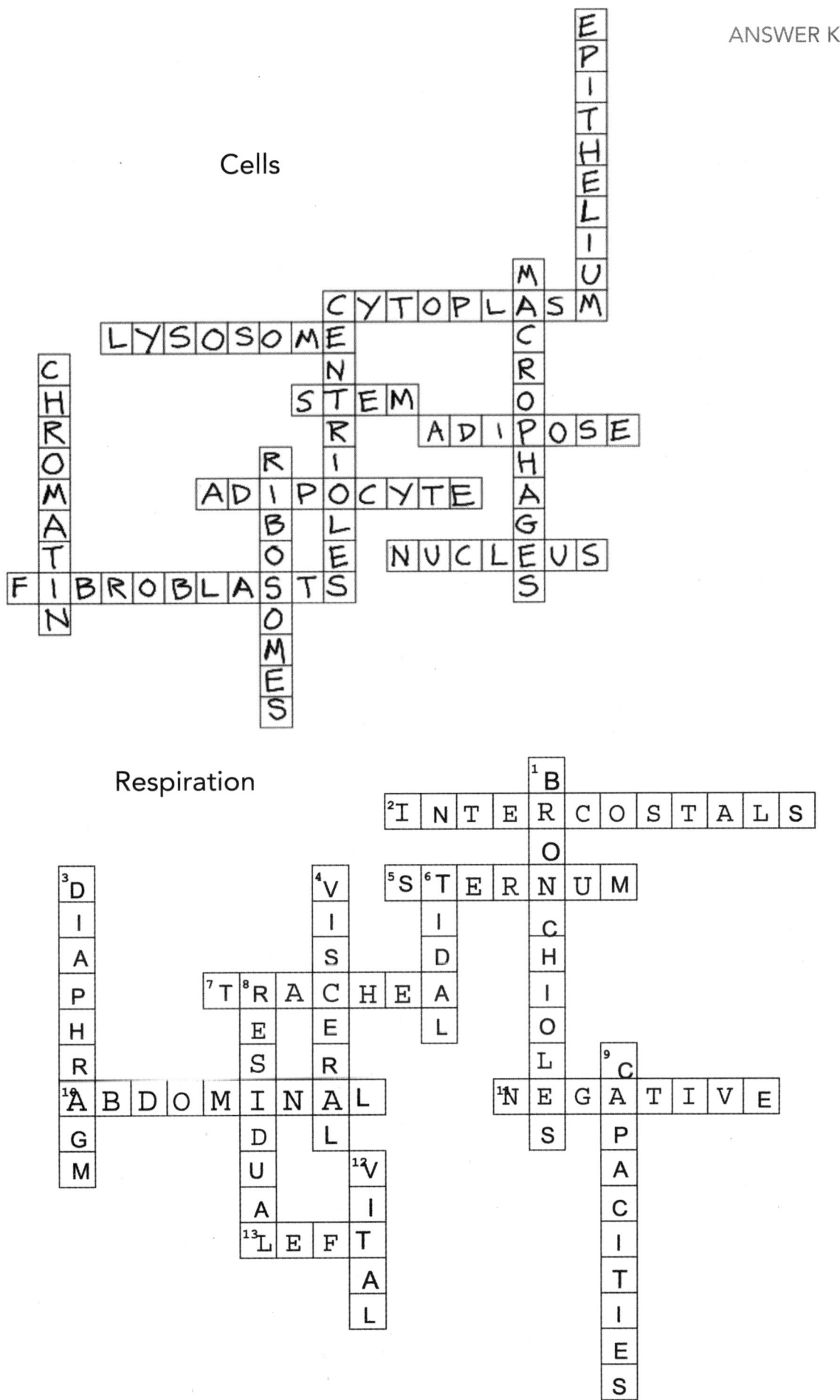

Respiration

Muscles of the Larynx

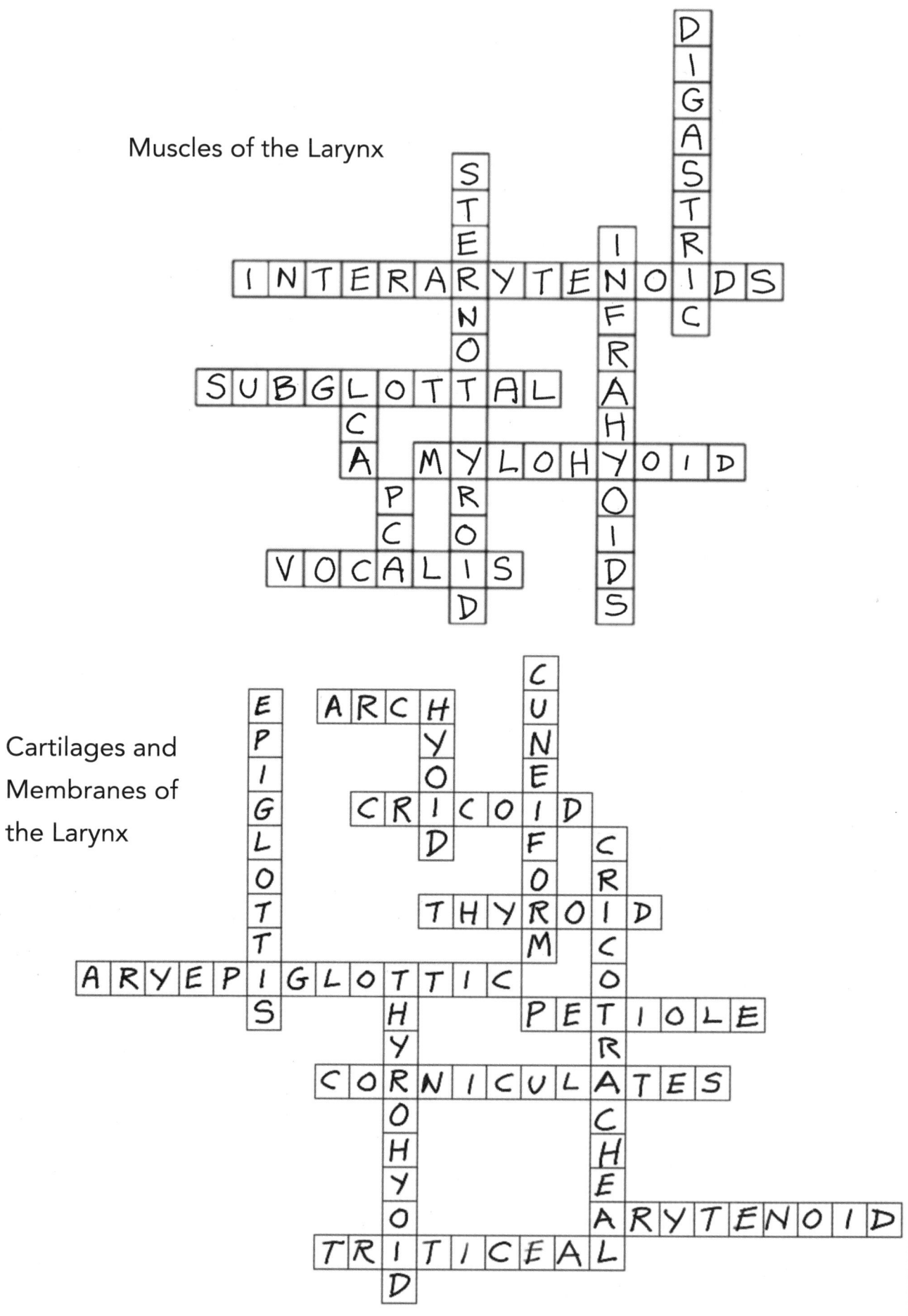

Cartilages and
Membranes of
the Larynx

Joints and Folds of the Larynx

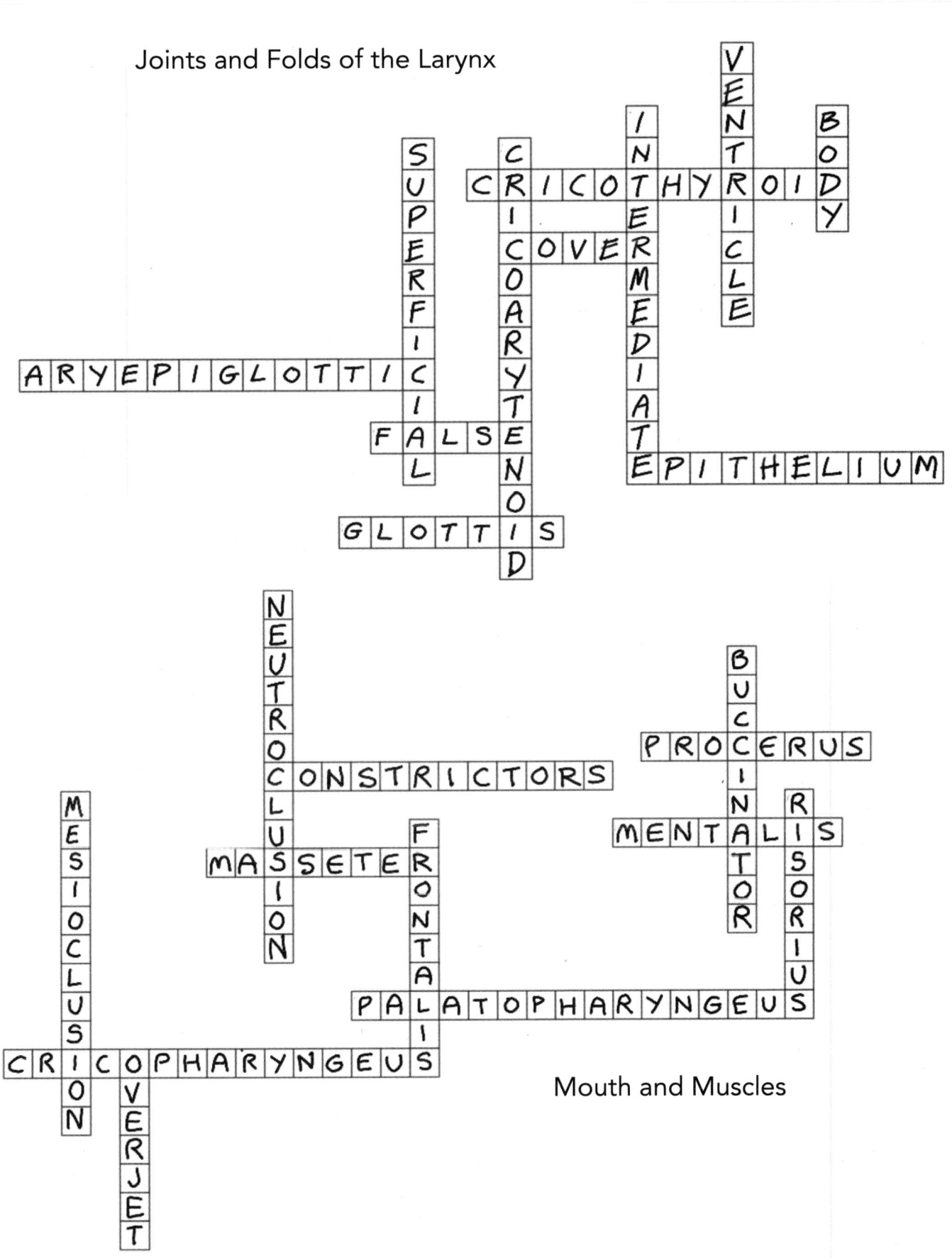

Mouth and Muscles

Tongue

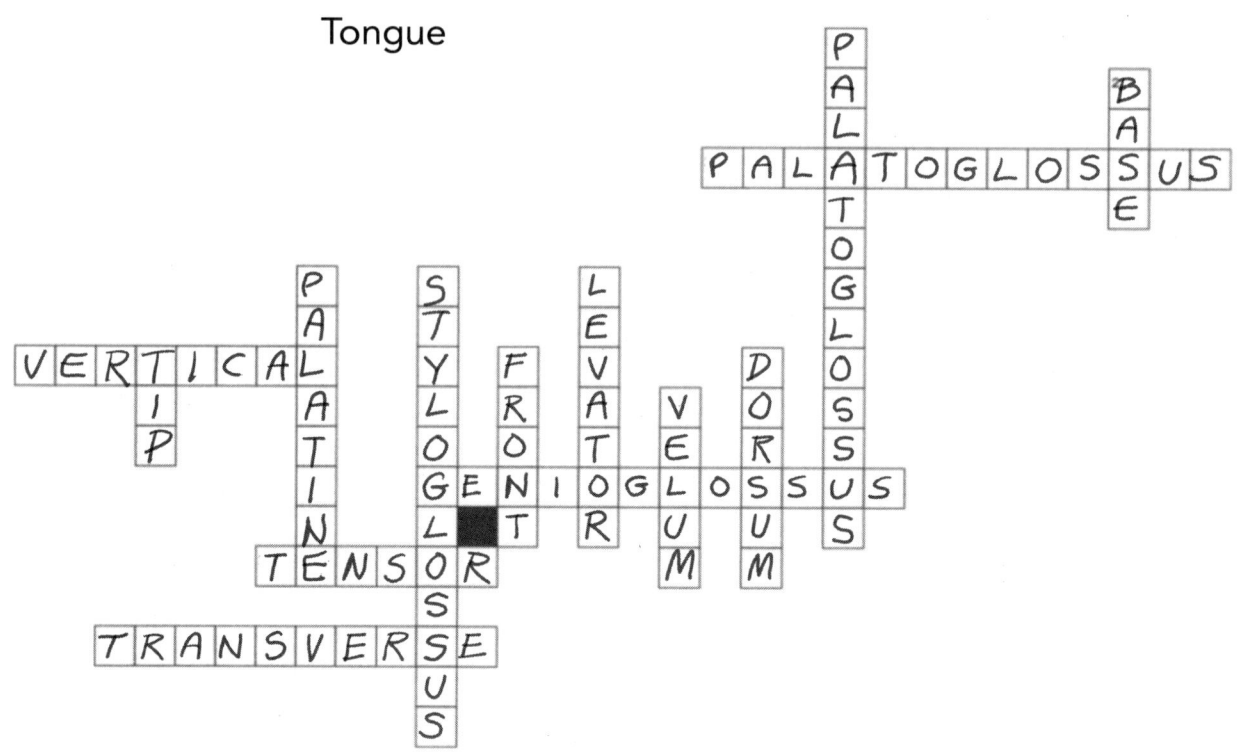

Cranial and Facial Bones

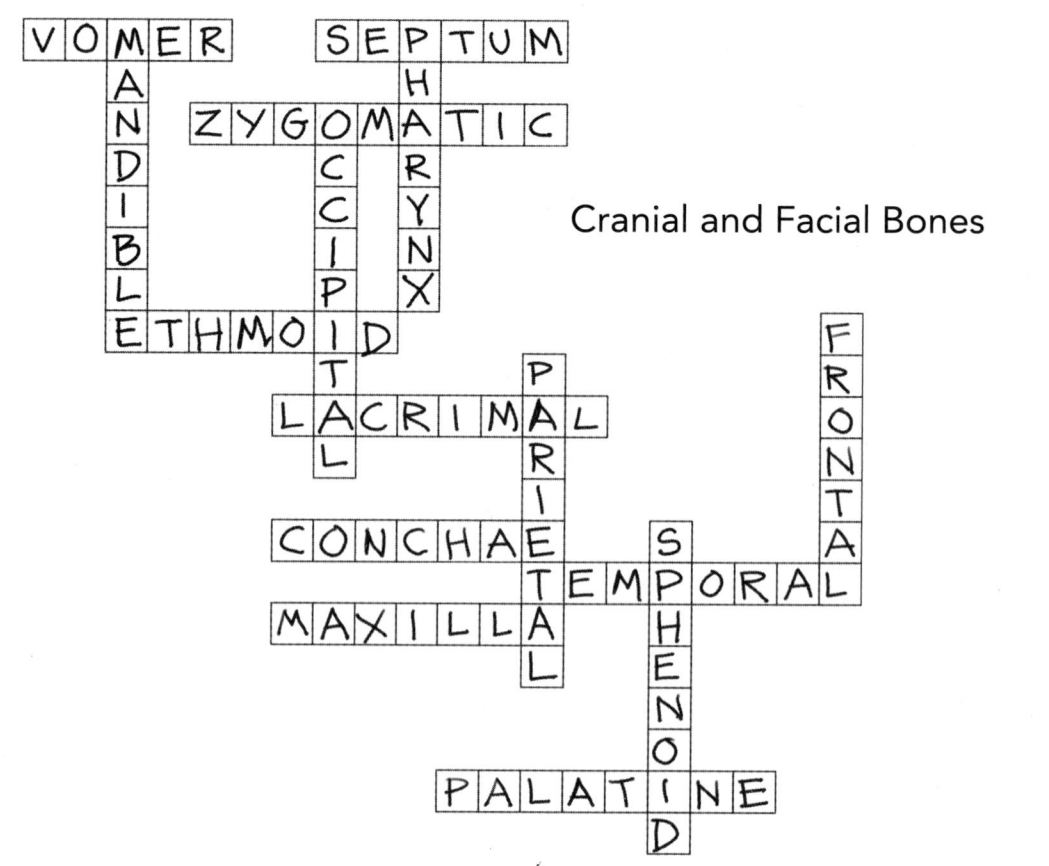

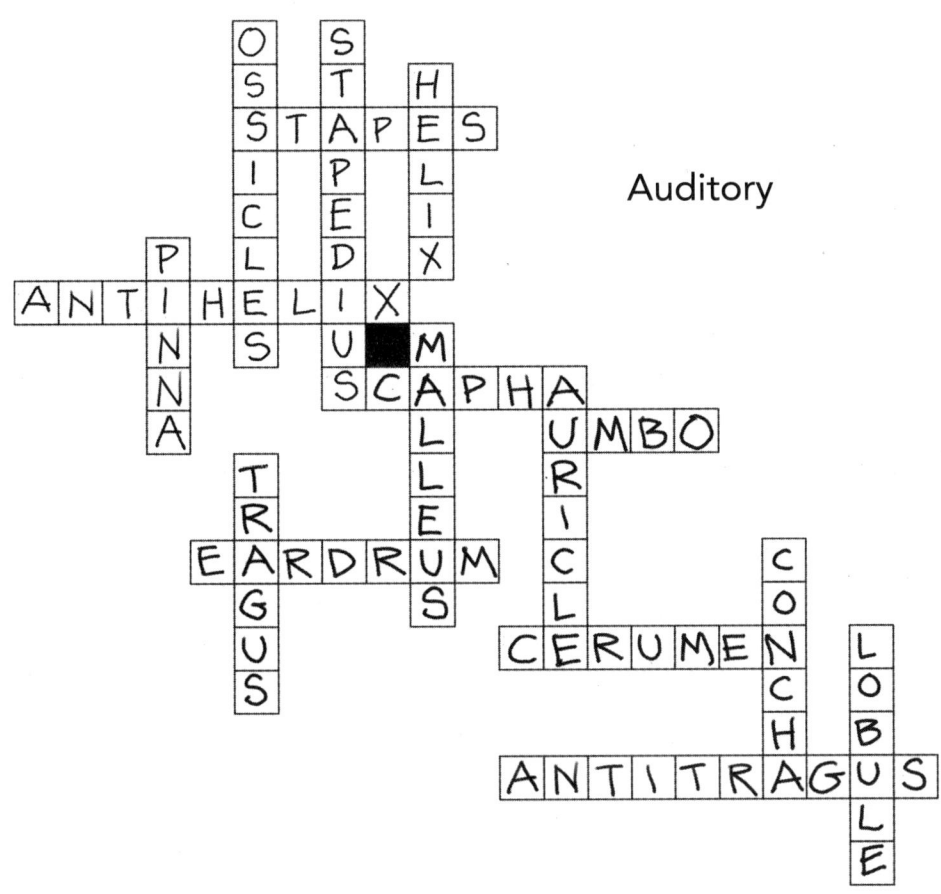

Auditory

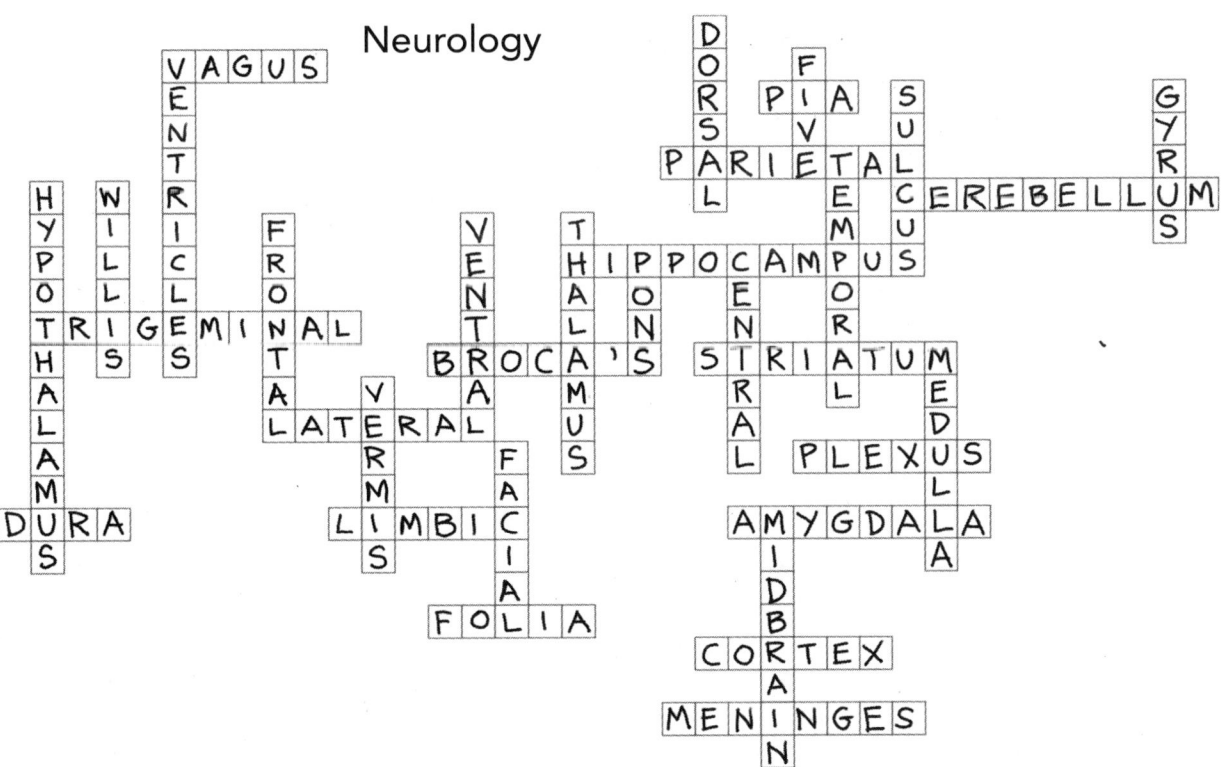

Neurology

Neurology 2

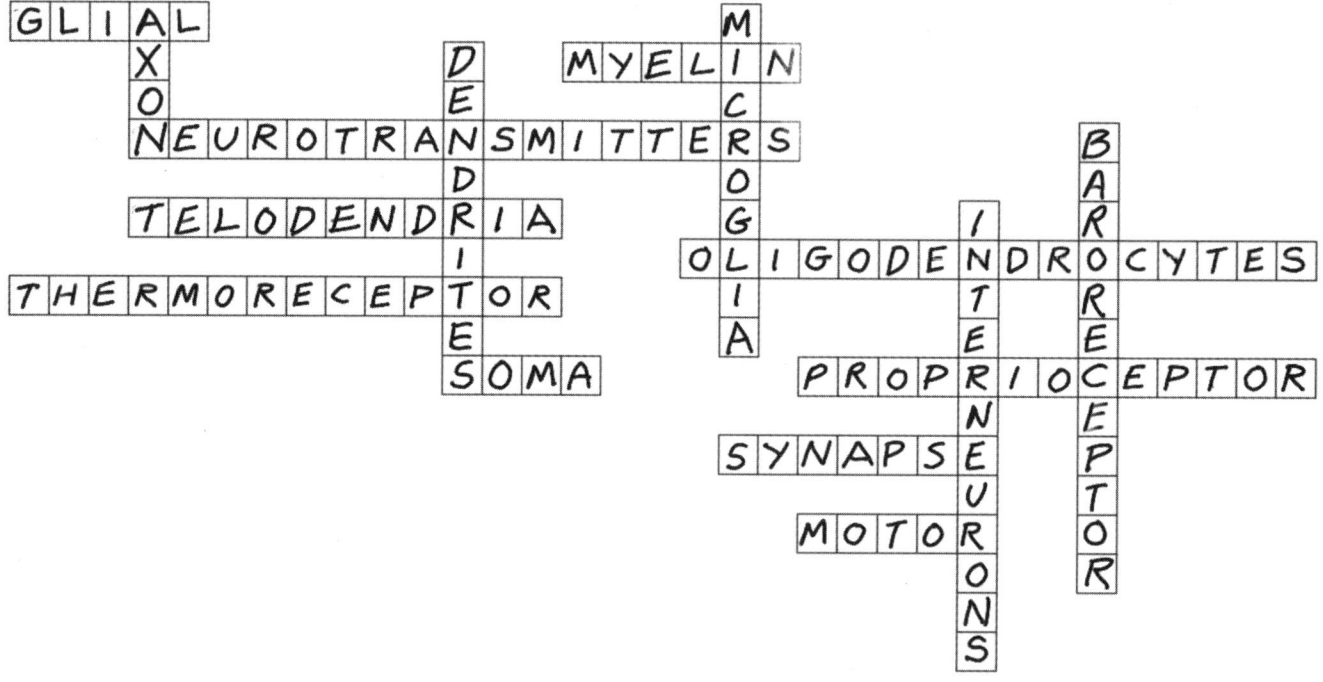

This workbook can be ordered at:

Aplusanatomy.com

Made in the USA
Las Vegas, NV
22 May 2025

22564641R00044